Overcoming Infertility

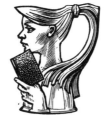

By the Author

Be Fruitful and Multiply:
Fertility Therapy and the Jewish Tradition

Richard V. Grazi
OVERCOMING INFERTILITY
A Guide for Jewish Couples

The Toby Press

For my patients,
without whom I could not know what I know,
do what I do,
or be what I am.

Overcoming Infertility

First Edition, 2005

The Toby Press LLC, 2004
POB 8531, New Milford, CT. 06676-8531, USA
& POB 2455, London W1A 5WY, England
www.tobypress.com

ISBN 159264 1067, hardcover original

A CIP catalogue record for this title is
available from the British Library

Illustrations by Joseph Grazi

Typeset in Garamond by Jerusalem Typesetting

Printed and bound in the United States
by Thomson-Shore Inc., Michigan

Contents

Foreword, Lord Immanuel Jakobovits, ז״ל, *xi*

An Explanation of Rabbinic Terms
Used in this Book, *xvii*

Note on the transliteration, *xxi*

Introduction, *xxiii*

PART I. INFERTILITY IN PERSPECTIVE

Introduction, *3*

A Brief History of Fertility Therapy
Richard V. Grazi, 5

The Rabbinic Conception of Conception
Edward Reichman, 31

PART II. THE RELIGIOUS JEWISH INFERTILE COUPLE

Introduction, *65*

The Longing for Children in
the Traditional Jewish Family
Yoel Jakobovits, 67

The Rabbinic and Medical Partnership
Hershel Billet, 73

Infertility: Issues from the Heart
Sara Barris and Joel Comet, 79

A Rabbinic Response to Infertility
Allen Schwartz, 95

On Adoption
Rabbi Joseph B. Soloveitchik, ל"ז, 101

**PART III. DIAGNOSTIC EVALUATION
OF THE INFERTILE COUPLE**

Introduction, *107*

The Couple, the Physician and the Rabbi:
A Triumvirate Partnership
Richard V. Grazi, 111

The Physiology of Conception
Richard V. Grazi, 121

General Aspects of Female Infertility
Richard V. Grazi, 131

Diagnostic Procedures in the Female Patient
Richard Weiss, 189

A General Overview of Male Infertility
Yoel Jakobovits, 227

PART IV. THERAPEUTIC INTERVENTIONS

Introduction, *247*

Evaluation and Treatment of Male Infertility
Nahum Katlowitz, 251

Halakhic Considerations in the Treatment
of Female Infertility
Richard V. Grazi, 277

Assisted Reproduction
Richard V. Grazi, 311

PART V. SPECIAL CONSIDERATIONS FOR
THE INFERTILE JEWISH COUPLE

Introduction, *367*

Fertility Treatment on the Sabbath and Festivals
Gideon Weitzman, 369

Rabbinical Supervision during Fertility Therapy
Rabbi Avrohom Friedlander, 391

PART VI. ETHICAL ISSUES

Introduction, *407*

New Ethical Issues
Richard V. Grazi and Joel B. Wolowelsky, 409

ix

Future Directions
Joel B. Wolowelsky and Richard V. Grazi, 425

PART VII. RESOURCES

A Glossary of Medical Acronyms and Terms, 443

Acronyms, 479

Glossary of Halakhic Terms, 481

Useful Organizations, 487

Bibliography, 491

Index, 499

About the Author, 501

Lord Immanuel Jakobovits, ז״ל

Foreword

The biblical account of the human story begins with the imperative to "be fruitful and multiply" as the first of the Torah's 613 commandments. And Jewish history opens with the yearning to overcome the disability of childlessness. Abraham and Sarah were barren for most of their lives, to be granted the gift of a child only in hoary old age, while Rachel in her despair pleaded, "give me children or I am dead."

In biblical times, only recourse to prayer and reliance on divine assurances could counter infertility. Today, thanks to the spectacular advances of medical science and technological skills, effective aids are available to triumph over many natural impediments, whether physical or psychological, on both the male and the female side.

But often these innovations raise new problems, particularly for observant and morally sensitive Jewish doctors and patients. Some of these difficulties may be of a purely religious or ritual character, such as possible clashes with the laws of family purity (*niddah*) when invasive procedures cause vaginal bleeding, or when treatments such as insemination or in vitro fertilization are required during the period of abstention. Other new techniques may encounter grave moral objections, such as when donated sperm or eggs are used to secure a successful impregnation. The resultant questions range from possibly violating the marriage bond by a quasi-adulterous relationship to establishing the true identity of a child born without certainty as to father, mother, and other blood relatives.

Of course, Jewish teachings not only create problems; they often help to solve them. Lives sanctified by strict adherence to moral precepts tend to be superior lives, less prone to erosion of faithlessness, the alienation of children from their parents, or the subversion of society by indiscipline and selfishness.

This book—the first of its kind to deal specifically with infertility—provides an extensive survey of the relevant medical and halakhic data, based on professional expertise and the verdicts of many leading rabbinical authorities. Readers will be interested not only in their sometimes diverse rulings, but equally in the sources and thought processes leading to their conclusions.

Not least valuable, I hope, will be the deep concern of Judaism and its administrators to overcome the trial of infertility evinced in these papers, together with the encouragement given to persons who are perplexed or distressed.

May the children to be born out of the application of Jewish insights into scientific wonders of modern medicine personify the intentions of this valuable volume's authors to increase life and to hallow it.

For the pillars of the earth are the Lord's, and upon them he set the world.

Hannah's Prayer, *Samuel 1, 2:8*

Rabbi Yohanan said: Three keys the Holy One blessed be He has retained in His own hands and not entrusted to the hand of any messenger, namely, the Key of Rain, the Key of Childbirth, and the Key of the Revival of the Dead.

The Key of Rain, for it is written, *the Lord will open unto you His good treasure, the heaven to give the rain of your land in its season*; the Key of Childbirth, for it is written, *And God remembered Rachel, and God hearkened to her, and opened her womb*; The Key of the Revival of the Dead, for it is written, *And you shall know that I am the Lord, when I have opened your graves.*

Babylonian Talmud, *Ta'anit 2a*

...for what we engender by the soul, the children of our mind, of our heart and ability, are provided by a nobler part than the body and are more our own...

Montaigne

The author wishes to thank the following contributors for their invaluable contribution to this book:

Sara L. Barris, PsyD
Clinical Psychologist
Co-director, American Fertility Association Support
Group Services
Queens, NY

Hershel Billet
Rabbi, Young Israel of Woodmere
Woodmere, NY

Joel Comet, PhD
Clinical Psychologist
Coordinator, Trauma Treatment Unit
Shiluv Institute
Israel

Avrohom Friedlander
Rabbi and Chief Chaplain
Maimonides Medical Center
Brooklyn, NY

Yoel Jakobovits, MD
Assistant Professor of Medicine
Johns Hopkins University School of Medicine
Baltimore, MD

Nachum Katlowitz, MD
Director Male Sexual Dysfunction and Male Infertility
Staten Island University Hospital, Staten Island, NY
Maimonides Medical Center, Brooklyn, NY

Edward Reichman, MD
Assistant Professor of Emergency Medicine
Montefiore Medical Center
Assistant Professor of Philosophy and
the History of Medicine
Albert Einstein College of Medicine
New York, NY

Allen Schwartz
Rabbi, Congregation Ohab Zedek
New York, NY

Richard Weiss, MD
Rabbi, Young Israel of Hillcrest,
Flushing, NY

Gideon Weitzman
Head, English-Speaking Section
Puah Institute
Jerusalem, Israel

Joel B. Wolowelsky, PhD
Dean of Faculty, Yeshivah of Flatbush
Joel Braverman High School
Associate Editor, *Tradition*
Brooklyn, NY

An Explanation of Rabbinic Terms Used in this Book

Halakha is the legal and ethical system of rabbinic Judaism. Biblical law generally refers to rulings found in the Pentateuch (the first five books of the Hebrew Bible). It also includes rulings not explicitly mentioned in the Bible but which are part of the oral tradition accompanying the Bible and are viewed as biblical by the rabbis. Generally, rabbinic authorities have very little leeway in modifying biblical laws.

Rabbinic law refers to requirements and restrictions imposed by the early rabbinic authorities and codified in the Mishnah and Talmud, which, together with the Bible, form the primary texts of rabbinic Judaism. Rabbinic authorities have some extra leeway in modifying the application of rabbinic laws, but cannot amend them at will or dismiss them.

The basic sources for the investigation of halakhic positions on any ethical or legal issue are the Bible, the Mishnah and Talmud, and universally accepted codifications such as Maimonides' medieval *Mishneh Torah* and Rabbi Yosef Karo's later *Shulhan Arukh*.

But rulings on contemporary issues cannot be promulgated by any central authority, as there is no formal hierarchical structure to the various rabbinic authorities and courts currently functioning. Positions on contemporary issues are developed by circulation of responsa (rabbinic rulings) to questions posed to various rabbinic authorities. These responsa are issued individually and eventually are published in a volume or series of volumes, sometimes posthumously. While collegial review and community acceptance eventually allow for specific opinions to emerge as authoritative, individual rabbis or layman will often defer to their local authority, whose position is considered decisive.

Peru u'revu is the Hebrew phrase for "be fruitful and multiply," the commandment/blessing contained in the first chapter of Genesis.

Niddah is the state induced by the onset of a woman's menstrual period and which continues until she immerses herself at the specified time in a natural body of water or a specially constructed pool called a *mikvah*. Biblical and rabbinic law prohibit a woman who is in a state of *niddah* from having any physical contact (including but not limited to intercourse) with her husband. After immersion in the *mikvah*, she achieves a state of *tahara*, or purity, and all prohibitions regarding physical contact are then lifted. *Taharat hamishpa'ha* refers to the entire body of halakhic law that governs spiritual purity within the family, and includes all of the laws of *niddah* and *tahara*.

Generally, any type of uterine blood flow induces a state of *niddah*, even if it is not a result of the woman's normal menstrual flow, while an artificially induced wound (a *makkah*) does not. The consequences of these halakhic categories are discussed in detail in this book. While the concept is foreign to most non-observant people, it is a core value in halakhic Judaism that has great impact on an observant couple's married life.

Halakhic Sabbath and holiday laws include a number of prohibited activities; *muktzeh* refers to those objects that cannot be handled because of their association with these prohibited activities.

*A complete glossary of the Hebrew terms used
in this book is found in Section VII.*

Note on the transliteration

The Sephardic pronunciation has been used to guide the English spelling of all Hebrew words. Commonly known Hebrew terms have not been italicized, such as "mitzvah," "halakha," "Mishnah," "Midrash," "Aggadah."

Introduction

Anyone who has experienced infertility first hand knows the overwhelming sense of sadness and fear that it brings. Sadness, because it signifies that something very important remains out of reach; fear, because there is no certainty about when the predicament will end. Unfortunately, the complexities of human reproduction do not always lend themselves to a reliable or quick fix. The only thing predictable about infertility is that, over time, it will precipitate a true crisis in the life of a couple.

This book will not solve that crisis. It will not eliminate the sadness or the fear. For most couples who struggle with infertility, only the arrival of a baby can accomplish that. But it is important to empower those who live with infertility to take control of their condition. Infertile couples who abide by the guidelines of Jewish law and ethics, collectively referred to as 'halakha,' commonly encounter challenges that complicate the standard solutions to infertility. Just as their religious observance adds a unique dimension to their lives, so it may add a unique set of problems. This book comes to address the needs of this particular audience. If there is one overriding lesson to be learned in the pages that follow, it is that there is a solution to nearly every one of those problems.

Traditional and Orthodox Jewish couples who live in large communities sometimes have the advantage of being cared for by physicians familiar with the imperatives of halakha. Those who do not but who must, nevertheless, confront fertility treatment are often at a loss to explain to their physicians exactly why their treatment may be problematic or how accommodations might be made to make it less so. Many of the chapters in this book are meant to stand alone, to be shown to physicians who are new to this subject. In a similar vein, couples with infertility do not always have access to rabbinical authorities who are conversant with the intricacies of reproductive halakha. Couples so challenged may use certain chapters in this book to sensitize those advising them to their situation and to help explain the medical and physical challenges with which they must grapple. Of course, no work of this type can be truly comprehensive, and generalizations about so complex a topic as infertility inevitably will be off the mark for some readers. It is my hope, however, that the impressions and advice offered in this book will ring true for many, be they physicians, rabbis, or the couples themselves.

My work with infertile couples over the last eighteen years has kept me ever vigilant of the ways that couples function separately and together as they confront their infertility. Some couples, unfortunately, experience a psychological "disconnect" that impedes their ability to cope, ultimately resulting in marital discord, psychological separation, and the loss of any real opportunity to solve their infertility. In healthy relationships, however, the experience of infertility can be an opportunity to grow ever-closer, as the quest for parenthood compels each partner to confront and share feelings and thoughts that would otherwise remain hidden, laying the groundwork for a lasting, healthy family. Fortunately, the latter mode of interaction is the rule among Torah-observant couples. The vast majority of them will overcome infertility, either naturally or with treatment, and emerge successfully as parents. This book will be useful to them in the interim, helping them to navigate their way to a successful resolution.

All infertile couples are at risk for succumbing to the profound difficulties of their situation. In this sense, infertile couples who live by the rules of halakha are no different. But the very fact that in the halakhic community only a married couple can experience infertility is, in another sense, a potent salve for the psychological pain that infertility brings. Individuals who find themselves in the midst of this challenge have already completed one of the major passages of life. They have, by definition, found another with whom to share the rest of their lives, and know first hand the bonds of love. As the Torah tells us in Genesis, "this is why a man will leave his father and mother and bond to his wife." If the next passage—parenthood—is delayed, at least there is someone else with whom to share the wait. During that waiting period, no Torah-observant Jew should forget that other obligations such as pleasing one's spouse and enjoying this world are still there to be fulfilled.

⁊⃀

A substantial part of *Overcoming Infertility* appeared in my original work on this topic, *Be Fruitful and Multiply: Fertility Therapy and the Jewish Tradition*, which was published in 1994. The genesis of that book was spelled out clearly at the time. Technological advances in treating infertility were developing at an astounding pace, to the point where it seemed that nearly every clinical problem had a solution. Yet, within the traditional Jewish community, couples were largely unsure about the appropriateness of using this technology to their advantage. To complicate matters, their rabbinical advisers were often unclear about just what these treatments involved, and so they could offer no clear guidelines for approaching them. Physicians involved in treating observant Jewish couples were typically uninformed about the restrictions under which these therapies could be offered.

My position as the Director of Reproductive Medicine at

Maimonides Medical Center placed me in the center of these issues on a daily basis. The medical center is located in Boro Park, Brooklyn, home to one of the largest Orthodox Jewish communities in the world. In the surrounding neighborhoods, having children is not just a casual consequence of being married—it is a serious life calling. As a result, the couples with whom I consulted saw themselves as grappling not with a straightforward medical problem, but rather with an all-encompassing and devastating illness. Against this backdrop, my personal religious commitment, combined with my familiarity with both the culture and language of halakha and my practical knowledge of the medical issues involved, served to set me squarely in the middle of many a dramatic circumstance.

As we struggled to address the issues of the day, the important "players" in the clinical management of infertility began to define themselves. Requests for consultation came not only from patients but also from their rabbis. Conversations with the latter were often frustrating in that there were few, if any, precedents with which to address certain issues and, at the time, many were not yet part of the halakhic vocabulary. Many calls also came from my physician colleagues. As a group, they understood the significance of their work and the consequences of success or failure for each couple. There was naturally some confusion, therefore, about aspects of care that were, medically, highly feasible and seemingly ethical, yet impermissible for halakhically technical reasons.

The audience for the original work was consequently not limited only to infertile Jewish couples. For the rabbinic community, it contained basic information about reproductive physiology and the ways in which it could be manipulated in order to overcome infertility. A summary of then-current halakhic discussions that had addressed the new reproductive technologies was also included, in order to serve as a basis for future problem-solving. For physicians who dealt with Orthodox infertile couples, a chapter dealing with the basic laws of *tahrat hamishpa'ha* (family purity) was crucial for giving insight into some of the important issues that confront their patients. On a very practical level, strategies that could be used to keep fertility therapy within the guidelines of halakha were presented in detail. Chapters on the special psychological and social problems faced by devout infertile couples were meant to benefit rabbis and physicians alike.

It was my hope, in publishing that first text, that a greater familiarity with these issues would heighten the sensitivity to infertile couples among those who care for them both physically and spiritually. Additionally, my intention was to alert medical and rabbinic professionals about the importance of their respective roles, and also about the boundaries to their areas of expertise. *Be Fruitful and Multiply* was intended to clarify those boundaries and to encourage the rabbinic and medical communities to interface more closely in assisting their common clients.

The forerunner to this book closed with some thoughts on the following words of Charles Duell, the commissioner of patents in 1899: "Everything that can be invented has been invented." That was before egg freezing, embryo biopsy, and cloning were first described. It was before posthumous parenting had become possible. It predated the time when the secrets of the human genome began to unravel. When it comes to the expansion of our knowledge and ingenuity, the only certain thing is that the future will bring changes and possibilities beyond our ability to imagine today.

My original attempt to describe some of the ways in which infertility and its cure affect the Jewish community has not been immune to this reality. So much has occurred in the past ten years that the original work feels old. Perhaps this was predictable. Keeping a work of this type current is very much a matter of hitting a moving target. Nevertheless, I have borne this burden since shortly after *Be Fruitful and Multiply* was first published.

The far reach of the original work was unanticipated, and it continues to grow. Good timing has been a blessing. The rapid pace of progress in reproductive medicine has not abetted. Public interest in the science and ethics of each new technique is intense. The Jewish community is no less affected than any other by the problem of infertility. Indeed, there are reasons why infertility looms larger, particularly for Jews who live according to halakha. Of necessity, *Be Fruitful and Multiply* has become a major resource for those who enter this territory for the first time. But it is no longer a comprehensive guide.

Overcoming Infertility is my attempt to keep Jewish couples informed about the current technology. With that as my goal, and knowing how rapidly this field changes, I am aware that this project can enjoy only fleeting success. Still, it is a good place to store another decade of experience in caring for infertile couples and some new knowledge that has accrued to me from my years as an author of some interest to my community. This book is, consequently, more than just a revision of my original work. The publication of *Overcoming Infertility* has provided me the opportunity to include topics that were missing in the original work.

As with *Be Fruitful and Multiply*, I have tried at all times during the writing to keep my threefold audience in mind. This new work is intended foremost for traditional Jewish couples who are struggling with infertility. For them I have taken care to update the chapters on medical treatment, to make them comprehensive and also to align their contents with the current technology. A new chapter specifically dealing with assisted reproduction has also been added. But like its predecessor, this book is also intended as a resource for the physicians and rabbis who care for these couples. To help bridge what is sometimes a wide gap in understanding between these two groups, other chapters have also been added. The first section of this work describes some history of medical interventions for infertility, because context is always important. A history of halakhic responsa on the subject is entirely new to this work, and should be of interest to rabbis, physicians and patients. Chapters on Sabbath considerations and rabbinical supervision in the fertility laboratories are also crucial to this topic. As several contributors deal with the same issues from different angles, there will be some unavoidable repetition. However, seeing the same facts from various viewpoints can help clarify and deepen understanding, and I hope that readers will bear with us and ultimately find it rewarding.

When *Be Fruitful and Multiply* was first published, it was the first in-depth examination of the topic of fertility therapy and the Jewish tradition. Since that time, this topic has become of great interest to many, and by now a voluminous literature on the subject exists. The purpose of *Overcoming Infertility* is not to reexamine everything that has been written on the subject, but rather to offer a single source where couples in need can find a straightforward discussion of the issues that confront them. To the extent that this information is shared with caregivers, including rabbis and counselors as well as clinicians, my goal will have been attained.

This book is intended to cover the broadest possible spectrum within the traditional (halakhic) Jewish community. It is not intended to serve as a halakhic source, just as it is not intended to serve as a source of medical advice. Its purpose is to open up for all parties involved new dimensions to their labors. Ultimately, the material it presents should create better educated consumers as well as better informed caregivers.

❧

Those who collaborated with me on this project have brought together a diverse experience with the problem of infertility in the traditional Jewish community. What has bound us together is the unusual fence which each of us has to straddle. That is, we continually see professionally interesting clinical problems on one side confront a strict set of religious mores on the other. Throughout the preparation of this work and, to a certain extent, throughout our careers, we remain perched on that fence. What we have gathered together is a description of some of the problems we face and some of the solutions that have emerged from our involvement.

There are numerous individuals whom I would like to thank for helping me to put together this work. Lord Immanuel Jakobovits, *zt"l*, the pioneer in presenting halakhic medical ethics to the broader community, was kind enough to write an introduction to *Be Fruitful and Multiply*. As the same spirit and purpose has suffused the current text, I have taken the liberty of reproducing it here. I also thank Tova Lichtenstein for allowing me to include an excerpt on adoption from the manuscripts of Rabbi Joseph B. Soloveitchik, *zt"l*.

xxxi

Sara Barris and Joel Comet shared with me the conception of this type of book. In 1989, we led a workshop at a symposium which focused on the special problems of Orthodox Jewish couples with infertility. As each couple related the particulars of their personal despair, we were left feeling that something needed to be done. Together, we conceived of a book which would bring together the halakhic issues pertaining to infertility. Their chapter "Infertility: Issues From the Heart," which deals with the psychological and social problems that affect Jewish infertile couples is especially insightful and should be helpful not only to those couples but also to the physicians and rabbis who work with them.

Dr. Yoel Jakobovits presented the first essay for *Be Fruitful and Multiply*. His discussion of the halakhic issues pertaining to the diagnosis of male infertility was thorough in its scope and set a scholarly tone for those that followed. This work has already appeared as a separate piece in *Tradition*. I would also like to thank the editors of *Tradition* for allowing me to reprint this material.

Like Dr. Jakobovits, Dr. Richard Weiss also combines the qualities of a *talmid hakham* (Torah scholar) and physician. His chapter on the laws of *niddah* is thoroughly detailed and referenced and should serve as essential reading for gynecologists who care for Orthodox women. He and I want to thank Rav Hershel Schachter, Rosh Kollel at Yeshiva University, for reviewing the material.

Rabbi Allen Schwartz contributed a thoughtful essay; his involvement with infertile couples and deep concern for them is obvious throughout. I must also thank Rabbi Heshie Billet for his interesting analysis.

All of the original authors included in *Be Fruitful and Multiply* have checked and revised their original work to reflect the passage of a decade. To their ranks have been added some new contributors, whom I thank as I acknowledge. Rabbi Avrohom Friedlander is the Chief Chaplain at Maimonides Medical Center, where I continue to serve as the Director of Reproductive Medicine. In consultation with Rabbis Menachem Burstein and Gideon Weitzman, of Machon Puah in Israel, Rabbi Friedlander implemented a program of full rabbinical supervision for Orthodox couples at Genesis Fertility & Reproductive Medicine, the program for assisted reproduction at Maimonides. With his help, thousands of Orthodox couples who otherwise would not have had access to treatment have been able to build their families through advanced reproductive techniques. The program at Genesis continues to be the only program of its type in the United States. Specifics of rabbinical oversight are presented in his chapter with the hope that the program may be duplicated in other settings that offer fertility services to this clientele. Complementary to this work is Rabbi Weitzman's chapter explaining the challenges that Sabbath observant Jews encounter during fertility therapy. These difficulties should also be considered by their caregivers.

Dr. Edward Reichman's historical review of the ways in which rabbis understood reproduction has become a classic in this genre since its original appearance in *Tradition*. This book is better for its inclusion. I again thank the editors of *Tradition* for allowing me to reprint this material.

Dr. Nachum Katlowitz has written a chapter on the treatment of male infertility. It perfectly complements the chapter on the diagnostic evaluation of male infertility already mentioned.

The transition from the original, shorter work on this topic to the current text was made possible with the help of many others. Rabbi Benjamin Kramer was invaluable as my assistant during this project. Donna Wach helped type some sections of this manuscript. My son, Joseph Grazi, was my artist in residence, painstakingly producing every drawing that I requested to help clarify the details of the accompanying narrative. May he continue to use his talent in other worthy pursuits. Joseph and I thank Tim Peters and Company and Dr. Mark Goldstein for allowing us to draw from some of the medical artwork that they have previously generated.

The professionals at *The* Toby Press could not have been more helpful to me in bringing this work to completion. Aloma Halter had overall responsibility for production of this manuscript, and offered many helpful suggestions and comments. Tani Solow

designed the artwork, and Raphaël Freeman, at Jerusalem Typesetting, supervised all the production aspects. I am especially indebted
to Batnadiv Weinberg, who did me the extraordinary favor of agree-
ing to edit this work. The breadth of her knowledge of secular and
Jewish sources, her dogged pursuit of clarity, her insight, and her
willingness to challenge me on virtually every aspect of the book, all
served to make this work more accurate, readable and user-friendly.
Above all, I thank Matthew Miller, my publisher and good friend,
for taking on this project and for encouraging his talented staff to
help me produce a book worthy of *The* Toby Press.

ॐ

There is a tradition in Judaism of *hakarat hatov*, acknowledging a
favor. This book would not have been possible without the many
favors done for me by Dr. Joel B. Wolowelsky, who continues to
be my teacher as well as my friend. His greatest favor has been
his broadening of my contacts with scholars in the halakhic community. The perspective this has given me in my work has helped
me in innumerable ways. Joel has continued to take an interest in
this and other topics in Jewish medical ethics. He has been kind to
include me in new thoughts and concerns, some of which we share
in a completely revised chapter on the ethical issues that stem from
the new reproductive technologies. His influence on this work is,
however, not confined to that one section. Indeed, he has continued
to guide me at each step during the production of this work. I am
forever grateful for his friendship and guidance.

My children Sally, Joseph, Ariel, Rebecca, Evan and Tamar
have grown up understanding what it means to have a father with
serious commitments beyond his family. Knowing that my commitment to them stands above all else, they have allowed me the
space and time to pursue my professional goals. My wife, Leslie,
has been and continues to be my main source of strength. She is
the wellspring of boundless energy and unconditional love that fills
our home and which compensates for me wherever I fall short. As
is painfully clear to all of my patients, there is no substitute for a

family. My love and thanks go first and foremost to my own. May they be fruitful and multiply, not only in their physical lives but also in their good deeds and commitment to their spiritual heritage.

Tov shem mi'shemen tov.

RVG, 2005

Part I
Infertility in Perspective

Introduction

Infertility is not a new problem. Indeed, it is as old as the Bible itself. Only our perception of infertility and how we deal with it have changed. Where once it was considered a spiritual affliction, today it is seen as only one of many medical conditions that may visit a person during his or her lifetime. It may be simple or complex, amenable to intervention or resistant, temporary or permanent. What makes infertility different from most other physical conditions, of course, is the spiritual overlay with which it is experienced.

It is useful for couples dealing with infertility to understand the historical context of their predicament. For Jewish couples, this includes the approaches of the rabbis through the ages, and especially during the modern age of reproductive treatment. Rabbis who advise such couples may also benefit from an historical perspective, inasmuch as this brings current medical therapy into focus, not as the ultimate solution for any given problem, but rather as another step in an evolving scientific process.

The chapters in this section are meant as an overview that may assist all involved as they delve deeper into the intricacies of resolving infertility within the context of contemporary Jewish law and ethics.

Richard V. Grazi

A Brief History of Fertility Therapy

> *Our Rabbis taught: There are three partners in the creation of man, God, the father and the mother. The father seminates the white substance, from which are derived the bones, vessels, fingernails, brain and the white of the eye. The mother seminates the red substance, from which are derived the skin, flesh, hair and the black of the eye. God provides the spirit, the soul, the beauty of the features, vision for the eyes, hearing for the ears, speech for the mouth, movement for the legs, understanding and intelligence. When the time comes for a man to depart this world, God rescinds his contribution, leaving behind the contributions of the mother and father.*
>
> Babylonian Talmud, Niddah 31a

The Talmudic description of the creation of man is well known because of its profound spiritual connotations. At its essence, it explains the Jewish concept of childbearing somewhat differently than what was set forth in the Torah. While man is commanded to "be fruitful and multiply," he cannot do so without the assistance of the Creator. Although the union of man and woman may be blessed, that union alone is insufficient to bring about the blessing of children. God's benevolence is also an integral part of conception and birth.

The integration of fertility with a spiritual force is not unique to the Jewish tradition. Historically, the process of conception was so shrouded in mystery that the only possible explanation was a mystical one, involving a power greater than the sum of man and woman alone. Such thinking was ingrained in nearly all ancient cultures and religions, and vestiges of it survive to this day in much of the cultural lore surrounding infertility.

It is somewhat difficult, from the high perch of our detailed scientific knowledge, to appreciate just how poorly our ancestors understood the reproductive process. It is instructive, nonetheless, to consider what was thought to control reproduction and how our knowledge about fertility and infertility evolved over time. Discussions about infertility that follow in this book are better understood with proper historical perspective. To be complete, some mention will be made of the seminal events and issues that confront the Jewish community and which currently beg a halakhic response. The newness and complexity of modern fertility therapy must be grasped in order to completely fathom the challenges it poses to observant Jews.

Infertility through the Ages

Observation was ancient humanity's sole scientific method. Following the only available clues, they recognized only the maternal contribution to reproduction. A professor describes the times wistfully: "At that stage the union of the sexes was a natural, simple pleasure entailing no responsibility whatever to either partner. Women bore children, and oaks bore acorns, but the intrusion of a fertilizing male element in either case was undreamed of."[1] In this matriarchal paradigm, menstrual flow was thought to be the precursor of children, explaining the observation that the cessation of menses was a prelude to pregnancy and that a woman who did not menstruate could not bear children. It was believed that blood was stored up over a nine month period to be transformed into a small human being.

Hippocrates, who lived in Greece in the fifth century BCE, at the end of the period of the First Temple, was among the first to explore and document the physiology of reproduction. The Hippocratic corpus is replete with writings specific to women, including treatises on conception, pregnancy, and infertility. In these works, Hippocrates hypothesized the existence of discrete male and female roles in conception. He thought, incorrectly, that impregnation occurred shortly before or after menses. Hippocrates also hypothesized that there exists a female seed. The derivation and location of this seed, as well as its exact purpose, were unknown, but he conjectured that male and female seed each produced different structures in the developing fetus. The Talmud as quoted above is consistent with this theory. Although the basic elements of the Hippocratic theory are correct, it would take nearly 2,000 years to prove this particular notion.

A contrasting view was put forth and popularized by Aristotle (384–322 BCE), whose life coincided with the early years of the Second Temple. Aristotle ascribed to the female no distinct role in the formation of the fetus. He conjectured that the male seed, which was readily visible, was "planted" in the womb, much the same way that farmers plant seeds in the ground. The purpose of the seed was to provide form to the matter that eventually produced the fetus, i.e. the accumulated menstrual flow. This view was adopted by Pliny, a first century Roman, who wrote that menstrual flow "is the material for human generation, as the semen from the males acting like rennet collects this substance within it, which thereupon immediately is inspired with life and endowed with body."[2]

Although the function of the testes and the pathway of seminal fluid were somewhat understood, there were many theories about the source of the male seed. Hippocrates believed that the seed was a derivative of other crucial parts of the body, especially the brain, from which it drew its formative powers. The extent to which each part contributed would determine if a male or female child was produced. This view is echoed in the writings of many philosophers of the time. Aristotle, in contrast, pinpointed the soul as the source of the male seed; others hypothesized that it was derived from the spinal marrow or other blood components.[3] This idea is also found in the epic work of Lucretius, (96–55 BCE), who describes the journey of the seed through every part of the male body, concentrating in the genitals and finally ejecting "in the direction in which tyrannical lust is tugging."[4]

The nature of the uterus was the subject of much speculation. Hippocrates believed that the uterus is bicornuate, like those of rodents, with the right side reserved for female fetuses and the left for males. He therefore predicted that a unilateral uterine abscess, though not a barrier to fertility, would allow an affected woman to bear children of only one sex.[5] Many popular myths attributed to the uterus an independent existence, capable of wandering about and leaving the body. Plato (c. 428–347 BCE) is known to have championed the idea that a uterus deprived of pregnancy could meander about the body, causing anxiety and respiratory difficulties.[6] The idea that the uterus was independently animated was taken as medical gospel for centuries and was influential even in relatively recent theses on hysteria.[7]

The earliest complete work on the subject of gynecology is considered to be Soranus' description of female anatomy, written in the second century CE. (It was a well known text in its day, and it seems reasonable to assume the *amoraim* were aware of it.) After this treatise was refined by Aetius in the sixth century, the practice of gynecology changed little for the next thousand years. During that time, female infertility was treated mainly with dilatation, local applications of various plant parts, fumigation and rectification of malpositions. It was only in the sixteenth century that Gabriele Fallopius (1523–1562), a professor of anatomy in Pisa, first described the tubes leading from the ovary to the uterus, which were subsequently named for him. He failed, however, to grasp the function of the Fallopian tubes.

Treatment for male infertility consisted of the prescription of innumerable aphrodisiacs to impotent males. Male infertility in the presence of sexual competence was not recognized as a medical problem at all, and the affected were wont to use magic instead.

In this confusion over reproductive organs and processes, no consistent theory of infertility was possible. Most doctors did feel, however, that it was a disease, and not a symptom of one. Common folklore relegated this disease, even more than others, to the will of the gods. But Western medicine was of no better help in properly deciphering and addressing the causes and treatments of infertility. Throughout the Renaissance and early industrial age, medicine as a discipline had about as much to offer infertile couples as the more mystical or religiously oriented cures. Both modalities resulted in sporadic pregnancies among previously infertile couples. As no rigorous scientific method had yet been developed with which to determine cause and effect, such "successes" led to the proliferation of many potions and procedures. Though these had little, if any, basis in physiology as we now understand it, they gained the attention and respect of their adherents just as the magic of primitive societies had a hold on its people and, for that matter, just as modern science captivates its current audience. It would take many centuries until medical and surgical cures would replace the more popular methods aimed at dispelling demons and placating a deity. Many modern day superstitions surrounding infertility are holdovers from this particular history.

With this as background, it is obvious that all of the early rabbinic literature that discusses fertility and infertility developed at a time when the true nature of reproduction was shrouded in mystery. The Mishnah was codified in approximately the year 200 CE. The Babylonian Talmud was codified in approximately the year 500 CE. The *rishonim*—Rashi, Rambam and the Rosh[8]—all lived between the years 1000 and 1300 CE. The *Shulkhan Arukh*, which initiated the era of the *aharonim*, was completed by Rabbi Yosef Karo in 1532, prior even to Fallopius' work on female anatomy.

To reflect a more accurate picture of reproduction, the writings of the *aharonim* would need to await further elucidation of reproductive anatomy and physiology. This began in earnest in the seventeenth century. In 1651, William Harvey, best known for his description of the circulation of blood, postulated that all living beings must derive from eggs. Using gross anatomical dissection, Reinier de Graaf first described the egg follicle in the ovary in 1672 (the mature egg follicle is still referred to today as the Graafian follicle). But the seminal event in the understanding of reproduction occurred in 1650, with Antonie van Leewenhoek's invention of the microscope. In 1677, the existence of sperm was discovered by Luis Namon in Germany. When these were examined microscopically by van Leewenhoek and Spallanzani, both agreed that what they saw were "animalcules," or precursors of human beings.[9] Their drawings indicate that prior beliefs were very prejudicial to their visual findings for, among their drawings, they included depictions of a small "homonculus," a completely formed human being lying within the head of the sperm. They were careful to include details such as digestive tracts in what we now know to be simply spermatozoa. These reports were used to support the theory of preformation, a

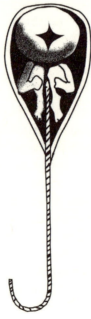

Homonculus

popular notion about conception that lasted another two hundred years. Rabbinic responsa, both of *rishonim* and *aharonim,* are replete with references to this theory and should be understood in their proper context.[10]

Preformation, later called the homunculus theory, replaced the notion of menstrual blood derivation. This theory proposed that a tiny human being, complete with rudimentary organs, was secreted in the semen and grown in the uterus. Predictably, a contrary school of thought developed around the ovarist theory. This stated that certain "germes" preexisted in the ovaries since the commencement of the world, boxed one within the other, developing themselves successively with each generation. These "germes" were supposed to have contained all the lineaments of the new being, and contact with semen was all that was needed to begin their growth.

Although few could dispute the words of eminent scientists, there were some doctors who were not satisfied. In 1777, Andrew Wilson wrote the following: "After all that is known of animalcules, and ova and of embryos found in the Fallopian tubes, etc. the act of generation, and what individually each sex contributes to it, remains still a mystery. Whether one sex furnished the rudimental organ of an individual, and the other excites the first determinate action of what ethical principle that is to animate and possess it, I will not determine. However, I must say that I think the learned and sagacious Dr. Harvey's theory on that subject has still more verisimilitude in it than the doctrine of animalcules and their nidi, or ova; which to me carries this absurdity in it, that ultimately it makes generation the work of the male alone; and which is still more absurd, it reduces the generation of living animals to the mere secretion of a gland or glands."[11]

Uterine function was less debated but equally misconstrued. Menstruation, which retained in western cultures a primitive mystique, was believed by physicians to be a healthy purging of the body's plethora of blood. This was based on the notion of natural phlebotomy, originally proposed by Galen in the second century.[12] A woman who did not menstruate was therefore subject to a variety of curative attempts. The famous Dr. Herman Boerhaave, who also described anatomical impediments to menstruation, explains the treatments available in 1724: "But when occasioned from the Stagnation of the Liquid, then ought it be made to flow, 1. By fomenting and rubbing the Feet, Legs, and Thighs 2. By opening a Vein in the Foot, and letting out a moderate quantity of Blood. 3. By giving Purges that will work upon the Womb. 4. By administering Emmenagoga. 5. By Plaisters to the Belly, Fomentations, Liniments, Steams to the privy Parts, and received into the Vagina through a Funnel, and by Heat. 6. By strengthening the very Vessels weakened by the Plethora with Chalibeats and Astringents."[13]

In 1769 Giovanni Batista Morgagni published a series of letters which dealt with, among other things, "the Impediments to Venery, and of Sterility in both Sexes."[14] It is significant that, in the entire essay, only anatomical impediments to conception are mentioned, for only these could usually be directly observed. Ingenious contraptions and procedures are described, with enthusiastic reports of success. However, sterility in a couple who could properly mix semen and menstrual flow is not considered. It is probable that such couples still utilized the services of priests and magicians.

Prior to the 1800s, the ovum was thought to be discharged at intercourse, as a result of orgasm, for it was well known that male orgasm caused the discharge of semen. In fact, even as late as 1855, a French physician published a treatise on sterility that maintained that frigidity was a major cause of female sterility. A year later, however, Dr. A.K. Gardner offered a different view of the problem: "I am convinced that but one questioned is to be asked, viz. if healthy spermatozoa are brought into contact with healthy ova, to decide this question."[15] He proposed that ovulation occurred during menstruation, independent of sexual activity, and that in order for conception to occur, the ovum had to be fertilized before entering the uterus. Although he was close to the mark physiologically, his recommended treatments for female sterility were the usual cantharides and mercurials.

The difficulty in understanding and treating infertility can be observed in the classic nineteenth century overview of the subject, Mondat's *Sterility in the Male and Female,*[16] with its characteristic mixed bag of theories concerning the causes of infertility and its list of largely useless medical and surgical procedures. In the first section, a variety of anatomical anomalies in the male and their surgical corrections are described. Anaphrodesia, however, is implicated as the major cause of male infertility. The etiologies of this condition are many. These include excessive abstinence, as well as excessive masturbation, both of which were considered abusive to the body. Affections of the mind, especially as a result of extreme passions such as hatred and jealousy, are also implicated. This tendency toward negative value judgments of the sterile male is somewhat offset by Mondat's contention that the pursuit of genius may also be enervating, for it attracts the entire attention of the nervous system. As an example, he notes that Newton is said to have died a virgin. Recommended treatments include exercise, improved diet, malaxation, shampooing, and some less soothing remedies such as electricity and application of leeches to the neck.

The causes of infertility, however, were thought to preside primarily in the woman. Abnormalities of the female reproductive tract are described in the second section of Mondat's book. Again, anaphrodesia is heavily implicated in female infertility. However, nymphomania is also suspected. "Thus an erotic, ardent temperament…seems to be less favorable to fecundation than a temperament less sensitive to the enjoyments of love. If fecundation requires on the part of the man ardent desires, it demands of the female only pleasant complaisance and tender affections." Mondat goes even further in arousing suspicion of the infertile female by suggesting that her condition may be due to a rejection of traditional femininity. Observing that most women who are serious students of science are sterile (sic), he remarks that "the sanguino-lymphatic temperament with which it [the female organization] is generally endowed appears also to be more favorable to conception, and hence it has been remarked that those females who vary the most from this temperament are most subject to sterility."

In regards to medical and surgical procedures, the interventions suggested are probably about as efficacious as the fertility rites of primitive societies. What is more, it is questionable whether even contemporaries viewed these fertility treatments as anything other than Western man's version of magic and exorcism.

From our modern perspective, Mondat's pronouncements regarding infertility seem ludicrous, and it is convenient to think that we have now achieved a more objective, non-judgmental approach to the problem of infertility. But folklore does not easily disappear. A telling example is the evaluation of the male fertility factor. In 1909, semen analysis was first advocated as a routine procedure. The author who introduced this test explained that "[T]his examination, which is of comparatively recent introduction, is becoming recognized by the public, and will be, perhaps, before long expected by them. Many, however, are still unaware that a man who is sexually vigorous is ever barren"[17] Nearly a century later, it is still not uncommon for physicians to perform lengthy, expensive, and sometimes painful infertility workups on women without first addressing the male factor. Halakhically, there may be compelling reasons to do so. But it remains an important cultural myth that barrenness is mainly a problem of women. As will be demonstrated later in this book, this could not be further from the truth.

Fertility Therapy in the Modern Era

The first artificial insemination using sperm from the husband was performed and described by John Hunter in 1785. The use of fresh semen from a donor for artificial insemination is first described by William Pancoast in 1884. This technique remained essentially unchanged for 100 years, until HIV/AIDS made the use of such material too risky.

During the nineteenth century, modern scientific methodology was further developed. It underwent important developments, and physicians were able to incorporate many scientific advances into the practice of medicine. Anesthetics, antiseptics, and aseptic techniques allowed for the comfortable and safe performance of surgery. By the beginning of the twentieth century, the process of ovulation was understood, as were the proper function of the sperm, the egg, the fallopian tubes, and the uterus. Many novel methods were subsequently developed by which physicians could diagnose and surgically treat infertility. Some of these are listed here:

A Chronology of Developments in Modern Reproductive Medicine[18]

	Ephraim McDowell performs first abdominal surgery
1827	Ernst Von Baer proves the existence of a human egg, or oocyte
1842	Crawford Long introduces ether anesthesia
1845	Ignaz Philipp Semmelweis develops aseptic technique
1849	Marion Simms becomes the first gynecologic surgeon
1902– 1933	Robert Dickinson, MD, a Brooklyn gynecologist, draws and sculpts accurate presentations of the female anatomy
1920	Isadore Rubin develops tubal insufflation for detecting tubal infertility
1944	Founding of the American Fertility Society (AFS)
1948	J. Macleod describes washed sperm
1950	First issue of *Fertility & Sterility*, official publication of the AFS
1955	AFS endorses donor insemination
1960	First oral contraceptive pill approve by the US Food and Drug Administration (FDA)

1962	Clomiphene introduced
1965	Varicocelectomy reported as helpful for male infertility
1968	Human menopausal gonadotropins approved by the Food and Drug Administration (FDA)
1970	Laparoscopic surgery introduced by Kurt Semm
1977	Microsurgery of the fallopian tube described by Victor Gomel Nobel Prize in Medicine awarded to Rosalyn S. Yallow, PhD, developer of radioimmunoassay for measuring hormones
1978	First birth from in vitro fertilization, England
1981	First birth from in vitro fertilization, US
1984	Gamete intrafallopian transfer (GIFT) is described
1986	First Ethics Committee Report of the AFS, *Ethical Considerations of the New Reproductive Technologies*
1987	Society for Assisted Reproductive Technology is formed

In 1878, the first attempts at in vitro fertilization using mammalian eggs were performed in Vienna by Schenk. Building on his techniques, Walter Heape showed that unimplanted fertilized eggs from rabbits could be collected and transferred to recipient rabbits, which would then bear offspring. (This exact technique was later adapted for egg donation in humans, as described by John Buster.)[19]

The techniques of culturing mammalian eggs, in vitro fertilization, and embryo transfer were perfected in the early decades of the twentieth century and eventually laid the foundations for later work in humans. The first successful IVF pregnancy in rabbits was described by Chang only a few years after Landrum Shettles first suggested the idea of human in vitro fertilization (IVF). From these achievements, it became clear that oocytes, or eggs, required maturation before fertilization was possible, and that sperm were required to undergo a process called "capacitation" before they were capable of fertilizing the oocytes. The first successes using embryo freezing were also reported in the 1950s, and this work was later adapted to human IVF.

No work on the development of modern infertility techniques would be complete without the mention of Dr. Robert G. Edwards, a British reproductive biologist whose pioneering work has profoundly influenced the current generation of reproductive scientists and physicians. Dr. Edwards began his work in the early 1960s, studying the process of fertilization in small mammals and then, in the latter half of the decade, moving on to human oocyte physiology. In 1968, he first met Patrick Steptoe, a British gynecologist who was a pioneer in the use of the laparoscope. The laparoscope is a thin telescope that can be used to peer inside the pelvic cavities of women in order to diagnose and cure certain illnesses. With his laparoscope, Steptoe was easily able to see his patients' fallopian tubes and ovaries. If tubal blockage was the cause of his patient's infertility, Steptoe would retrieve oocytes, which Edwards would then fertilize and culture in vitro. But human fertilization in a Petri dish was more finicky than what had been observed in rabbits. It took a decade of persistence, working on hundreds of patients, until, on July 25, 1978, Steptoe and Edwards reported the birth of Louise Brown, the first human being born after fertilization and conception in vitro.[20]

It is an important historical note that, after the announcement of the world's first "test tube baby," there followed a worldwide outcry over the ethics of the procedure. Although it was clear that the technique opened up a whole new avenue of treatment for women who were hopelessly sterile because of blocked tubes (the potential for the use of IVF to cure other causes of infertility, including male problems, was not yet appreciated), religious leaders and ethicists of the day denounced the technique as exploitive and predicted that it would begin a "slippery slope" in the devaluation of life. As a result of popular sentiment, Steptoe and Edwards lost their support from the National Health Service of the United Kingdom and found an equally cold reception from their university colleagues. Having no other choice, in 1980 they set up a private clinic—Bourne Hall. Today, Bourne Hall remains one of the world's most outstanding research facilities in the field of human reproduction.

The following events followed quickly after the first few years of experience with IVF:

Historical "Firsts" in Human Assisted Reproduction

1982	First use of ovarian stimulation prior to egg retrieval
1982	First use of transabdominal ultrasound for egg retrieval
1983	First use of transvaginal ultrasound for egg retrieval First pregnancy using uterine lavage for egg donation First birth from a cryopreserved (frozen) embryo
1984	First pregnancy using egg donation with IVF
1986	First pregnancy from a cryopreserved egg
1988	First pregnancy from micromanipulation of sperm and eggs
1989	First birth after preimplantation genetic diagnosis
1992	First birth from intracytoplasmic sperm injection
1993	First cloned human embryos
1996	First birth of a mammal (sheep) cloned from a somatic cell
1997	First birth from a cryopreserved egg
2004	First pregnancy from cryopreserved ovarian tissue

This explosion of information and rapid development of technologies related to fertility and infertility is not expected to abate. The recent decoding of the human genome will open up completely new possibilities, not only in alleviating infertility but also in preventing and curing genetic diseases. What is clear about cloning—which by now has been performed successfully in numerous mammalian species—is not just that it can be done in humans but that inevitably it will be done. Despite the grave problems and concerns of living in today's world, the quest to have children remains powerfully constant, and the experience of infertility is as devastating as ever. While no one can negate the power of prayer to beseech the heavens for a swift solution, many couples must now and in the future turn to medical science to open the gates of parenthood. Scientific progress will continue and, over time, heretofore unexpected solutions will undoubtedly arise. Jews committed to the authority of the halakha trust that problems will be met squarely, proper analyses will be done and, over time, consensus will emerge for the benefit of the community.

Halakhic Responses to Fertility Interventions

Jewish law takes very seriously the *yihus* of a person—that is, his or her genealogical history. One reason is the natural assumption shared by many people that personality traits run in families. But much more important is the fact that *yihus* must be established in order to allow two people to marry. Under Jewish law, both parties must be Jewish and not have a first degree relationship (sibling, filial) between them. In addition, *mamzerim* (sg. *mamzer*: the halakhically illegitimate) can only marry among themselves. If the genetic father of a child is unknown, he or she might not be able to marry freely, as Jewish legal authorities must consider the possibility—even though it may be remote—that the couple before them share a genetic father, making them half-siblings and ineligible for marriage.

19

Historically, only halakhic paternity could be in doubt, as maternity was the obvious and recognized consequence of a woman's pregnancy and delivery. With the advent of certain types of assisted reproduction, however, genetic conception and birth can now be separated. This medical achievement has forced a re-examining of the halakhic determinants of maternity and paternity.

Unlike secular law, which can define and alter parental relationships, for halakha, once established, parenthood is immutable. The halakha, therefore, is more concerned with *discovering* maternity and paternity. In response to various developments in reproductive medicine, the halakha has explored the issues, using precedent to determine whether or not each procedure is permissible, and who would be the halakhic parents in each situation. The earliest halakhic literature of this type addressed the permissibility of undergoing artificial insemination. Rabbinic responsa dealing with every imaginable consequence of artificial insemination proliferated as more and more couples found the need to undergo this procedure.

All rabbinic writings dealing with artificial insemination rely on a widely held belief, dating back to antiquity, that a woman may conceive without intercourse if she bathes in water into which sperm has been emitted. Two sources for such "bathhouse insemination" exist in classic Jewish literature. The Talmud, in Hagiga 14b, discusses whether the *Kohen Gadol* (high priest) could marry a pregnant woman who claims to be a virgin. Bathhouse insemination explains her predicament. The second is the *Alphabet of Ben Sira*, an apocryphal text detailing the life of Shimon Ben Sira, widely believed to be the son and grandson of the prophet Jeremiah. The prophet's daughter conceived from his emission when she inadvertently entered the same bath.

Although the veracity of Ben Sira's conception as well as the Talmudic description of bathhouse insemination are matters of some controversy, they are extensively cited by *rishonim* and *aharonim*. Ben Sira's story is also noteworthy in that his lineage and legitimacy are never questioned. Noting the case of Ben Sira, Rabbi Pertetz ben Eliyahu of Corbeil, author of *Sefer Mitzvot Katan*, states that a woman who is *niddah* may conceive from the remnant sperm of her husband if she lies on his sheets, but that the child would not be considered a *ben niddah*.[21] The halakhic implications are twofold. First, the child born from conception without intercourse is considered the legitimate offspring of whoever produced the sperm. Secondly, the prohibition of *arayot* (illicit relations) refers only to the physical act of intercourse. Without it, a child cannot be considered a *mamzer*.

These sources have been used to permit procreation by artificial insemination, though the halakhic paternity of a child born by such means has been a matter of controversy. The use of donor sperm for insemination is a more complex matter that will be discussed later in this book.

The earliest responses to IVF, on the other hand, were negative. The dominant views followed the argument put forth in 1982 by Rabbi Eliezer Waldenberg, Chief Justice of the Beit Din (rabbinical court) in Jerusalem and author of the *Tziz Eliezer*.[28] Although in an earlier responsum he had allowed artificial insemination using the husband's sperm, he maintained that he did so with misgivings, and only under extraordinary circumstances. He could not apply his leniency with artificial insemination to IVF for several reasons. First, he maintained that the medical establishment could not be trusted to use only the husband's sperm, as their primary concern is to increase success and not necessarily to adhere to any ethical guidelines. Halakhic oversight of the process notwithstanding, Rabbi Waldenberg felt that it would be easier to switch the husband's sperm for a donor's in the context of IVF, because the materials being manipulated necessarily spend more time outside of the body than with insemination. Secondly, he reasoned that, with insemination, all of the sperm are returned to the woman, independent of the outcome. With IVF, on the other hand, no sperm is returned, evoking a concern for *hoza'at zera levatala* as well as potentially leaving leftover sperm available for misuse. With regard to *hoza'at zera levatala*, he could find no room for leniency when the main reason for the husband to produce the semen was not to overcome a problem of fertility in himself, but rather to overcome a problem in his wife, e.g. tubal blockage. Thirdly, there is an historic disagreement among *poskim* (rabbis who have authority to issue halakhic rulings) regarding halakhic paternity when conception occurs with artificial insemination. Because Rabbi Waldenberg regarded the insemination procedure as a simple matter of assisting the process of fertilization to occur in its natural location, he took the lenient view of assigning paternity. However, as IVF entails separating the gametes and the embryo from their natural locations, he held that evidence of both paternity and maternity were compromised. As a result, neither the mitzvah of *peru u'revu* or *lashevet yitzrah* were fulfilled when a child was born through IVF. Fourth, Rabbi Waldenberg anticipated that the use of IVF technology would lead to complete development of the fetus in vitro, to cloning, to the eventual breakdown of the marital relationship, and that the halakhic concept of *yihus* (lineage) would be tainted. Finally, Rabbi Waldenberg felt that IVF was not amenable to proper halakhic oversight, and it therefore held the potential for misuse, leading to situations where siblings might marry, or the transgression of *gilui arayot*. Having considered all of these matters, his conclusion was that IVF was not permissible.

Not all authorities, however, fell in line with Rabbi Waldenberg. Those who permitted IVF, most notably Rabbi Yosef Elyashiv and Rabbi Ovadia Yosef, did so on the basis of three principles: (1) the obligation to fulfill the commandment of *peru u'revu* which, in keeping with our understanding of biology and also the normative view, is fulfilled as long as the sperm and eggs are those of the husband and wife, (2) the value of *gemilut hasadim* (loving-kindness) according to which it is improper to prolong the suffering of an infertile couple by withholding from them an available treatment, and (3) the preservation of *shalom bayit* (family integrity) which has a position of such high importance in Jewish tradition that it can tip the scales in favor of leniency whenever halakhic uncertainty arises.[23]

Today the dominant halakhic view of standard IVF using gametes from the husband and wife is one of permissibility. Lone dissenters are confined to the *poskim* of the *haredi* (the so-called ultra-Orthadox) communities, and even they may give a *heter* (halakhic permission) privately when the circumstances so warrant. However, many questions in reproductive halakha remain unresolved as of this writing. These include the use of IVF when it entails the use of gametes—egg or sperm—from a third party, or when a gestational surrogate is used to carry the fetus. Such "third party reproduction," as well as the "spin-off" technologies of cloning, nuclear transfer, preimplantation genetic diagnosis and others will be considered in detail later in this book.

Difficult Issues

Although it would be easy to dismiss the concerns of the *poskim* about the switching of gametes from one couple to another, any complete discussion of the development of modern reproductive medicine must include the mistakes and abuses that have peppered its otherwise exemplary history.

In William Pancoast's original 1884 description of successful donor insemination, he reported unabashedly how he used a semen specimen from "the best looking medical student in the class" to inseminate his patient without the knowledge of her husband. Interestingly, he states that when this was revealed to him, the husband was pleased. It is difficult to believe that this was so, as such intentional cuckoldry would have been appalling to most men. (While some rabbis permit donor insemination, most would agree that a woman who does this without the consent of her husband is forbidden to her husband after the event, and must divorce him and forfeit the rights of her *ketubah* [marriage contract].)[24] This dishonorable aspect of donor insemination reached its climax in the case of Dr. Cecil Jacobson who, throughout the 1970s and 1980s, used his own sperm to inseminate his patients. DNA testing eventually confirmed that as many as 75 children were born from these inseminations. Dr. Jacobson was eventually convicted and sent to prison. The effects on those families established as a result of his criminal activities have not been addressed. In 1995, investigators

revealed that Dr. Ricardo Asch, a well-know reproductive specialist in Irvine, California, had used the eggs of women undergoing
IVF without their knowledge to produce embryos for other women
who had requested egg donation. Dr. Asch and his collaborators
escaped the United States as fugitives from the law and currently
practice medicine in South America.

Although these cases are striking and horrifying, they represent the only known intentional abuse of gametes in the application
of modern fertility technology, which has otherwise been used successfully to produce millions of babies in the last 25 years. But the
intentional misuse of reproductive materials is not the only fuel for
rabbinic misgivings. In 1996, scientists in Holland reported to the
world the first acknowledged mistake in an IVF lab. According to
their account, a stray sperm from one couple's treatment cycle was
used to inject an egg from another couple. The woman conceived
and delivered twins, one white and one black. The mother kept both
children. Racially discordant twins were also born in New York City
in 1995 after an embryologist mistakenly transferred embryos to the
wrong patient. In this case, each child was subsequently given to its
genetic parents. However, such events are, again, the rare exceptions
to the rule, which is that IVF is generally done uneventfully the
world over, in hundreds of thousands of patients annually.

In light of the above, it is fascinating to consider just how pre-
scient were the concerns of those rabbis who wrote their responsa
in the early days of IVF. On the other hand, it should be noted that
most of the early concerns have been addressed by professional
societies and, in many countries, by governmental authorities that
have set standards for the safe operation of embryology laboratories. The many rules, regulations, processes, and inspections to
which the modern-day reproductive laboratory is subjected make
it exceptionally unlikely that mistakes can occur. *Intentional* deceit
would now require a sophisticated and highly secretive conspiracy
among physicians and laboratory staff, the stuff of fictional novels.
Still, because the halakhic consequences are so grave,[25] many *poskim*
have required as condition of their *heter* for IVF that independent,
rabbinically sanctioned supervision be present in the laboratory.

These *mashgihim* add a layer of religiously sanctioned comfort to Orthodox couples who avail themselves of modern reproductive care. This solution to rabbinical concerns is discussed in more detail later in this book and is an example of halakhic problem-solving at its best.

The Problem of Consenus

The ways in which Jewish couples presently confront and solve their infertility are as diverse as the Jewish people themselves. There is not one unified approach. Secular and non-observant Jews tend to live comfortably with modern reproductive technologies, and use them liberally in order to achieve their family building and community expanding goals. However, *haredi* Jews may rely more on prayer, and use medical intervention sparingly and reluctantly. Between these two groups, and with a more complicated response to the problem of infertility and its treatment, lives a large and like-minded community of traditional Jews who on the one hand view infertility as a spiritual challenge, and on the other view modern medical technology as just another manifestation of divine solutions. This group will use technology willingly, but only insofar as it meshes with what is perceived to be ethically and spiritually proper.

 The opposing viewpoints may be summarized by two principles rooted in halakhic lore. The first is the principle of *hadash assur min haTorah*,[26] "that which is new [literally] is forbidden by the Torah." The actual Mishnaic statement refers to the "new" harvest, which, until the *Omer* grain-offering was brought to the Temple, was not permitted for consumption. In later times, however, rabbis have used it to prevent changes in local customs. Reproductive technologies certainly fit the rubric of *hadash*, so it would be simple to conclude that their newness renders them impermissible. On the other hand, there is a competing Mishnaic principle of *kal d'aved rahamana l'tav aved*,[27] "everything that the Merciful One has created He has created for good." Thus, for example, Jews of all traditions have willingly adopted broadcast and computer technology to enhance their Torah learning and teaching capabilities. With this principle in mind, reproductive technology is no different: it must be harnessed to further the needs of the Jewish community. Finding a balance between these two principles is the difficulty: Can it be said that everything that is new is permissible? May it be permissible, but not desirable?

As the Jewish community confronts the emerging reproductive technologies, it would be useful if there were one authoritative voice that could provide *the* answer to every question. In this way, clear lines could be drawn between acceptable and unacceptable medical decision-making. But this is not in keeping with Jewish tradition. "There are seventy faces to the Torah," the Talmud states.[28] Within the accepted framework of halakhic principles, interpretation of the law is left to the discretion of the local *posek,* or rabbi whose understanding of halakha is comprehensive enough to enable him to issue the final word. *Mutar* or *assur*, permissible or not, is up to his judgment, which must withstand the scrutiny not only of the questioners but also of his peers. It is understood—indeed it is expected—that different *poskim* may reach different conclusions about the same matter. So it is, for example, that in one community a certain product is considered kosher, while in others it is not.

Still, the problems brought to bear by fertility technologies differ in certain ways. If two neighbors observe different standards of kashrut, there are no serious implications. They may, perhaps, not eat at each other's homes, but their relationship is otherwise unaffected. If, however, those same neighbors adhere to different halakhic views about reproductive technologies, there may be serious implications. For example, one may believe a certain reproductive procedure to be impermissible according to halakha. He might even consider the procedure akin to an adulterous relationship, and the resultant child therefore a *mamzer*. But his neighbor may disagree, believing that the procedure in question is perfectly permissible, and that the child is kosher for all intents and purposes. If the second neighbor now brings such a child into the world, the first would not consider such a child marriageable within his own family. Fearing a problem of lineage and legitimacy, lines would be drawn between otherwise like-minded neighbors who may even live and worship in the very same Jewish community. Furthermore, unlike holiday observance or adherence to the dietary laws, the use of fertility therapies usually occurs in secret. Infertile couples understandably guard their privacy. When they are successful, they will rarely divulge the details of how their long-awaited offspring came to be. Some may even consider such discussions immodest. The lineage of all Jews will therefore become suspect. How future generations of halakhically committed Jews will look to issues of lineage is currently unclear.

Conflicting views among groups of individuals who follow the same religious guidelines may be confusing to health care providers. It is important for them to understand that the halakha is a living and evolving legal construct, continuously responding to a rapidly changing science. Because there are so many vastly different scenarios of the use of reproductive technology, there is not as yet any uniform halakhic response. At the same time, uncertainty regarding the halakhic permissibility of certain treatments exacerbates the already intense pressures that couples encounter during medical therapy. The treatment of infertility is often experienced as an invasion into the Jewish values of physical privacy and sexual modesty. It also may bring unanticipated demands on the halakhot that govern marital life. These medical, logistical, and spiritual challenges are best met when the couple is confident that decisions are being made on solid halakhic foundations.

Nevertheless, most traditional Jews today find themselves living at the crossroads of modern medicine and traditional halakhic values. In trying to square the demands and potentials of both, each may find a different comfort zone. Just as each person interprets the spiritual challenges differently, each may draw the road to resolution slightly differently. Because the halakha is constantly reacting to change, the choices made by individuals will also change with time. It is crucial for Jewish couples confronting infertility to be aware of the possibilities that are available to them within the guidelines of contemporary Jewish law and ethics. Likewise, their caregivers—rabbis and doctors alike—must be sensitive to the complex demands with which they struggle in their quest for parenthood.

Endnotes

1. D. McKenzie, *The Infancy of Medicine*, (London: MacMillan & Co, Ltd., 1972).
2. C.C. Mettler, *History of Medicine*, (Philadelphia: The Blakiston Co., 1947).
3. C.V. Mondat, *Sterility in the Male and Female,* (Boston: Saxton, Pierce & Co., 1844).
4. Lucretius, *On the Nature of the Universe*, (New York: Penguin Classics, 1951).
5. Mettler, 1947.
6. McKenzie, 1927.
7. A. Wilson, *Medical Researches*, (London: Hooper and Robinson, 1777).
8. Respectively, Rabbi Shimon Yitzhaki, Rabbi Moshe ben Maimon (Maimonides) and Rabbi Asher—See Glossary of Halakhic Terms. They each compiled commentaries on the Talmud that hold special significance in halakhic literature.
9. R.D. Amelar, L. Dubin and P.C. Walsh, *Male Infertility*. (Philadelphia: W.B. Saunders Co., 1977).
10. See the following chapter for a more comprehensive discussion of historical views on fertility and their impact on rabbinic writings.
11. Mettler, 1947.
12. See note 7.
13. H. Boerhaave, *Aphorisms: Concerning the Knowledge and Core of Disease*, (London, 1724).
14. G.B. Morgagni, *The Seats and Causes of Diseases*, (London, 1769).
15. A.K. Gardner. *Sterility*, (New York: DeWitt & Davenport, 1856).
16. Mondat, 1844.
17. G.N. Champneys, *Sterility in System of Gynaecology*, C. Allbutt, U.S. Plavtain, and T.W. Eden, eds., (London: MacMillan & Co, Ltd., 1909).
18. W.E. Duka, A.H. DeCherney, *From the Beginning: A History of the American Fertility Society 1944–1994,* (American Fertility Society, 1994).
19. J.E. Buster, "Embryo donation by uterine flushing and embryo transfer," *Clinics in Obstetrics and Gynecology*, 12(4):815, 1985.
20. R.G. Edwards, P.C. Steptoe, *A Matter of Life—The Story of a Medical Breakthrough*, (London: Hutchinson and Co., Ltd., 1980).
21. Although a child conceived while his mother is a *niddah*—a *ben niddah*—is

considered fully legitimate, spiritual and mystical considerations ascribe to such children a special status that is considered problematic by some halakhically observant couples.

22. Rabbi Eliezer Waldenberg, *Tzitz Eliezer* xv, no. 45, in Assia vol. 9, no. 1, 5742.

23. M. Halperin, "In vitro fertilitzation, embryo transfer, and embryo freezing," *Jewish Medical Ethics* 1(1):25–30, (1988).

24. For a more detailed discussion, see Abraham S. Abraham, *Nishmat Avraham*, vol. iii, siman 1. (Brooklyn: Mesorah Publications, Ltd., 2004).

25. See opening of section.

26. Mishna Orlah 3:9.

27. *Babylonian Talmud*, Berakhot 60b.

28. Midrash Bamidbar Rabbah 13:15.

Edward Reichman

The Rabbinic Conception of Conception

The extraordinary technological advances of this century have been applied with full force to the field of science and, in particular to the specialties of genetics and reproductive medicine. Man now has more control over his own reproduction than ever before in history, such that the old notion of the doctor playing God has taken on new meaning. In the ultimate form of *imitatio dei*, just as God creates, now, it appears, so does man. We currently have the capability to isolate a single sperm, unite it in vitro with an egg, and test the resultant embryo for genetic abnormalities before subsequent implantation into a human being for the completion of gestation.[1] Sperm and fertilized embryos are routinely frozen for later use, menopause is no longer a barrier to pregnancy and artificial wombs are on the horizon.

Although all acknowledge the value of this technology, it is not without its cost. Whereas the Talmud mentions only three partners in creation—"the father", "the mother", and God—current reproductive practices have expanded the list of potential partners to include the sperm donor, egg donor, cytoplasm donor, surrogate mother, and soon, with the application of genetic splicing to human gametes, the partial gene donor. If our limited past experience is any measure, then introducing more partners into the process of procreation clearly introduces more complications, be they emotional, financial, legal or ethical.

To solve these ethical dilemmas, secular ethicists utilize philosophical principles, some with historical precedent, others simply a recent product of the human imagination. In either case, ethicists are in no way bound to the ideas of the past. Orthodox Jews who subscribe to the halakhic process and live by the words of *Hazal*, however, turn to their predecessors for both halakhic and supra-halakhic guidance, employing the past to solve the dilemmas of the present and future.

As with any halakhic discourse, all contemporary halakhic discussions of reproductive technology cite sources spanning from antiquity to the Renaissance to modern times. As the understanding of reproductive anatomy and physiology has changed throughout the centuries, each source, depending on its historical period, bases itself upon a different understanding of embryology and reproductive medicine. Therefore, an awareness of the embryological theories contemporaneous with each author may aid our understanding of his discussion of medical or scientific ideas. Furthermore, if the context of the source is halakhic, it may enhance our appreciation of the halakhic issues with which each source is dealing. This knowledge can perhaps assist current *poskim* in their utilization of rabbinic source material for incorporation into medical halakhic responsa. It is useful, therefore, to pause for a moment from addressing modern halakhic dilemmas of reproductive technology and turn our eyes backward to analyze our predecessor's conception of conception.[2]

This chapter will explore selected passages from Jewish literature from antiquity to modern times that explicitly address or allude to theories relating to reproduction. These sources will be discussed in their own right as well as placed in a medical-historical context. Although rabbinic sources cover the gamut of issues of reproduction and heredity, two major topics have been chosen for the purpose of illustration, each highlighting a different aspect of reproductive medicine. The first topic addresses the very nature of the male and female seeds, focusing largely on embryology: who contributes what to the fetus. The second section traces the history of artificial insemination, a matter of reproductive physiology, and contains sources that are oft quoted in contemporary halakhic discussions. Therefore, the rabbinic sources in this section will receive disproportionately greater treatment than the secular. In each section, the secular sources are discussed separately.

Male and Female Seed

SECULAR SOURCES

Almost all major figures in the history of science in antiquity devoted time to the study of animal and human embryology.[3] As the knowledge of anatomy and physiology was limited, the theories were based on simple observation and philosophical intuition.[4] For example, analogies were often made to agriculture, the male seed being compared to the plant seed and the uterus being compared to the nourishing earth.[5] The male contribution to conception was readily observable, as the male seed was emitted outside the body (more on the male seed below). The nature of the female contribution, however, was a matter of intense debate.

Female Seed
Since the female seed was not visible to the naked eye, and is not emitted externally, its very existence was a matter of conjecture. As a result, two competing theories evolved in antiquity which coexisted until premodern times.[6] Galen (130–200 CE),[7] following in the footsteps of Hippocrates (circa fifth century BCE),[8] maintained that both the male and female contributed seed. The exact identity of the female seed was in question, but he conjectured it might be

located in the uterus. He also claimed that the male semen provides the material for the development of the nerves and the walls of the arteries and veins, whereas the menstrual fluid is the source of the blood.[9] Aristotle, on the other hand, denied the existence of a female seed, claiming that only the male possessed seed. This seed provided the "form" and the "principle of the movement" of the fetus, whereas the female provided the material from which the fetus was formed. The menstrual blood was identified as this material.[10]

Which of these theories predominated throughout the Middle Ages is arguable, but the falsehood of Aristotle's theory was decisively demonstrated by William Harvey. Harvey (1578–1657), known best for his description of the circulation of the blood, was also a pioneer in the field of embryology. While the ovum was not yet described in his lifetime, he nonetheless postulated that all living beings must derive from eggs.[11] Aside from placing the first nail in the coffin of the theory of spontaneous generation,[12] Harvey superseded Aristotle and paved the path for Reinier de Graaf who in 1672 first described the egg follicle.[13] The microscopic female human egg, as we now know it, was not described until 1827, when Ernst von Baer published his classic description of the mammalian ovum.[14]

Male Seed

There were three Greek theories regarding the origin of the sperm.[15] The encephalo-myelogenic doctrine claimed that the sperm ultimately derived from the brain, and it traversed the spinal cord on its way to the male genital organs. The second theory, of which Hippocrates was an advocate, was called the pangenesis doctrine and contended that the sperm derived from the entire body. The sperm extracted from each limb would yield the corresponding limb in the fetus. Aristotle supported the hematogenic doctrine, claiming that the seed originated from blood, and was in fact nothing but blood in a certain state of coagulation.

Although a male seed was always acknowledged, it was not

until 1677 that Antonie van Leewenhoek first visualized the human spermatozoa under the microscope.[16]

Preformation and Epigenesis[17]

The discovery of the egg follicles by de Graaf and of spermatozoa by van Leewenhoek gave birth to two opposing theories regarding the embryological development of the fetus in utero. Some maintained that the fetus formed in a stepwise fashion with the development of one organ or limb preceding the next, i.e. epigenesis. Others believed that within the seed, either male or female, there existed a minuscule complete preformed being that simply enlarged during the course of gestation. These so-called preformationists were split into two camps, those claiming that the preformed child was within the female egg (ovists) and those claiming it was within the male sperm (animalculists).[18]

So convinced of this belief was one animalculist that he drew a diagram of a completely formed child crouched within the confines of one human sperm. This figure became known as the homunculus.[19] It is unclear exactly when the theory of preformation was disproved, but it had its supporters up to the late nineteenth century.

JEWISH SOURCES[20]
Now equipped with the historical background we can approach the Jewish sources throughout the ages that address, both explicitly and implicitly, embryological theories. For the sake of clarity, the sections on male and female seed are seperated as above. Since the same sources often discuss both seeds, there will be, by necessity, limited repetition. For the repeated sources, the bibliographical information will be referenced the first time the source is mentioned.

Female Seed
The Talmudic source which serves as the foundation of all subse-

quent rabbinic discussions on embryology, especially with regard to the female seed, is found in the Talmud, *Niddah* 30a:

> Our Rabbis taught: There are three partners in the creation of man, God, the father, and the mother. The father seminates (*mazria*) the white substance, from which are derived the bones, vessels (*gidim*),[21] fingernails, brain, and the white of the eye. The mother seminates (*mzara'at*) the red substance, from which are derived the skin, flesh, hair, and the black of the eye.[22] God provides the spirit (*ruach*), the soul (*neshama*),[23] the beauty of the features, vision for the eyes, hearing for the ears, speech for the mouth…and intelligence. When the time comes for a man to depart this world, God rescinds his contribution, leaving behind the contributions of the mother and father.

It seems clear that the Rabbis, similar to Galen and in contrast to Aristotle, clearly acknowledged both a male and female seed, the female seed appearing to be identified with the menstrual blood. It is interesting to note that the list of organs that are derived from the respective seeds roughly resembles that of Galen. However, even though Galen was a contemporary of Rabbi Yehuda HaNasi, the compiler of the Mishnah, there is absolutely no mention of Galen, or Hippocrates for that matter, in the entire text of the Mishnah and Talmud.[24] As a result, any suggestion of cross-cultural borrowing is purely speculative.

The next detailed source appears in the biblical commentary of Rabbi Moses ben Nahman, (Ramban, 1194–1270). Although Ramban is best known for his exceptional Talmudic scholarship, he was also a practicing physician, purportedly at Montpellier,[25] the major center of medicine in the Middle Ages.[26] As a matter of fact, one of the few references we have to the Ramban's medical practice states that he treated a non-Jew for infertility.[27]

The reference is found in the Ramban's comments on the phrase in Leviticus, 12:2 *"isha ki tazria v'yalda zachar."* The root of the word *"tazria"* is *"zera"* or seed, hence the translation could be, "when a woman emits seed." Whereas most biblical commentators interpret this phrase to mean when a woman conceives, and thereby ignore the issue of the existence of the female seed, the Ramban takes this opportunity to address rabbinic theories of embryology:

> ...Although it says "when a woman emits seed"...the implication is not that the fetus is made from the female seed. For even though a woman has ovaries (*beitzim*) analogous to those of the male (*beitzei zakhar*) [testicles], either no seed is made there, or the seed has nothing to do with the fetus. Rather the term "*mzara'at*" refers to the uterine blood...that unites with male seed. In their opinion [*Talmud Niddah* quoted above] the fetus is created from the blood of the woman and the white [semen] of the man, and both of them are called seed...and likewise is the opinion of the doctors regarding conception. The Greek philosophers thought that the entire body of the fetus derives from menstrual blood, and that the man only provides...form to the material.

The mere fact that the Ramban mentions this embryological debate reflects that it still was a topic of discussion in his time. Here the Ramban accepts the contribution of a female seed and identifies that seed with the uterine blood, based on the passage in the Talmud. He states that this is also the position of the doctors. As we know that the Ramban was himself a physician, we can accept this statement as having some authority. Although he mentions no names of specific doctors, he may be aligning the Talmudic position with the teachings of Galen. The Ramban also clearly rejects what we know to be Aristotle's position.

Rabbi Bahya ben Asher (1255–1350) follows the Ramban in his interpretation of the phrase in Leviticus, but adds a novel explanation of the term "*tazria*." It means, he says, "when a woman gives over the *zera*." The *zera*, he maintains, is a deposit, which is given to the woman by the man for safe keeping as a plant seed is deposited in the ground. In both cases the matured seed is to be returned from its repository when the time is right.[28] As already mentioned above, the agricultural analogy is one that has been used since antiquity.

While the Ramban claimed that a woman may or may not have her own seed independent of the menstrual blood, Rambam (Maimonides, 1135–1204)) also a famous physician, clearly acknowledges the existence of a female seed.

> Between the *heder* [room] and the *prozdor* [passageway][29] lie the two ovaries of the woman and the pathways [fallopian tubes?] wherein her seed matures.[30]

The Rambam does not, however, address whether this seed has any role in conception.

Rabbi Shimon ben Tzemach Duran (1360–1444), known as Tashbetz, devotes a significant section of his philosophical work *Magen Avot* to the anatomy and physiology of reproduction. In this citation he confronts the issue of the female seed:

> Regarding whether the female seed has a role in conception, this has been debated by Aristotle and Galen. We have explained that *Hazal* say it has no role whatsoever in conception…The philosophers have concluded that the female seed has no role in conception…and they reached the same conclusion that was received by *Hazal* from the prophets and teachings of the Torah.[31]

He proceeds to identify the menstrual blood as the contribution of the female.

In contradistinction to the above source, which although acknowledging the existence of an independent female seed gives this seed no role in conception, the following reference grants a prominent role to this seed. This passage is excerpted from *Shevilei Emunah*, the work of Meir ben Isaac Aldabi, also known as the Tashbetz (1310–1360), the grandson of Rabbi Asher ben Yehiel.[32]

> …and next to the uterus are the woman's two ovaries…and from them the female seed flows into the cavity of the uterus. When the

male seed is emitted into the uterus the female seed also is emitted from the ovaries and joins with the male seed [to form the fetus].[33]

This appears to be the first Jewish source that ascribes such significance to the female ovarian seed, and thus ends our discussion of Jewish sources prior to the works of Harvey and van Leewenhoek.

In summary, all the Jewish sources espouse the doctrine of the two seeds, both male and female, yet opinions differ as to the identity and contribution of the female seed. These sources are better understood in the context of the ongoing scientific debate in the secular world regarding the existence and nature of the female seed.

We now turn to some Jewish references to embryology at a time when the scientific world had recently undergone major upheaval. The sperm had been identified, the existence of a female egg was universally accepted although the egg itself had not yet been observed, and the theories of preformation and epigenesis were being debated.

Tobias Cohn (1652–1729),[34] a graduate of the famous University of Padua,[35] was educated in this scientific milieu. His classic work, *Ma'aseh Tuvia*, covers topics including botany, cosmology and medicine, and the following passage on embryology reflects the climate of his time. As Cohn was well educated in rabbinic as well as scientific literature, his words are of particular interest to this discussion.

Aristotle, who rejected the Torah of Moses, brought a number of disappointing proofs that the menstrual blood is in place of the seed, and besides this, a woman has no other seed. However, recent physicians, who accept our holy Torah, have…brought other proofs which contradict his disappointing proofs…. The first proof is that one cannot deny the existence of a female seed, for it was not for naught that a woman was created with *beitzim* and pathways that transmit seed similar to a man.

….There is almost no need for the proofs brought by the great physician Harvey on the existence of a female seed…. The great

physicians of late maintain that the purpose of the ovaries (*beitzim*)
is to give rise to tiny eggs (*beitzim*), similar to fish eggs, which have
been seen with the microscope.[36]

This is likely the first Hebrew source that uses the term *beitzah* to
describe the female egg as we understand it today. In all previous
sources the term *beitzim* is used to refer to the ovaries or testicles
interchangeably, and the female seed is called simply her *zera*. Given
an understanding of the history of embryology, this observation
makes perfect sense, as it is only during this period that Harvey's
theory of the existence of a female egg was developed.

A more detailed physiological description of conception
is found in *Tiferet Adam*, the anatomical work of Baruch Schick
(1744–1808),[37] who is perhaps best known for translating Euclid's
Geometry into Hebrew for the Vilna Gaon.[38] In this excerpt, the
author, after discussing the passage from *Niddah*, mentions the
single egg.[39]

> ...in the body of the woman are found the ovaries...the seed emit-
> ted by the man...induces the emission of a single egg from the
> ovaries...

Our next passage alludes to another embryological theory
and stems from a question entertained by Rabbi Ya'akov Emden
(d. 1776) regarding whether it was possible for a virginal woman
to conceive in the absence of conjugal relations, e.g. bathhouse
insemination (more on this topic below). In this passage he invokes
the theory of preformation, in particular that of the animalculists,
to answer the above question in the affirmative. Quoting the references to the male and female seeds:[40]

> ...such a thing is decidedly not in the realm of the impossible...as
> *Hazal* said "maybe she conceived in the bathhouse?" [*Hagiga* 14b]...
> and this is compatible with the ideas of the scientists, who describe
> only a limited role for the female seed in conception ...but it is now

clear that the female seed provides no material contribution to the fetus whatsoever…and this does not contradict what is written in the Torah, "*isha ki tazria v'yalda.*" (See the commentary of the Ramban on this verse and you will see that it is not a contradiction.)[41] They have found through the use of the glass [microscope] and other experiments that man, like birds and fish, is created from an egg in the ovary of the woman. And in the male seed they have seen…the image of a tiny human being, complete with its limbs…

Rabbi Emden goes on to explain that the preformed fetus in the male seed receives its nourishment and sustenance, including warmth and moisture, from the female seed. It is interesting to note that he accepts the notion of the homunculus (preformation) and claims that this is in consonance with the commentary of the Ramban. As mentioned above, the Ramban granted no role to a female seed independent of the menstrual blood. However, the Ramban does maintain, based on the Talmud in *Niddah*, that the menstrual blood does contribute materially to the fetus. This latter notion would not be compatible with the theory of preformation. In any case, Rabbi Emden incorporates the contemporary embryological theories into his halakhic discussion.

The final selection in this section comes from the work of Pinhas Eliyahu Hurwitz (1765–1821), *Sefer HaBrit*. This work is a compilation of medical and scientific theories culled from sources in many languages and it served as a valuable resource for its Jewish audience, to whom many of these ideas were inaccessible. This fact accounts for the book's popularity and multiple printings. This selection gives a balanced view of the opposing embryological theories while at the same time incorporating the teachings of *Hazal*:

Some scholars have written that all the features of the entire human body, complete with its limbs, are found within the egg of the woman…and some scholars have written that within the seed of the man is the form of a minuscule human being, for when male seeds…are viewed under the microscope small creatures can be seen

> within them moving to and fro…God knows the truth of this matter. However, it is known in truth that the woman also emits seed, as the verse explicitly states, "*isha ki tazria*." And her seed is not white, but red as *Hazal* have said "the mother emits the red substance."[42]

In conclusion of our discussion of the female seed, it is apparent that these sources do not reflect a consensus of opinion regarding the identity and nature of the female seed. Many of the sources, irrespective of the theories they espouse, attempt to align their positions with the words of *Hazal*, in particular the passage from Talmud *Niddah*.

Male Seed

The following section presents a selection of Jewish sources that address theories regarding the origin and nature of the male seed. Some of these sources were already encountered in the above section on the female seed. It begins with a passage from the Talmud, from which can be inferred the understanding of the origin of the male seed:[43]

> Levi was sitting in a bathhouse and observed a man fall and strike his head. He said, "his brains were agitated (*nitmazmez*)"…Abaye said "he has lost the ability to procreate."

The implication is that an injury to the brain somehow affects the male seed, an allusion to the encephalo-myelogenic theory of the origin of the sperm. This interpretation of the passage is also advocated by Rashi.[44]

In *Sefer HaBahir*, a kabbalistic work attributed to Rabbi Nehunia ben HaKana (a first century *Tanna*), the reference to the encephalo-myelogenic doctrine is more explicit.[45] "The spinal cord, which comes from the brain, enters the male organ (*amma*) and from there comes the seed."

Meir ben Isaac Aldabi, mentioned above, mentions both the encephalo-myelogenic and the pangenesis doctrine, but does not indicate which one he advocates:

The scientists have debated. Some say the seed comes from the brain, via the spinal cord, to the testicles, and there it matures and whitens. The proof to this is that pain in the spine will sometimes heal with emission of seed, and also that one whose spinal cord is severed cannot procreate. However, Hippocrates maintains that the seed is an extract from all the limbs of the body.[46]

The Tashbetz, mentioned above, refers to the pangenesis doctrine: "We must ascertain…if the seed derives from the entire body or not. Behold, the ancients have said this…."[47] However, he ultimately rejects this in favor of the hematogenic doctrine of Aristotle, which he claims *Hazal* also espoused.

> …and this is their intent *[Hazal]* when they said "the seed is inter-mixed (*m'balbel zarei*)." The meaning of this phrase is that from all the limbs there is a combined power, not that each limb yields its corresponding limb [pangenesis doctrine]…this is their opinion *Hazal*, in agreement with the opinion of the philosopher [Aristotle].[48]

In summary, up to this point we have seen that there is no consensus regarding the origin of the male seed, and that Jewish sources refer to all three theories.[49] Let us now, as above, shift our attention to the period following the discoveries of van Leewenhoek and Harvey, when the theories of epigenesis and preformation were prevalent.

Pinhas Eliyahu Hurwitz, in the passage cited above, refers to the theory of preformation and mentions the position of the animalculists as well as the ovulists. In the following quote he invokes the position of the animalculists in a novel interpretation of a Talmudic passage.

> …and they have seen with a microscope that in the seed of a man…exist tiny creatures, whose form resembles that of man, and that are alive and move within the drop. With this we see how all the words of *Hazal* are to be believed and how all their words are truthful and just…even regarding those matters which seem far

fetched or inconceivable.... Our Talmud treats this sin [*hotza'at zera l'vatala*] harshly, equating it to murder, as it is written, "Rabbi Eliezer ben Ya'akov said that one who emits seed wastefully is considered as if he killed a soul..." and so said Rabbi Yitzchak and Rabbi Ami in tractate *Niddah*. This statement seemed far fetched in the eyes of the philosophers amongst our people...who were unaware of the looking glass mentioned above [microscope]. How could it be considered murder prior to the conception of the child...when the human being had not yet appeared? ...[For] the seed at this time is only fluid from the brain[50] and is still substance without form.... But now, after it has been seen with the aforementioned instrument that living beings in the image of man move to and fro within the seed, it is remarkable...to hear such a thing. Every intelligent person would judge such a sin as truly equivalent to murder.[51]

While most Jewish sources accepted the theory of preformation, Baruch Schick (1744–1808) (see above) stood alone in rejecting the theory of preformation in favor of epigenesis:

The limbs of the body are not all formed at once, rather they grow one by one like a tree.... Some have said that the form of a small human being is found within the egg, and there is no place for their words. Still others have said that within the male seed is found the image of a tiny living being, their proof being that when the male seed is viewed under the microscope moving objects, like worms, can be observed.[52] They therefore say that these worms are in fact little human beings...This assertion is also baseless. First, if they are correct, why are there so many worms [sperm]? Second, the very form of the worm attests that it is not the likeness of a man.[53]

Despite Schick's refutation of the theory of preformation, it was still perpetuated by rabbinic sources, especially with reference to the prohibition of destroying male seed (*hotza'at zera l'vatala*).[54] This may be due, in part, to the fact that while *Sefer HaBrit* was a popular, widely read work, *Tiferet Adam* was more obscure.

In summary, there are Jewish sources that cover the gamut

of embryological theories regarding the origins of the male seed. As with the female seed, attempts were made to align these theories with the words of *Hazal*, including areas of halakha. An historical understanding of the various embryological theories contemporary with each of these sources gives us a better appreciation of each authority's context and scientific frame of reference.

Artificial Insemination[55]

Artificial insemination is a commonly practiced procedure for the treatment of infertility. Although the procedure has grown tremendously in popularity and application over the last few decades, the concept of intentionally injecting sperm into a woman for the purpose of impregnation dates back to at least the mid-eighteenth century, when John Hunter successfully inseminated a woman whose husband had a severe form of hypospadias.[56] Hermann Rohleder wrote the first history of the artificial impregnation of human beings as early as 1934.[57] However, since the widespread application of this procedure is, as stated, only relatively recent, it is in this period that we find the proliferation of rabbinic responsa dealing with every imaginable halakhic consequence of artificial insemination.[58] But what sources could there be in the Talmud or *Rishonim* that could possibly aid in the halakhic explication of this seemingly novel procedure? To answer this question we must understand that the belief in virginal or non-natural conception dates back to antiquity and antedates Christianity.[59] Various modes of non-natural conception were described. Specifically we must mention one indirect form of artificial insemination: There was a widely held belief, dating back to antiquity, that a woman could become pregnant in a bathhouse, for it was thought that when a woman bathes in a bath into which a man has previously emitted sperm, she may become pregnant. The following section will briefly trace the history of the notion of artificial insemination in secular and Jewish sources from antiquity to the present.

SECULAR SOURCES

Though the notion of virginal or non-natural conception dates back to antiquity, explicit reference to the phenomenon of artificial insemination is found only in sources from the Middle Ages.[60] Avicenna (980–1037) in his *Canon* on medicine and Averroes (d. 1198) in his *Colliget* acknowledge the possibility of artificial impregnation. Thomas Aquinas (d. 1274) relates that a woman became pregnant from lying in a bed into which sperm was previously discharged.[61] (Rabbi Peretz of Corbeil (c. 1295), a contemporary of Aquinas, accepted this possibility and therefore dealt with the halakhic ramifications). Amatus Lusitanus quotes Avicenna and Al-Jazzar (10th cent.)[62] as authorities who accept artificial insemination.[63]

In 1750, a pamphlet entitled "Lucina Sine Concubito" by Dr. Abraham Johnson was published in London.[64] It was submitted by Johnson to the Royal Society, the preeminent scientific body in England, and is comprised of a personal account of a patient of Johnson's, whom the latter believed had conceived by artificial insemination. In this fantastical essay, Johnson postulates the means by which this insemination was achieved. He believed, based on classical sources, that the reproductive seed derived from the western winds and was accidentally ingested by his female patient. He further claimed that he tested his theory experimentally on his house maid, without her consent, and achieved positive results (i.e. the maid became pregnant). He therefore submitted his results to the Royal Society with suggestions for wider applications of his technique.

While the belief in artificial insemination persisted into the twentieth century,[65] it was not without its detractors. Paolo Zacchias (1584–1659), physician to Pope Innocent X and prominent medical legal writer,[66] rejects the possibility, as did the great scientist Albrecht Haller (1708–1777). [67]

JEWISH SOURCES

As with the secular sources described above, the Jewish belief in the possibility of artificial insemination persisted into the twentieth century, though not without its detractors. There are two early references to artificial insemination, which have served as the source for virtually all contemporary halakhic discussions on artificial insemination. The first case is mentioned in Talmud *Hagiga*[68] in the course of a discussion about whether a *kohen gadol*, who is prohibited from marrying any woman who is not virginal, may marry a pregnant woman who claims she is still a virgin.[69] How, after all, could a woman become pregnant if not through normal intercourse? Shmuel attests to the fact that it is possible to have intercourse without perforating the *betulim* (hymen). But the Talmud entertains another possibility, that of impregnation in the bathhouse, in which case, the woman, in fact still being a virgin, would be permitted to marry a *kohen gadol*.

The second case is mentioned in the *Alphabet of Ben Sira*[70] in reference to the nature of Ben Sira's birth. This narrative work, of questionable date and authorship (some date this work from the Geonic period), details the life of Shimon Ben Sira (second century BCE), the author of *Divrei Shimon Ben Sira* ("The Wisdom of Ben Sira"). The relevant passage appears in the first section of this work, which is a biography of Ben Sira from his conception to the age of one year. The passage, apparently omitted in many editions, describes how the prophet Jeremiah was simultaneously both the father and grandfather of Ben Sira. Ben Sira's mother was Jeremiah's daughter. Jeremiah was forced by evil men to perform an act of onanism in a bathhouse, and his daughter conceived from his emissions when she inadvertently entered the same bath. Ben Sira was then born seven months later, the product of artificial insemination.[71] The text further mentions that it is no mere coincidence that the numerical value of the Hebrew letters (*gematria*) of Sira equals that of Jeremiah, thereby hinting that Ben Sira is, in fact, the son of Jeremiah.

Not everyone accepted the veracity of the aforementioned story of Ben Sira's birth. Solomon ibn Verga (15th to 16th century) states in his historical narrative *Shevet Yehuda* that Ben Sira was the grandson of Yehoshua ben Yehotzadak, making no mention of any relation to Jeremiah.[72] Rabbi David Ganz, the seventeenth century chronicler, claims that this story is mere exaggeration, as "I have not found it anywhere in the Talmud, and I have not heard from my teachers that it is found in any Aggadah or Midrash."[73]

Assuming for our discussion the veracity of the passage in the *Alphabet of Ben Sira*, some important halakhic points can be derived, which explains why it has been so extensively quoted by subsequent *Rishonim* and *Aharonim*. Ben Sira is clearly assumed to be the product of Jeremiah and his daughter. Whether this was known to Jeremiah by *ruach hakodesh* (divine inspiration) or whether this was because Jeremiah's daughter was trusted to have been a virgin is unclear. In either case, despite the fact that Ben Sira is the product of a halakhically illicit relationship, nowhere do we find aspersions cast on his lineage, and never is he referred to as a *mamzer*. The legal implication is that only the marital act can create the prohibition of *arayot* and the labeling of the resultant child as a *mamzer*. The relevance of this to artificial insemination with donor sperm is obvious. Secondly, Ben Sira was known as the son of Jeremiah. This implies that a child born from artificial insemination may be considered halakhically related to the sperm donor.

One of the earliest references to the case of Ben Sira is by Rabbi Peretz ben Eliyahu of Corbeil (c. 1295) in his glosses on *Sefer Mitzvot Katan* (also referred to as *Amudei Gola*).[74] He states that a woman need not refrain from sleeping on her husband's sheets while she is a *niddah* out of the concern that she might bear a child from the remnant seed on the sheet and the child will be *a ben niddah*. However, Rabbi Peretz does warn that a married woman should not sleep on the sheets of a strange man. Why Rabbi Peretz differentiated between these two cases is a matter of halakhic import, but implicit in these statements is that Rabbi Perez acknowledged that a woman could indeed become pregnant in this manner. He brings proof from the case of Ben Sira who, despite being the product of a halakhically illicit union, was not considered a *mamzer* because no conjugal relations (*biah*) actually took place. Jacob Moellin (1360?–1427) also mentions the case of Ben Sira in the *Likutei Maharil*, where it appears as a statement without particular halakhic context.[75]

More elaborate treatment of this topic is found in the

responsa of Tashbetz,[76] to whom a question was posed about a woman who claimed to have had a virginal conception. Rabbi Duran, who was also a physician, was asked to determine whether this was in fact possible, and, if so, what would be the halakhic ramifications. Whether this so-called bathhouse impregnation was actually feasible or simply contrived for the sake of halakhic analysis was a matter of intense debate among the *Aharonim*, as we shall soon see. The Tashbetz was one of few *Rishonim* who addressed this topic. He concludes that it is feasible, marshalling evidence from the aforementioned passage in *Hagiga*, as well as from the case of Ben Sira. With respect to the latter he prefaces with a disclaimer: "If we believe the apocrypha then we have proof from Ben Sira." What is particularly interesting is the Tashbetz's reference in a gloss to two of his contemporaries, one an unnamed gentile, and the other named Rabbi Abraham Israel, both of whom claimed to have been familiar with actual cases of virginal women who had conceived.

The next Jewish reference to artificial insemination is not rabbinic in origin, but appears in the case studies of the famous Marrano physician Amatus Lusitanus (1511–1568).[77] This discussion, like the aforementioned passage of Ben Sira, is not found in all versions of Lusitanus' classic work, the *Centuria*, as it was expurgated by the censors.[78] (Lusitanus invokes the notion of artificial insemination [*sine concubito*] to exonerate a nun with a uterine mole who was accused of impropriety.) He adduces his proofs from the case of Ben Sira, as well as from other scientific sources, discussed above.

Yet another famous Jewish physician makes mention of artificial insemination in his work,[79] though this particular work is halakhic, not medical in nature. Rabbi Isaac Lampronti (1679–1756),[80] in his magnum opus *Pahad Yitzhak*, poses the following riddle. A child is the son of a woman who was impregnated by her father, yet he is not a *mamzer*. How is this possible?[81] He answers, "this is Ben Sira," after which he recounts the incident in the bathhouse, "as is written in *ketubot*." This reference is clearly not to the Talmudic tractate, as we have already mentioned that the story derives from the *Alphabet of Ben Sira*. The term *"ketubot"* is likely to be translated as "the writings," in which case it may refer to the apocrypha.[82]

We consider the scientific question of whether bathhouse impregnation is even possible. Implicit from all the above sources is that they accepted the possibility of this unique form of artificial insemination. However, few of them address the question specifically, with the exception of the Tashbetz and Lusitanus, both of whom accept the possibility. One of the first to expressly deny the possibility of such an event was Rabbi Judah Rosanes (d. 1727), who articulates his position in his glosses to the Rambam's *Mishneh Torah*, entitled *Mishnah L'Melech*.[83] Rabbi Rosanes maintains that a woman can only become pregnant through the completion of the natural marital act (i.e. *gemar biah*). He brings support for this notion from Talmudic sources, and also discusses the Talmudic teaching that a woman cannot become pregnant from the first intercourse (*biah rishona*). Based on these as well as other sources he concludes that bathhouse impregnation is impossible.

This passage from the *Mishneh L'Melech* is cited widely by subsequent authorities, some with approbation,[84] others with condemnation, as we will soon see. Although a number of *Aharonim* mention the *Mishneh L'Melech* approvingly, including Rabbi Moses Schick, perhaps his most enthusiastic advocate was Rabbi Solomon Schick. In a responsum to Rabbi Yoseph Edinger, Rabbi Solomon Schick states assuredly, with no ambiguity, that bathhouse impregnation could never happen. In addition to quoting Rabbi Rosanes and Rabbi Moses Schick in his support, he interprets the passage in *Hagiga* in a novel fashion. The aforementioned passage follows the story of the four rabbis who entered *"pardes"*(however it is to be defined), one of whom is the same Ben Zoma of our relevant passage. As this Ben Zoma was harmed by his journey into *"pardes,"* Rabbi Schick maintains that the Talmud is making folly of him. Never, according to Rabbi Schick, did the Talmud believe that bathhouse insemination could occur.[85]

Other authorities subsequent to Rabbi Rosanes have independently questioned the possibility of bathhouse impregnation. Rabbi Yosef Hayyim (1833?–1909), author of the *Ben Ish*

Hai, espouses a novel position in his work *Torah Lishma*.[86] Rabbi Hayyim was asked whether he would allow sperm procurement from an ill man to facilitate a proper medical diagnosis. The questioner maintained that since the sperm could subsequently be used to impregnate a woman, this should mitigate the prohibition of *hashhatat zera*. Rabbi Hayyim contends that "nature has changed" (*nishtaneh hateva*)[87] with respect to artificial insemination. Whereas insemination through an intermediary medium (e.g. bathhouse impregnation) was possible in the times of the *Tannaim*, owing to greater bodily strength and potency of seed, such is not the case from the time of the *Ammoraim* and onward. If it were at all possible, it would be an extremely rare occurrence, as, he maintains, was the case mentioned by the Tashbetz. He answers, therefore, that as the likelihood of impregnating a woman with the remaining seed is so remote, sperm procurement is not to be allowed.[88] (It is interesting that around the time this responsum was written, John Hunter performed the first successful artificial insemination of a human being. However, his success was not known to the world at large, let alone the rabbinic community.)[89]

Along a similar vein, a number of *Aharonim* also maintained that bathhouse impregnation was not possible in their time due to changed nature. However, it was the changed nature of the bath, they maintained, not that of the seed, that explained why insemination was no longer possible.[90] According to this opinion, since the baths in Talmudic times were heated from below[91] it was theoretically possible for insemination to occur, either because a man was more likely to emit seed in this kind of bath, or because this particular heat source was more conducive to the survival of the seed.[92]

While these approaches also questioned the possibility of bathhouse impregnation, it was Rabbi Rosanes who was always hailed as the main opponent to this notion. His position did not remain unopposed, as a number of *Aharonim* refuted his contention.[93] There were three different approaches in response to Rabbi Rosanes. Rabbi Yehonatan Eybeschutz (1690–1764) argued against Rabbi Rosanes based on a re-analysis of the Talmudic passages that Rabbi Rosanes cites, concluding that the latter's interpretations were incorrect, and that hence, artificial insemination is possible.[94] Rabbi Haim Yosef David Azulai (1724–1806) mentioned on three separate occasions in his writings that bathhouse impregnation was possible because it was accepted as fact by the Talmud, as well as by a number of prominent *Rishonim*.[95] The third approach of refutation is scientific in nature and was taken by Rabbi Barukh Mordekhai ben Ya'akov Libschitz (1810–1885). Rabbi Rosanes had stated that conception could only be accomplished with *gemar biah*. Rabbi Libschitz responded that with respect to bathhouse impregnation, the waters of the bath could transport the seed to the internal organs of the woman, thereby effectively accomplishing the same result as *gemar biah*.[96]

In conclusion, since the possibility of bathhouse insemination would be difficult to disprove, whether it has or can actually occur remains a mystery.[97] Contemporary *poskim*, in their discussions on modern therapeutic artificial insemination, refer to some of the aforementioned sources to establish paternity. However, as the possibility of non-coital conception is, at least in the modern medical context, an accepted fact, little space is devoted to the scientific question of feasibility.[98] More time is instead apportioned for the resolution of attendant halakhic dilemmas.

Endnotes

1. See, for example, Jiaen Liu, et al., "Birth after preimplantation diagnosis of the cystic fibrosis F508 mutation by polymerase chain reaction in human embryos resulting from intracytoplasmic sperm injection with epididymal sperm," *Journal of the American Medical Association* 272:23, (Dec. 1994), pp. 1858–60. Since this early paper, preimplantation diagnosis has been widely applied to many genetic diseases, including Tay Sachs disease.

2. For another example of the application of a medical historical approach to halakhic sources, see E. Reichman, "The halakhic definition of death in light of medical history," *Torah U'Maddah*, 4, (1994), pp. 148–74.

3. For an overview of the history of embryology, see J. Needham, *A History of Embryology*, (New York, 1959); H. Adelmann, "A brief sketch of the history of embryology before Fabricius" in his trans. of *The Embryological Treatises of Hieronymous Fabricius of Aquapendente* (Ithaca, 1967), I, pp. 36–70.

For references to embryology in Jewish sources, see Samuel Kottek, "Embryology in Talmudic and Midrashic literature," *Journal of the History of Biology* 14:2 (Fall, 1981), pp. 299–315; David I. Macht, "Embryology and obstetrics in ancient Hebrew literature," *John Hopkins Hospital Bulletin* 22, 242 (May, 1911), pp. 1–8; W.M. Feldman, "Ancient Jewish eugenics," *Medical Leaves* 2 (1939), pp. 28–37; D. Shapiro *Obstetrique des Anciens Hebreus* (Paris, 1904); W.M. Feldman, *The Jewish Child* (London, 1917), pp. 120–44; H.J. Zimmels, *Magicians, Theologians and Doctors*, pp. 62–64; Needham, op. cit., pp. 77–82; Julius Preuss, *Biblical and Talmudic Medicine* (New York, 1978), pp. 41–138; Ron Barkai, *Les Infortunes De Dinah:Le Livre De La Generation-La Gynecologie Juive au Moyen Age* (Paris, 1991). I thank Mr. Tzvi Erenyi for bringing the latter book to my attention.

4. There are no clearly documented human dissections from the time of Rashi, although scattered references to autopsies and dissections appear in the thirteenth and fourteenth centuries. Mundinus (1270–1326) is recognized to have been the first to incorporate human anatomical dissection into the medical curriculum. See, for example, C.D. O'Malley, *Andreas Vesalius of Brussels* (Berkeley, 1964), pp. 1–20; Ludwig Edelstein, "The history of anatomy in antiquity," in *Ancient Medicine* (Baltimore, 1967), pp. 247–302; Charles Singer, *A Short History of Anatomy and Physiology from the Greek to Harvey* (New York, 1957); Mary Niven Alston, "The attitude of the Church toward dissection before 1500," *Bulletin of the History of Medicine* 16:3 (Oct., 1944), pp. 221–38; Nancy Sirasi, *Taddeo Alderotti and His Pupils* (Princeton, 1981), pp. 66–69.

5. Hippocrates, in his essay "The seed and the nature of the child" devotes a lengthy section to agriculture. He says "you will find that from beginning to end the process of growth in plants and humans in exactly the same." G.E.R. Lloyd, ed., *Hippocratic Writings* (New York, 1978), p. 341. See also A.J. Brock, trans., *Galen On the Natural Faculties*, (London, 1916), p. 19.

6. See Joseph Needham, *A History of Embryology*, (New York, 1959) for extensive discussion of ancient theories of embryology. The most complete account of pre-Aristotelian theories of sexual generation is Erna Lesky, *Die Zeugungs und Vererbungslehre der Antike und ihre Nachwirkung*, (Mainz, 1950). This work is widely quoted. See also Monica Green, *The Transmission of Ancient Theories of Female Physiology and Disease through the Early Middle Ages*, PhD dissertation, Princeton University, 1985 and Sarah George, *Human Conception and Fetal Growth: A Study in the Development of Greek Thought from Presocrates through Aristotle*, PhD dissertation, University of Pennsylvania, 1982.

7. Galen discusses his theories of generation in many places. See, for example, Margaret Talmadge May, trans., *Galen: On the Usefulness of the Parts of the Body*, (Ithica, 1968), vol. 2, pp. 620–54. See also Anthony Preus, "Galen's Criticism of Aristotle's Conception Theory," *Journal of the History of Biology*, 10:1, (Spring, 1977), pp. 65–85.

8. Modern scholarship has revealed that the Hippocratic corpus is not the work of one author. For ideas of conception see, for example, G.E.R. Lloyd, ed., *Hippocratic Writings* (New York, 1978), pp. 317–46, chap. entitled "The seed and the nature of the child".

9. Preus, op. cit., 83. See also Needham, op. cit., 78, who quotes a similar idea from Hippocrates.

10. See A.L. Peck, trans., *Aristotle:Generation of Animals*, (Cambridge, 1942), p. 71, pp. 100–101 note a, pp. 109–12.

11. *Exercitationes de Generatione Animalium* (Amsterdam, 1651), later translated and annotated by Gweneth Whitteridge, *Disputations Touching the Generation of Animals* (Oxford, 1981).

12. The belief in spontaneous generation in Jewish and secular sources merits its own article. A passage in the *Babylonian Talmud*, Shabbat 107b, seems to indicate that the Rabbis believed that lice could spontaneously generate. This passage, as well as others that conflict with our current understanding of science, have been the subject of many a heated discussion. Francesco Redi (1620–97) was the first to scientifically study spontaneous generation, and he dealt the theory its first major blow in his work, *Esperienze Intorno Alla Generazione Deg'lisetti* (Florence, 1668). Louis Pasteur (1833–93) laid the theory to rest. For treatment of this topic in Jewish sources see Isaac Lampronti, *Pahad Yithak*, (Bnei Brak, 1980), s.v. *Tzedah ha'asura*; Arye Carmel ed. Eliyahu Dessler, *Mikhtav MeEliyahu*, (Jerusalem, 1984), vol. 4, 355, n. 4; Arye Carmel and Yehuda Levi, "R'ot haenayim bikviut hahalakha," *HaMaayan* 23:1, *Tishri*, (1983), pp. 64–9; David Ruderman, "Contemporary science and Jewish law in the eyes of Isaac Lampronti of Ferrara and some of his contemporaries," *Jewish History*, 6:1–2, (1992), pp. 211–24.

13. See his *De Mulierum Organis Generationi Inservientibus Tractatus Novus* (Leyden, 1672).

14. *De Ovi Mammalium et Hominis Genesi*, (Leipzig, 1827).

15. See Pieter Willem Van Der Horst, "Sarah's seminal emmission: Hebrews 11:11 in the light of ancient embryology," in *Greeks, Romans and Christians: Essays in Honor of Abraham J. Malherbe*, David Balch, ed. et al., (Minneapolis, 1990), pp. 287–302. I thank Dr. Shnayer Leiman for directing me to this source, which places a number of rabbinic sources into the context of Greco-Roman theories of embryology. Horst provides a nice summary of these three theories. See also Sarah George, op. cit.

16. A.W. Meyer, "The discovery and earliest representation of spermatozoa," *Bulletin of the Institute of the History of Medicine* 6:2, (Feb., 1938), pp. 89–110.

17. Needham, op.cit., 205–11; A. Du Bois, "The development of the theory of heredity," *CIBA Symposia* 1:8, (Nov., 1939), pp. 235–46.

18. According to the theory of preformation, either Adam or Eve, depending on whether one is an ovulist or animalculist, contained within them the preformed bodies of all the people that would populate the earth. Within

each preformed seed must exist preformed seed of the next generation, and so on.

19. Regarding the origins of this depiction and its initial false attribution to Antonie van Leewenhoek, see A.W. Meyer, op. cit.

20. See David Feldman, *Marital Relations, Birth Control and Abortion in Jewish Law*, (New York, 1974), esp. chaps. 6 and 7 for his excellent treatment of these topics. Some of the sources from this section derive from this book.

21. The term *"gidim"* can mean either blood vessels or nerves, and has been used interchangeably in rabbinic literature. The clarification of Hebrew medical terms, especially in the Middle Ages, has plagued many a doctor and historian throughout history. The confusion stemmed from differing etymologies of medical terms, ranging from Latin, to Greek and later Arabic, as well as the fact that these terms were not easily rendered into Hebrew. Some terms were transliterated, others translated and often entirely new words were devised. This confusion led many Jewish physicians to include a glossary of medical terms in their books. On Hebrew terminology see, for example, Juan Jose Barcia Goyanes, "Medieval Hebrew anatomical names," *Koroth* 8:11–12, (1985), pp. 192–201; A.S. Yahuda, "Medical and anatomical terms in the Pentateuch in light of Egyptian medical papyri," *Journal of the History of Medicine* 2:4, (Autumn, 1947), pp. 549–73. Multiple articles have appeared over the years in the journal *HaRofe HaIvri* on the topic of Hebrew medical terminology.

22. It is interesting that blood is not mentioned as one of the contributions of the female seed, especially since this seed, according to the Talmud, is itself comprised of blood. For a discussion about this discrepancy see *She'iltot D'Rav Achai Gaon*, She'ilta 56 and commentaries of Rabbi Isaiah Berlin (*She'ilat Shalom*) and Rabbi Naftali Tzvi Yehuda Berlin (*Ha'Amek Sh'aila*) on this passage. I thank Dr. Maier Halberstam for directing me to this source.

23. The terms *ruach, nefesh* and *neshama* are all abstract and difficult to define. They are often used interchangeably. See Samuel S. Kottek, "The seat of the soul: contribution to the history of Jewish medieval psycho-physiology," *Cliomedica* 13:3–4, (1978), pp. 219–46.

24. Rabbinic sources of the Middle Ages and beyond clearly knew of Galen. In addition, Galen himself was at least peripherally familiar with Jews and Jewish medicine. See Reichman, op. cit., esp. 166, n. 6.

25. We know of the Ramban's medical practice primarily from the responsa of his student, Rabbi Shlomo ibn Aderet (Rashba). Responsa numbers 177, 413 and 825 discuss the Ramban's use of an astrological figure of a lion to cure a kidney ailment. The Rashba discusses the halakhic issues involved in using astrological figures. See also Rabbi H.Y.D. Azulia, *Shem HaGedolim Ma'arekhet Gedolim*, s.v. *Ramban*. Medical historians have mentioned that Ramban practiced in Montpellier. See Isaac Alteras, "Jewish physicians in Southern France during the thirteenth and fourteenth centuries," *Jewish Quarterly Review* 68, (1977–78), p. 218. No Jewish sources that I have found place the Ramban as a physician in Montpellier.

26. On the University at Montpellier in the Middle Ages see Sonoma Cooper, "The medical school of Montepellier in the fourteenth century," *Annals of Medical History*, new series 2, (1930), pp. 164–95; CIBA *Symposia* 2:1, (April, 1940), entire issue devoted to Montepellier.

     Regarding the Jewish presence at Montepellier see Luis Garcia-Ballester, "Dietetic and pharmacological therapy: a dilemma among fourteenth century Jewish practitioners in the Montepellier area," *Clio Medica* 22, (1991), pp. 23–37; Joseph Shatzmiller, "Etudiants Juifs a la faculte de medicine de Montepellier dernier quart du xiv siecle," *Jewish History* 6:1–2, (1992), pp. 243–55.

27. Rashba, responsum 120, also quoted in Rabbi Yosef Karo, *Bedek HaBayit* on Yoreh De'ah 154.

28. Commentary on Leviticus, 12:2.

29. These terms derive from the Mishnah in Niddah 2:5 and have been the source of much discussion regarding their anatomical identification.

30. *Hilkhot Issurei Bi'ah* 5:4.

31. *Magen Avot* 40a.

32. This book is a compilation of theories in philosophy, theology, psychology, and medicine. The material was culled from the existing literature of that time, as stated by Aldabi in his introduction, but unfortunately there are no references, for which Aldabi apologizes. This book was first printed in 1518 in Riva di Trento, but because of its immense popularity it has been reprinted many times over the centuries, most recently in Jerusalem, 1990.

33. *Shevilei Emunah*, (Jerusalem, 1990), pp. 177–8.

34. For biographical information on Tuvia Cohn see his introduction to *Ma'aseh Tuvia*. See also Dr. D.A. Friedman, *Tobias Cohn*, (Tel Aviv, 1940); *Encyclopedia Judaica*, s.v. Cohn, Tobias.

35. On the Jews of the University of Padua see, for example, Cecil Roth, "The medieval university and the Jew," *Menora Journal* 9:2, (1930), pp. 128–41; Jacob Shatzky, "On Jewish medieval students of Padua," *Journal of History of Medicine* 5, (1950), pp. 444–47; Cecil Roth, "The qualification of Jewish physicians in the Middle Ages," *Speculum* 28, (1953), pp. 834–43; David B. Ruderman, "The impact of science on Jewish culture and society in Venice (with special reference to Jewish graduates of Padua's medical school)," *Gli Ebrei e Venezia*, (Venice, 1983), pp. 417–48.

36. (Cracow, 1908) p. 118. Note his mention of the microscope, which was first designed in the late-seventeenth century.

37. Note that this author has been variously referred to as Baruch of Shklov, Baruch Shklover or Baruch Schick, the latter name under which he is listed in *Encyclopedia Judaica*. For biographical information see David Fishman, "Science, Enlightenment, and Rabbinic Culture in Belorussian Jewry, 1772–1804," PhD dissertation, Harvard University, (1985); ibid., "A Polish rabbi meets the Berlin haskalah: The case of Rabbi Baruch Schick," *AJS Review* 12:1, (Spring, 1987), pp. 95–121; Noach Shapiro, "Rabbi Baruch Schick MiShklov," *HaRofe*

HaIvri 34:1–2, (1961), pp. 230–35; David Margalit, "Dr. Baruch Schick V'Sifro 'Tiferet Adam,' " *Koroth* 6:1–2, (Aug., 1972), pp. 5–7.

There is debate in the above sources as to whether Baruch Schick was a physician. See also Israel Zinberg, *A History of Jewish Literature: The German-Polish Cultural Center,* (New York, 1975), pp. 271–74.

38. (Hague, 1780). In the introduction to this book appears the oft-quoted notion, in the name of the Vilna Gaon, that scientific knowledge is needed for the study of Torah.

39. *Tiferet Adam,* (Berlin, 1777), p. 3. This book was printed together with *Amudai Shamayim,* an astronomical work by the same author. As this latter work appears first in the combined volume, the book is often referenced by its name only.

40. This is a loose translation from *Igeret Bikoret,* (Zhitomer, 1868), 25b.

41. Parentheses are in original text.

42. *Sefer Habrit,* (Jerusalem, 1990), vol. 1, chap. 2, p. 240.

43. Hullin 45b.

44. loc. cit. s.v. *she'aino moleid.*

45. *Sefer HaBahir* has also been referred to as *Midrash Rabbi Nehunia ben HaKana.* The Ramban refers to it by this title in his biblical commentary. This citation is from chap. 51 and is quoted by Moshe Perlman in his *Midrash HaRefuah,* (Tel Aviv, 1926), p. 23.

46. *Shevelei Emunah,* (Jerusalem, 1990), netiv 4, 211.

47. *Magen Avot,* 38b. The Tahbetz mentions some of the proofs to this doctrine. These proofs make fascinating reading and reflect the medieval understanding of heredity, particularly the inheritance of acquired characteristics. The concept of heredity in *Hazal* is another topic that merits medical/historical analysis.

48. ibid., 39a.

49. The encephalo-myelogenic doctrine was also mentioned by Rabbi Yehiel Michel Epstein in his halakhic work *Arukh HaShulhan,* Even HaEzer, 23:3.

50. This is a reference to the encephalo-myelogenic doctrine.

51. *Sefer HaBrit,* (Jerusalem, 1990), article 16, chap. 3, pp. 232–3.

52. Many scientists of that time referred to sperm as seminal worms. See for example, William Cullen, trans., *Albrecht Haller, First Lines of Physiology,* (Edinburgh, 1786), p. 205.

53. *Tiferet Adam,* (Berlin, 1777), 3b–4a. Other arguments against the preformationists are cited in Needham, op. cit., 210. It appears from the last sentence of this quote that Schick may himself have viewed the sperm under the microscope. There is debate among historians whether Schick had a laboratory where he performed medical experimentation. See Shapiro, op. cit., pp. 234–5; Israel Zimberg, op. cit., p. 282.

It is also interesting that this entire passage is strikingly similar to the writings of Albrecht Haller, whose works were very popular in the scientific world at the time Schick was writing. Compare the passage below with the one by Schick:

> To the father some have attributed everything; chiefly since the seminal worms, now so well known, were first observed in the male seed by the help of the microscope.... But in these animals there is a proportion wanting betwixt there number and that of the fetuses; they are also not to be constantly observed throughout the tribes of animals. (From Cullen, op. cit., pp. 205–6)

A broader comparison between *Tiferet Adam* and the works of Haller may yield interesting results.

54. Rabbi Yosef Hayyim ben Eliyahu, *Rav Pe'alim,* vol. 3, Even HaEzer 2; Rabbi Yehiel Michel Epstein, *Arukh HaShulhan,* Even HaEzer 23:1; Rabbi Eliezer Waldenberg, *Tzitz Eliezer,* vol. 9, 51.

55. A number of authors have previously written on this topic from an historical perspective. See H.J. Zimmels, *Magicians Theologians and Doctors,* (London, 1952); Immanuel Jacobowitz, *Jewish Medical Ethics,* (New York, 1959), pp. 244–50. This essay treats the topic more comprehensively.

56. John Hunter (1728–1793) was a prominent scientist and comparative anatomist who is known for his self experimentation with venereal disease. His original manuscripts detailing his application of artificial insemination are currently housed at the Hunterian Museum in London, where one can also see on display thousands of human and animal anatomical specimens, which Hunter collected during his lifetime.

57. *Test Tube Babies,* (New York, 1934).

58. See, for example, Fred Rosner, *Modern Medicine and Jewish Law,* 2nd ed., (New York, 1991), pp. 85–100; Abraham Steinberg, *Encyclopedia Hilkhatit Refuit,* (Jerusalem, 1988), pp. 148–61. For a bibliography of responsa on this topic, see Rabbi Ya'akov Weinberg and Rabbi Maier Zichal, "*Hazra'ah Melakhutit,*" *Assia* 55, (Dec., 1994), pp. 75–89.

59. See Robert Graves, *The Greek Myths,* (Baltimore, 1955), p. 51 for descriptions of non-natural methods of conception. I thank Dr. Louis Feldman for this reference.

60. For the material on artificial insemination in medieval times I have relied on secondary sources, primarily Preuss. The primary sources are in Arabic and Latin and, for the most part, remain untranslated into English.

61. Preuss, 464.

62. On this author see Gerrit Bos, "Ibn Al-Jazzar on women's diseases and their treatment," *Medical History,* 37, (1993), pp. 296–312. In personal communication, Dr. Bos says he is unaware of any reference to artificial insemination in the extant works of Al-Jazzar.

63. ibid. Preuss provides no reference for this statement.

64. This work was reprinted and appended to Hermann Rohleder, *Test Tube Babies*, (New York, 1934).

65. Preuss, p. 464, cites Stern, that the belief in bathhouse insemination was still prevalent in Turkey at that time, i.e. early twentieth century. See also George Gould and Walter Pyle, *Medical Curiosities*, (New York, 1896), pp. 42–45, who state that the possibility of bathhouse insemination was still being debated. They also relate an extraordinary, if not fantastical, story from the Civil War of how a woman, struck in the abdomen with a bullet that previously hit the testicle of a soldier, gave birth, after two hundred seventy-eight days, to an eight-pound boy.

66. On Zacchias and other medical legal writers, see Bernard Ficarro, "History of legal medicine," *Legal Medicine Annual*, (1979).

67. Both Zacchias and Haller are mentioned in Preuss, op. cit., p. 464.

68. 14b–15a. Some have construed this passage to be a sarcastic allusion to the Christian doctrine of immaculate conception. See Rabbi Yehoshua Boymel, *Emek Halakha*, 1:68; Jacobowitz, op. cit., p. 359, n. 31. Preuss, op. cit., p. 477, has already pointed out that this cannot be, as the doctrine of the immaculate conception was not yet known at the time of Ben Zoma (first century CE).

69. See Tosafot, loc. cit., s.v. *betula*. Whether it is only claimed or actually verified that the woman is a virgin is a matter of discussion.

70. I referred to the text based on an Oxford manuscript, which was published in A.M. Haberman, *Hadashim Gam Yeshanim,* (Jerusalem, 1976), pp. 125–7.

71. The text also mentions that the *Ammoraim* Rav Zeira and Rav Pappa were born by artificial insemination, but unlike Ben Sira, the identity of their fathers was unknown. Yechiel Halprein, in his *Seder HaDorot,* (Jerusalem, 1988), section 2, p. 118, quotes *Sefer Yuhsin* by Abraham Zacuto, who, in turn, quotes this notion from *Sefer Kabbalat HaHasid*. Halprein then cites the original source of this idea from the *Alphabet of Ben Sira* and subsequently refutes the belief that Rav Zeira and Rav Pappa were products of artificial insemination. He does not, however, assail the belief that Ben Sira was a product of artificial insemination.

72. Pietrikov, 1904, introduction.

73. *Tzemach David*, sec. 1, *eleph rvi'i*, 448. See also *Tzitz Eliezer*, vol. 9, no. 51, gate 4, chap.1, letter *tet*.

74. This reference is mentioned by the *Bayit Hadash* (R.Y. Sirkes 1561–1640) in Yoreh De'ah 195 (s.v. *v'lo*) as appearing in the "*hagahot Semak yashan*" of Rabbi Peretz. The glosses of Rabbi Peretz first appeared in the printed text of *Sefer Mitzvot Katan* in the mid-1500s and all subsequent editions invariably contained these glosses. I consulted the 1556 Cremona edition and could not find this particular gloss. It seems that this gloss remained in manuscript form and was never printed, hence the term "*yashan*" of the Bach likely refers to an old manuscript edition. This fact is further evidenced by the comment of Rabbi Haim Y.D. Azulai (*Birkei Yosef,* Even HaEzer 1:14) that after much

effort he was finally able to locate this particular gloss of Rabbi Peretz in an old manuscript.

A passage similar to that of Rabbi Peretz' appears in the *Shiltei HaGiborim* on the Rif (Babylonian Talmud *Shavuot* 2a) attributed to an author referred to by his acronym, HR"M. Rabbi Eliezer Waldenberg (*Tzitz Eliezer,* vol. 9, no. 51, gate 4, chap. 1 letter het) has postulated that this may be a misprint, and the text should actually read HR"P, an acronym for HaRav Rabbeinu Peretz.

75. *Sefer Maharil*, Shlomo Spitzer, ed., (Jerusalem, 1989), pp. 611–12.

76. Vol. 3, no. 263.

77. On Lusitanus see essays in Harry Friedenwald, *The Jews and Medicine*, vol. 1, Baltimore, (1944), pp. 332–90. The section relevant to our discussion is on page 386. Preuss, op. cit., 464, also quotes Lusitanus in discussing the Talmud, *Hagiga*.

78. Friedenwald, op. cit., 363, n. 98.

79. See the work of another famous Jewish physician, Tobias Cohn (1652–1729), who mentions artificial insemination in his *Ma'ase Tuvia*, (Cracow, 1908), section 3, 118b.

80. Although known for his halakhic expertise, Lampronti was a prominent Italian physician and a graduate of the University of Padua. See Abdelkader Modena and Edgardo Morpurgo, *Medici E Chirurghi Ebrei Dottorati E Licenziati Nell'Universita Di Padova dal 1617 al 1816,* (Bologna, 1967), pp. 55–57. These authors mention that Lampronti consulted the famous physician Morgagni for assistance with his difficult medical cases. Saul Jarcho elaborates on these consultations in his article, "Dr. Isac Lampronti of Ferrara," *Koroth* 8:11–12, (1985), pp. 203–6. For a discussion on the interface between science and halakha in the work of Lampronti, see David B. Ruderman, "Contemporary science and Jewish law in the eyes of Isaac Lampronti of Ferrara and some of his contemporaries," *Jewish History* 6:1–2, (1992), pp. 211–24.

81. *Pahad Yitzhak* (Bnei Brak, 1980), s.v. *ben bito*. David Margalit does not mention this passage in his essay, "*Erkhim refui'im shebiEncyclopedia HaHilkhatit Pahad Yitzhak L'R.Y. Lampront,*" *Koroth* 2:1–2, (April, 1958), pp. 38–61.

82. Although the *Wisdom of Ben Sira* is included in the works of the apocrypha, the *Alphabet of Ben Sira* is not. See Rabbi Yehoshua Boymel, *Emek Halakha,* no. 68, regarding the quotation of Rabbi Lampronti: "...even though he did not cite his source for this, still his words are believed, and this *tzaddik* is free from iniquity."

Rabbi Boymel apparently thought the word "*ketuvim*" to be a generic reference, not a reference to a specific work or body of works.

83. *Hilkhot Ishut*, 15:4. See also *Mishnah L'Melech* on *Hilkhot Issurei Bi'ah* 17:15, where Rabbi Rosanes discusses these matters in great detail and states that the passage of Ben Zoma in Hagiga is not considered halakhic.

84. See, for example, Malakhi ben Ya'akov HaKohen (d. 1785–1790), *Yad Mal-*

akhi, (Berlin, 1857), *Klalei Hadinim* no. 247; Rabbi Moshe Schick, known as Maharam Schick, *Taryag Mitzvot* no. 1.

85. *Teshuvot Rashban*, Even HaEzer no. 8.

86. (Jerusalem, 1976), no. 481. Rabbi Hayyim wrote these responsa under a pseudonym.

87. The concept of *"nishtane hateva"* has been invoked many times in rabbinic literature. See, for example, *Tosafot* in the *Babylonian Talmud* Avoda Zara 24b, s.v. *para*; *Tosafot* in *Babylonian Talmud* Hullin 47a, s.v. *kol*; Even HaEzer 156:4 in the Rema. Two areas where authorities often discuss this principle are *hilkhot treifot* and *metzitza* in *mila*.

    For a comprehensive treatment of this topic, see Neria Gutal, *Sefer Hishtanut haTeva'im biHalakha* (Jerusalem: Maksshin Yahdav, 5755).

88. Rabbi Hayyim cites other reasons for forbidding sperm procurement in this case, such as, some seed might spill in the process of collection, or, even if they collect all the seed, it might not all be used for the purpose of insemination. These concerns have been voiced by current *poskim* in their discussions on artificial insemination.

89. See Rohleder, op. cit.

90. Rabbi Ya'akov Reischer, *Iyun Ya'akov*, (Wilhelmsdorf, 1725), on Hagiga 14b. See also Rabbi Pinhas Horowitz, *Pit'ha Zuta al Hil. Niddah U'Tevilla*, (London, 1958), 195:7, who explains the position of Rabbi Reischer. Both of these sources question why the Rambam omits the case of Ben Zoma from his code.

91. See Orach Haim 230:3 and *Mishnah Berura*, loc. cit.

92. Rabbi Yekutiel Greenwald, in his *Kol Bo Al Aveilut*, (New York, 1947), pp. 305–6, n. 8, states that the majority of poskim hold that bathhouse insemination could never happen. However, if it was ascertainable that such an event had occurred, the parents and children would be obligated to mourn for each other. Another halakhic question unique to a child born from bathhouse insemination is whether such a child could have his *mila* performed on Shabbat. See Rabbi Moshe Bunim Pirutinsky, *Sefer HaBrit*, (New York, 1973), p. 9, who states, based on the interpretation of Rabbeinu Hananel to *Hagiga*, that since such a birth is considered miraculous, and not by natural methods of conception, the *mila* should not be performed on Shabbat.

93. Many *Aharonim* still maintained the possibility of bathhouse impregnation without specifically addressing the *Mishnah L'Melech*. See Rabbi Ya'akov Emden *Iggeret Bikkoret*, (Zhitomer, 1868), and *Sheilat Ya'avetz*, vol. 2, no. 97.

94. *Bnei Ahuvah*, (Jerusalem, 1965), on Rambam, *Hil. Ishut* chap. 15.

95. *Birkei Yosef*, Even HaEzer 1:14; *Yair Ozen, ma'arehet* 1 no. 93; *P'tach Einayim* on *Hagiga* 14b. See also Rabbi Y.S. Nathanson, *Shai L'Moreh*, glosses on Even HaEzer 1;6; ibid., *Responsum Shoel U'Meishiv*, vol. 3, section 3, nos. 34 and 132 (end); Rabbi Eliezer Fleckles, *Teshuva Me'Ahava*, Yoreh De'ah no. 195.

96. *Brit Ya'akov*, (Warsaw, 1876), Even HaEzer no. 4. The author employs the same logic with respect to Rabbi Peretz' pronouncement about a woman becoming pregnant from seed remaining on the sheets. Here, too, he maintains that a

woman may use the sheets for internally cleaning herself, thereby bringing the seed into close proximity with the uterus.

97. Although I have been unable to find any contemporary medical references to bathhouse insemination, I have found an interesting case which attests to the viability of the human sperm. See Douwe A.A. Verkuyl, "Oral conception: Impregnation via the proximal gastrointestinal tract in a patient with an aplastic vagina," *British Journal of Obstetrics and Gynaecology*, 95, (Sept., 1988), pp. 933–4.

98. See Rabbi Shalom Mordechai Shvadron (1835–1911), *She'ailot U'Teshuvot Maharsham*, (New York, 1962), vol. 3, no. 268, who was asked whether it was permissible to undergo artificial insemination.

Part II
The Religious Jewish Infertile Couple

Introduction

In examining the problem of infertility, it is easy to become consumed with the complex details of diagnosis and treatment. The enormous need to be successful is felt not only by the affected couple, but usually by the physician as well. Together, they tend to focus their energies on the correction of certain physical problems. While this makes sense in regard to the specific medical treatment at hand, it should not preclude a discussion and evaluation of the couple's emotional status. Studies have repeatedly shown improved treatment outcomes in groups of patients who have received appropriate counseling. Certainly, the relief of stress can improve cyclic hormonal functioning in women and sexual performance in men. The improved result may also be due to those couples' ability to persist in therapy until the desired result is attained. No matter how highly functioning the couple appears to be or how straightforward their fertility problem, it is helpful for them to understand clearly the psychological and social context within which they experience their infertility.

For the couple who is committed to halakha and who lives in a community of like-minded people, the emergence of a fertility problem presents special difficulties and challenges. In this section we examine some of these, with specific emphasis on their origins and possible solutions. The material presented should help couples who are experiencing infertility to clarify some of the feelings and reactions which they often confront. Perhaps more importantly, it may prompt those who care for them to understand them more completely. Specifically, there is a great need for physicians to be sensitized to the cultural and religious framework within which such couples cope with their infertility. Likewise, rabbis and family members must be better attuned to the unique pressures—both physical and psychological—under which the couple is living. Especially when treatment is protracted, successful resolution of infertility is best achieved when patients, their caregivers, and their counselors all understand these issues.

Yoel Jakobovits

The Longing for Children in the Traditional Jewish Family

J udaism regards the gift of children as one of life's preeminent endowments—and challenges. Fecundity is among the most cherished of blessings, an attitude graphically amplified in Psalm 128 which speaks of "a wife as fruitful as a vine," whose "children are as olive plants around the table" leading to the ultimate joy of seeing "children to thy children." This is vividly emphasized by the belief that there are a predestined number of people who must be born before the Messiah can come.[1] Therefore, having more children hastens his arrival.

It has been postulated that the Jewish approach to procreation is, in addition, partially shaped by a legacy of lamentable historical conditions.[2] Frequent physical assault by massacres and pogroms coupled with equally devastating forced conversions and not-so-forced assimilation constitute an enormous—and, alas, persistent—depletion of Jewish demographics. A collective, subconscious instinct may exist to replenish these losses by achieving birth rates far in excess of the growth of the ambient society. Interesting and attractive as this theory is, its soundness as a historically valid social force remains conjectural, the thesis as yet untested by comparing different Jewish communities in separate periods.

The most distinctive defining characteristic of the observant Jew is, of course, loyalty to the dictates of Jewish law. Though not the only reason for marriage,[3] bearing children fulfills three specific religious imperatives—and sets the stage for many others—and is therefore the quintessential ambition of a religious couple. Indeed, the primacy of the mitzvah of procreation is reflected in its being first in the Torah.[4] And while the Mishnah regards the biblical references in Genesis as merely exhorting, as a minimum, the reproduction of the couple by having at least two children,[5] the Talmud explicates two supplementary ordinances. One, known as *lashevet*, is of biblical origin and based on the verse in Isaiah 45:18: "Not for void did He create the world, but for habitation (*lashevet*) did He form it." The second, known as *laʿerev* is of rabbinic derivation and is based on the verse: "In the morning, sow thy seed, and in the evening (*laʿerev*) do not withhold your hand." Subsequently these precepts were codified by Maimonides: "Although a man has fulfilled the mitzvah of *peru uʾrevu* (be fruitful and multiply), he is commanded by the Rabbis not to desist from procreation while he yet has strength, for whoever adds even one Jewish soul is considered as having created an entire world."[6]

The pressure, therefore, on devout Jewish infertile couples is often more intense than that which is found among the population at large. Indeed, opposite calculations may pertain. Whereas a modern, secular couple might choose to "protect" themselves against pregnancy during their first few years of marriage, the Jewish allegiant couple yearns for early parenthood. Actually, both prototypes are motivated to solidify their as yet tenuous relationships. But while a secular couple may believe that the premature arrival of children would likely undermine their vulnerable ties, the religious one believes that early parenthood is more apt to cement their marital bonds through the commonality of offspring. These divergent positions can be traced to fundamentally differing views of the marital covenant itself. On the one hand, many secular couples think of the *privileges* of marriage as paramount. On the other hand, the religious couple regards marriage's *responsibilities* as preeminent. Consequently, the secular view emphasizes the couple's fulfillment in one another; the religious view stresses their fulfillment in their offspring.

These sociologic features are ubiquitous in the religious Jewish community, fostering an unusual urgency to the resolution of infertility difficulties. It is common for childless couples to seek early counsel, perhaps even within the first few months of marriage. The urge to ignore such entreaties as premature must be tempered by the recognition that these cultural phenomena are deeply rooted in religious law and custom.

An ancient Talmudic axiom states that "a blessing is only effective on that which is concealed from the eye."[7] The psychological sensitivity of intimate human relationships cannot be over-emphasized. Great care must be exercised in advising a couple to embark on the trail of infertility investigation. A precise recommendation as to how much time should elapse before infertility investigations are begun cannot be made. Though, by convention, couples who remain childless after one year of regular, sexually active married life are called infertile, the point at which the diagnosis of infertility is earned is quite variable.[8]

Regarding the "right time" at which to initiate the various stages of infertility testing, the rabbinic opinions are quite variable. For example, while some allow semen analysis only after ten years,[9] others urge only a five[10] or even a two[11] year period. Rabbi Waldenberg underscores the need to tailor one's approach to the individual cases at hand.[12]

Even though the halakha may have no technical opposition to some investigations, there are some important psychological aspects to consider. An objective, scientific confirmation, particularly during the early months of marriage, of testicular failure in the male or ovarian failure in the female can have a devastating impact on the affected partner and hence on the marriage itself. Consequently great deliberation must be exercised when acquiescing to—or counseling—a couple asking for fertility testing.

Recurrent spontaneous abortions—miscarriages—can have the same outcome as infertility, albeit with much greater psychological repercussions. Therefore, counseling in instances of miscarriage must be conducted with commensurately greater sympathy and understanding. In general, young couples ought to be dissuaded from immediately undertaking costly, intensive investigations. Rather, they should be informed that it is estimated that up to a third of all human pregnancies end in spontaneous losses. As an application of the concept of survival of the fittest, early spontaneous miscarriages can be viewed as nature's (that is, God's) way of culling out the most feeble fetuses. Couples ought to delay formal investigations at least until after two or even three consecutive spontaneous losses. Both the couple and their adviser should also be aware that the earlier premature investigations are conducted, the greater the halakhic hurdles are likely to be.

We have already emphasized the degree to which an observant Jewish infertile couple may feel compelled to seek medical help. However, the mysterious[13] nature of the miracle of procreation instinctively prompts many infertile couples to first seek guidance and blessing from spiritual rather than medical sources, and the couple will often first seek the guidance of their rabbi. Indeed, infertility difficulties, in particular, are associated with prayer and spiritual exertions. The very concept of supplication in prayer to the Creator has its roots in the matriarchs, Sarah, Rebecca, and Rachel, all of whom were infertile through many years of marriage. The Bible chronicles their yearning for the blessing of children through anguished prayer, prompting the Rabbis to declare that "God is desirous of the prayer of the righteous."[14] These moving passages were eventually regarded as the paradigm of prayer and were therefore incorporated into the High Holiday services.[15] All who are involved in advising such people must be sensitive to these metaphysical aspects of their petitioner's needs.

Endnotes

1. Yevamot 62a, 63b; Avoda Zara 5b; Niddah 13b.
2. See D.M. Feldman, *Marital Relations, Birth Control and Abortion in Jewish Law*, New York: Schocken Books, 1974. p. 51.
3. See, for example, the series of expositions on the inherent value of marriage for the male partner in Yevamot 62b., where one who is unmarried is regarded as being without joy, blessing, good, Torah, protection, and peace. Likewise the Talmud (e.g. Yevamot 118b; Kiddushin 7a, 41a) often assumes that marriage is beneficial for the female partner: *"Tav l'metav tan du mil'metav arm'lu*—It is always to her advantage to be part of a tandem, married, rather than alone." Both reference focus on the companionship, non-procreative aspects of marriage.
4. Rashi and Tosafot (on Yevamot 65b) and Ramban (on Genesis 9:7) hold that the verses addressed to the Noachidic survivors of the Flood (Genesis 9:1 and 7) and to Jacob (ibid. 35:11) are the source of this injunction. Contrary to the common assumption, the charge to Adam and Eve (ibid. 1:28) is actually a blessing, not a commandment.
5. Yevamot 6 (61b).
6. *Mishneh Torah*, Hilkhot Ishut, 15:16.
7. Ta'anit 8b; Bava Metziah 42a. In fact several studies highlight the fact that pregnancy rates are fairly independent of treatment! See, for example, J.A. Collins, W. Wrixon, L.B. Jones, E.H. Wilson, "Treatment-independent pregnancy among infertile couples," *New England Journal of Medicine*, 309:1201, (1983).
8. See note 7. It should be pointed out that the authors report that 64% to 79% of women with infertility will conceive within nine years. Clearly, however, investigations should not be delayed until then.
9. Resp. *Minhat Yitzhak*, vol. 3. no. 108.
10. Resp. *Iggrot Moshe*, Even HaEzer, vol. 2, no. 16.
11. Hazon Ish cited by A. Avraham, *Nishmat Avraham*, Even HaEzer 23:2, p.113.
12. Resp. *Tzitz Eliezer*, vol. 9, no. 51:1.2.
13. E.E. Wallach, "The enigma of unexplained infertility," *Postgraduate Obstetrics and Gynecology*, 5:1, (1985) alludes to some of these unexplained phenomena. In general, it emphasizes that the shorter the duration of infertility is, the better the associated prognosis.
14. Yevamot 64a.
15. The Torah reading for the first day of Rosh Hashanah, taken from Genesis 21, recounts the realization of Sarah's plea upon the birth of Isaac. Similarly, the *Haftarah* (1 Samuel:1–2) relates how Hannah was ultimately blessed with the birth of Samuel. The Talmud (Megillah 31a) tells us that Sarah and Hannah were both remembered on Rosh Hashanah. Indeed, Hannah's prayer becomes a paradigm, serving as the source for many of the halakhot of prayer (See Berakhot 31a).

Hershel Billet

The Rabbinic and Medical Partnership

Rabbi Joseph B. Soloveitchik once observed that Jews must function in two dimensions. On the one hand, they share the universal human condition with all of mankind. On the other, they must confront life in their own unique, particularistic way. The instinct and ability to reproduce was implanted in mankind at the time of creation, and from this perspective Jews share with non-Jews the common problems associated with infertility. At the same time, though, they have unique religious rules relating to the biblical, prophetic, and rabbinic sources defining the special commandment to "be fruitful and fill the earth."

For a traditional Jewish couple, infertility is both a medical and a religious problem. As a medical problem, it requires the services of medical practitioners and the assistance of emotional support groups or professionals. As a religious problem, it requires a rabbinic consultation for clarification of halakhic and ethical issues which might be associated with each particular case.

The Bible includes many narratives, from the times of the

Patriarchs through the times of the prophets, concerning couples who had difficulty conceiving children. From the perspective of the Bible and the Talmud prayer is seen as a solution to this problem.[1] God is the Creator, the source of life, and He holds the keys to conception.[2] Rebecca, Isaac, and Hannah all succeeded through their prayers and were blessed with children. Judaism accepts that the metaphysical world directly affects the physical world. Therefore, prayer, an instrument of the metaphysical world, is seen as a means through which people can be helped to have children. Indeed, when the Rabbis formulated the daily essential prayer, they included a blessing for health. Prayer, then, is a vehicle which is designed to assist people in overcoming physical, health-related problems. Included in this category are problems related to procreation. Despite the fact that couples facing a problem of infertility are most often in good health, from a halakhic perspective infertility is a medical problem. As such, it is included under the license to heal that the halakha has given physicians.

The "License to Heal" and its Relationship to Infertility

Talmudic and rabbinic sources cite numerous precedents for allowing a physician to engage in the practice of medicine, with the goal of assisting people in overcoming their medical problems. Let us analyze the different sources on this subject and see how they lend themselves to the medical treatment of infertility.

The Talmud in *Bava Kama* 85a sees the verse "And he shall cause him to be thoroughly healed" (Exodus 21:19) as the source for a doctor's license to cure. Rashi and Tosafot both indicate that this license is necessary so that medical assistance not be seen as a human attempt to circumvent divine decrees. The Midrash Tanhuma further develops the point, seeing medical practice not only as licensed, but as an element of the partnership established between God and man in enhancing the quality of life in the world. Man is expected to fertilize, to plant, to harvest, to build, and to heal, to make God's world a better place in which to live. Maimonides sees man's search for medical help as a form of *bitahon*, trust in God.[3] From this point of view, the work of physicians who assist couples in their effort to conceive children certainly fulfills the stipulations of the divine mission of medical practice.

What is more, the Talmud declares that if any human being saves a single soul in Israel, it is regarded as if he had saved an entire world.[4] Although this statement refers to saving a life that already exists, it might be applied to assisting the birth of unborn or not yet conceived children as well. Certainly, Judaism believes that the destiny of Israel is bound with those not yet born as well as those already alive.[5]

Interpretations of Leviticus 19:16, "You shall not stand idly by the blood of your neighbor," transform a physician's license to practice into a demand, a duty. Rabbi Yosef Karo says that the physician as a healer saves lives, and withholding care is considered to be the shedding of blood.[6] In regards to infertility, Rashi says that someone without children is considered devastated[7] while the Talmud considers such a person to be without life.[8] From this perspective, a physician who helps a couple conceive is considered a restorer of life to the parents of the child.

Other sources highlight different aspects of a physician's responsibility. Maimonides, for example, sees the physician's responsibility to his patients as a function of the biblical verse requiring the restoration of lost property, "And you shall restore it to him" (Deuteronomy 22:2).[9] A person whose reproductive system needs medical intervention to restore it to proper function would fall under this category.

Nahmanides declares that the physician's medical practice is mandated by "Love your neighbor as yourself" (Leviticus 19:18). The implication of this commandment broadens the role of the physician to include other acts of kindness beyond healing. Hence, even if one were to argue that people who have a fertility problem are not technically ill, the physician would nevertheless be obligated to assist those people.

There are several other halakhic issues which might be raised by medical treatment for infertility. Among them would be the question of whether such treatment applies equally to a woman and a man, inasmuch as a woman is not commanded to fulfill the mitzvah of procreation. From the perspective of "love your neighbor," it might be argued that there is no difference between a man and a woman. A woman who yearns for a child is suffering both physically and emotionally, and "Love your neighbor" requires that we reach out to her as well. From the perspective of being devastated without children and having life restored with children, it would seem that there is no difference between a man and a woman. Indeed, Sarah is a biblical source of the notion of childless persons being devastated, as she declares, "Perhaps I will be rebuilt from her." A woman whose reproductive system needs repair would seem to fit the stipulations of "you shall restore it...."

Another question might relate to the form of the therapy. Risky, experimental, and non-therapeutic procedures pose halakhic questions. Percentage of success and consequences of failed treatment are all factors which have to be weighed according to different authorities. Also to be considered is that most authorities do not see infertility as a life-threatening circumstance. Despite Talmudic sources which suggest such an analogy, infertility is not really a physical threat to life and limb. The majority point of view would encourage couples to seek help. Yet it is important to understand the nature of all forms of treatment to assure that they do not contradict halakha.

A Note of Caution

Once it has been established halakhically that the medical community plays an important role in assisting couples along the road to parenthood, we must define the parameters within which this community may function in helping a traditional Jewish couple. If physicians or counselors wish to properly serve their religious patients, then they must accept that not all of the secular or ethical norms of their profession are acceptable to those patients. The professional must recognize that a local rabbi and/or halakhic authority may have to be consulted to help the couple resolve certain moral and halakhic issues which might arise in treating their problem. The physician/counselor must realize that, for these patients, resolving these questions in a halakhic way is as important as having a satisfactory result from their treatment. The infertility practitioner should therefore be sensitive to the patient's needs and interact in a positive manner with the patient's rabbi, deferring to him in halakhic matters.

The rabbi, on the other hand, has to be realistic about his role as well. Often, a religious couple will consult with their rabbi before seeking medical advice. The rabbi should be aware of the limitations of his role and should not try to dispense medical advice. Rather, a knowledgeable rabbi should see his relationship with the couple as a supportive one. The rabbi should know when the couple's fears are premature and when they are timely. He should be prepared to advise the couple about the relevant halakhic issues and should interact with the physician accordingly.

In summary, the appropriate treatment of the fertility problem of a traditional Jewish couple requires the interface of the medical community with the religious community. Such cooperative interactions would serve the couple in a positive way and hopefully will result in the "whole" patient being treated with sensitivity and dignity.

Endnotes

1. Yevamot 64a.
2. Ta'anit 2a
3. Rambam, *Commentary on the Mishnah*, Pesahim 4:10.
4. Sanhedrin 37a.
5. Deuteronomy 29:14, Yevamot 62a.
6. *Shulhan Arukh*, Yoreh De'ah 336:1.
7. Rashi, commentary on Genesis 16:2, s.v. *holekh ariri*.
8. Nedarim 64b.
9. Rambam, *Commentary on the Mishnah*, Nedarim 4:4.

Sara Barris and Joel Comet

Infertility: Issues from the Heart

In our years of working with infertile individuals, couples, and their families, we frequently heard these typical questions and comments: A parent-in-law asks, "Why are they making such a big deal about this? Thank God, it's not cancer. God will surely help!" A women a year into her infertility diagnosis bemoans, "Why do I feel like every time I come up for air, I'm drowning again?" A man five years into his infertility questions, "Why can't I get on with my life? It feel like everything is on hold."

For an outsider looking in, it is difficult to get a sense of how pervasive is the experience of infertility. For those going through the ordeal, it is often a shock to see just how powerfully infertility disrupts their lives. Much has been written to shed light on why infertility has such a far-reaching and profound impact.[1] The impact reflects the reality that infertility is a life-crisis which permeates one's sense of self, one's marriage, one's relationship to extended family, community and finally, to God. In this chapter, we will focus on how these issues are intensified for the Orthodox infertile couple.

There are two unique aspects in the interplay between infertility and Orthodoxy that make it a different experience from other medical illnesses. First, for those who are Orthodox, infertility directly challenges the first mitzvah, *peru u'revu*, be fruitful and multiply." This commandment has become one of the most pivotal and precious values in Jewish life, that of building a family. Child-free living is not as viable an option as it might be for other couples without this religious family life commitment.

Second, in traditional Jewish thought, the values of modesty, privacy, and a special sense of "holiness" (*kedusha*) are attributed to the body parts and physical behaviors involved with reproduction. These are suddenly thrown open to widespread scrutiny by physicians and to speculation by the community. It often requires a long and difficult transition for Orthodox couples to begin to deal with infertility issues more openly and comfortably. If they are unable to negotiate this transition, they may slowly withdraw from friends and community and enter a cocoon of embarrassment, shame, and lack of knowledge.

In the sections below, we will expand on the critical challenges that confront the Orthodox infertile couple and their family.

Personal

Growing up, people anticipate and prepare for the roles they are to play in life. These roles are derived from general culture and society and are accentuated by one's religious beliefs and practices. Whatever other professional or social roles women see themselves playing in society, being a mother remains an integral part of a religious woman's female identity. It is a role girls practice for and fantasize about from childhood onward. No woman expects to be infertile and the shock forces her to question her basic sense of self: What does it mean to be a woman who may not bear children? What does it mean to be a wife who may not be able to be a mother? As one is challenged to redefine the roles one has accepted and prepared for, new role definitions are not readily available. The woman suddenly finds herself in a state of limbo.

When an observant woman gets married, she thinks about starting a family and, accordingly, she makes critical decisions about other aspects of her life, such as continuing secular or religious education, accepting job offers or pursuing a career. With infertility, and the reawakening of the question of role definition, all of these decisions need to be thought through again. However, new roles and plans become difficult to pursue due to both logistical and emotional factors. The unpredictability, time, and effort involved in infertility treatment may require one to be available at various days of one's cycle, at specific times of the day, and at short notice. The emotional upheaval of infertility makes it difficult to focus on other facets of one's life. As one woman put it: "I'm miserable at my job, but how can I concentrate on looking for new possibilities when all my time and energy is consumed by my infertility?" A woman is left feeling empty: she is not a mother and she is too depleted to enhance and develop other parts of her identity.

Men frequently report that infertility attacks their sense of self on many levels. The Torah clearly defines a man's role in relationship to his wife. The man is expected to take on the responsibility of providing for his wife's material and sexual needs. The infertile man begins to doubt his ability to be an effective husband. He believes that he is disappointing his wife and feels like a failure. Furthermore, secular society shapes men's attitudes with messages that equate sexual performance with manhood. The naive general public often mistakenly equates male infertility with physical impotence. Infertile men who function well sexually may make that equation on an emotional level. They end up feeling like they are not "really men" and are often engulfed in a pervasive, vague sense of shame. A husband may begin to think that perhaps his wife would have been better off marrying somebody else.

The role of a father in relation to his child is also clearly defined and structured in religious society. A fundamental task is teaching one's children Torah. The childless Orthodox man is constantly reminded of his inability to fulfill this Torah mandate. When he attends Shabbat services, he feels empty as he is surrounded by other fathers praying along with their children. As he builds his Sukkah, he cannot help but notice that other men around him are aided by all their children. When he lights Hanukah candles, he is pained at being unable to share the recitation of the blessings. At the Passover Seder, he yearns to hear a small voice asking him the four questions; on Shavuot he craves to teach a child of his own during his night-long studies. Being unable to fulfill these expected roles of husband and father often leaves men feeling incomplete and anguished.

An integral part of a religious perspective is the value that is placed on constant improvement of one's character traits. It can be very difficult to feel that one is embracing this value in the face of the wide range of powerful emotions that are experienced and re-experienced at different stages of the infertility process. Anger, guilt, shame, depression, grief, and jealousy are all common feelings experienced by people going through infertility, yet people are frequently shocked at their presence and their intensity. They would never believe themselves capable of harboring these feelings which can seem so unacceptable at times, such as when one feels jealous and angry about one's close friend becoming pregnant. As these feelings arise, so does the guilt around one's failure to maintain a virtuous character. Many individuals feel that they are alone in experiencing these feelings and that these emotions reflect their own poor character. This leaves them feeling unworthy, isolated, and out of control.

Anger, which is often close to the surface and frequently directed at one's spouse, friends, family members, and doctors who are perceived as insensitive can be very unsettling. It may be directed at one's spouse for letting one down or for not being supportive. It is often directed at friends and relatives for failing to understand and for making well-intentioned but hurtful comments, such as "You know, you're not getting any younger!" or "Your poor sister, she just gave birth and had such a hard labor!" It may be felt toward physicians for not being successful, for building up expectations, for running their offices like factories, or for making their insensitive comments, such as "You're ruining my statistics!" It may also be directed at oneself as one searches out reasons to explain why one has been "punished" with this affliction.

Rather than berating themselves for experiencing these feelings, individuals must recognize that these feelings are common and normal. The Torah accepts these feelings as valid. For example, Rachel was jealous of her sister Leah, and Hannah, who was to become mother to the prophet Samuel, was inconsolably depressed. The Midrash recognizes these feelings as being positively motivated and acceptable. This does not mean that people are encouraged to immerse themselves and drown in their feelings, but rather that they not berate themselves for having these feelings and enter a cycle of self-blame that further intensifies their pain. Acknowledging these feelings helps the person gain a sense of validity and allows one to begin the process of letting go and moving on.

Resolving the emotions evoked by infertility is a process that takes place over time. Resolution does not mean that these feelings will never emerge again, even if couples are successful at having biological children. Like any wound that heals, it is more readily opened at vulnerable times in one's life, such as when one loses a family member. However, when healthy resolution begins to occur, couples can experience inner growth and strength of character. There can be increased sensitivity to others and an ability to be less judgmental about other's apparent negative behaviors. One knows first hand that surface behaviors do not necessarily reflect what the person is going through and one is better able to fulfill the traditional dictum of *dan lekhaf zekhut*, judging one's friend to his or her benefit.

It is not always easy to acknowledge these feelings as normal, especially when they relate to God. Many people question, Why is God punishing me? Am I so bad? Am I that much worse than the next person? This is particularly difficult for people who became observant later in life and who feel that they have made tremendous effort to elevate their religious functioning, but have been "rewarded" with infertility. It is often difficult and frightening for such individuals to question and doubt God's justice, especially when this is mixed with feelings of anger and fear of punishment. The traditional Jewish view that nothing in life is accidental can sometimes provide comfort. Using the models of the patriarchs and matriarchs who struggled with infertility, one can incorporate these difficult feelings into one's prayers to God. Many rabbis recommend that prayer for oneself and others and involvement in charitable activities can bring one closer to God and minimize feelings of alienation.

Profound feelings of grief and depression may occur and are often misunderstood by friends and family. It may be hard to understand the depth of these feelings because they relate to something vague, invisible, and potential. Couples may be grieving for many different types of losses: the unborn child, the pregnancy experience, sharing the birth experience with each other, bringing up a child steeped in Torah and good deeds, their own mortality, or the inability to compensate for the losses of the Holocaust with their own biological children. The loss may be different for each spouse. It is important for the couples to empathically understand both their own as well as their spouse's experience. Judaism does not provide rituals for mourning for these losses. Couples are left to mourn on their own, without the guidelines and structure that are available for other types of losses, such as *shiva* and *Kaddish*. It may be helpful for couples to mark these losses for themselves by giving to a special charity, by setting aside a special Torah topic to learn together, or by otherwise developing their own meaningful expressions of grief.

Marriage

Unfortunately, the effects of infertility are not contained within the individual but permeate his or her relationship with others, and a frequent casualty is the marriage. The marital relationship requires an enormous amount of energy, attention, and nurturance to keep it refueled from the constant draining demands that are placed on it. Many Orthodox couples begin trying to conceive immediately after they get married. These young relationships, without the benefit of a maturational process, are particularly vulnerable. In more mature relationships, communication skills have been improved, intimacy has deepened, and empathy has grown, thus better preparing the couple to deal with stressful events. On the other hand, couples who decided to postpone trying to conceive until later in their marriage may now need to additionally deal with a sense of guilt for having waited.

For all couples, the spontaneity and intimacy of sexual relations is compromised by the medical procedures and staff who often dictate the exact day, time, and position of intercourse. The laws of *niddah* that relate to a woman's menstrual cycle intensify these issues for the Orthodox couple. At a minimum, twelve days out of every monthly cycle is sexually off limits for the couple. On top of that, infertility procedures often further restrict the halakhically permissible time that a couple can be physically intimate with one another. A treatment procedure can cause a woman to become *niddah*, thereby prohibiting physical relations for at least an additional seven days. A doctor may also instruct a couple to abstain from relations until the woman is ovulating (which may be several days after the couple could otherwise have halakhically engaged in sexual relations) in order to increase the potency of the sperm.

The infertility treatment turns marital relations into a pressured, conflicting, and often unsatisfying experience. The Orthodox couple is left with very few days to engage in relaxed, physical intimacy. For newly married couples who are just beginning to learn to know one another and become comfortable on a physically intimate level, the problem is especially acute, and they can easily feel overwhelmed. Their sexual relationship becomes subject to scrutiny by themselves, doctors, nurses, lab staff and indirectly by parents, in-laws, extended family and community (who may be wondering why the couple is not pregnant). At times, they may feel that the "holiness" and intimacy of marital relations is gone, leaving in its place a mechanical and dehumanizing act. Instead of physical intimacy nurturing the young marriage, the marital relationship is replete with issues evoking feelings of disloyalty and betrayal. Wives may feel "violated" while husbands may feel estranged.

In addition, the complexity and high-tech nature of infertility treatments raises many halakhic issues which require the couple to consult a rabbi. These questions have become very complicated and require a halakhic authority who is knowledgeable and informed in this area. Even given this expertise, there is a range of different viewpoints, and tensions may occur in the relationship when a couple disagrees on whom to follow.

Rabbinic approval, as well as the family's and community's outlook, is also involved in the parenting options available to the couple. Rabbis differ in the degree to which they encourage adoption or egg or sperm donation as viable options, as well as do communities in the level of acceptance or stigma they apply to it.

These additional complexities confronting Orthodox couples can lead them to feel misunderstood and alienated from one another. Some couples may react to this by distancing and building barriers between themselves. Other couples may experience increased levels of stress, animosity, and fighting. Each spouse may end up feeling more alone and fragile. It is therefore especially important for them to make a conscious effort to develop ways of being mutually sympathetic and supportive. One way of coping is to learn when one's spouse is particularly vulnerable—as at the onset of the menstrual period, the pregnancy of a close relative, or the day when sperm has to be tested—and to take turns at being the stronger one at such times. Husband and wife may find that they react differently to infertility. They may experience the losses differently and have different ways of coping. It is helpful to place themselves in their spouse's shoes and to try to understand the loss experience from the other's point of view. (An excellent couples' exercise is to switch roles and see if one can accurately express a spouse's feelings.) It is also helpful to share the burden of gathering and analyzing the medical information so that one spouse does not feel overwhelmed and/or the other excluded. Couples should not choose one member to hear a doctor's recommendations and treatment plans. It is important to keep in mind that no matter which spouse is experiencing the primary medical problem or emotional reaction, infertility is always a shared couple's issue. When handled with care and sensitivity, the pain and trauma of infertility can ultimately serve to bring couples together and help them to develop a solid and loving marriage.

Family

Although families are traditional sources of support and comfort during crises, couples suffering infertility often experience family as a further strain. As mentioned above, modesty discourages people from discussing issues relating to the sexual relationship and parts of the body. Despite the fact that infertility is not a sexual issue per se, its association with marital relations can make it difficult and embarrassing to talk about. The intensity of emotions experienced—depression, anger, guilt, shame, and embarrassment—can also lead the couple to withdraw into themselves and away from support systems. When one spouse would like to seek the support of extended family but the other feels too ashamed to do so, marital tensions are heightened. This lack of communication and information exchange may lead to comments that are well-intentioned by the extended family, but can be experienced as hurtful by the couple. For example, "Is there a sexual problem?," "What's taking so long?," or "You're too tense! If you would just relax, you'd get pregnant."

Parents of infertile couples must also deal with difficult feelings. They may feel intense sadness about the pain and suffering of their children. Self-blame and guilt can emerge as parents try to make sense of their children's infertility. Parents are also mourning the potential loss of their own grandchildren. Given the importance of having children and the issue of family genealogy in the Orthodox community, family members may have a harder time accepting other options like adoption for building a family. Overall, these difficulties experienced by the couple and their parents can leave a void between them such that the couple is left without a vital support system and the extended family is left not knowing how to respond.

These kinds of issues may also occur even for couples who have a child. Those who attained parenthood through egg or sperm donation are usually secretive due to the stigma associated with it. They may feel unsupported and distressed when people assume that their infertility problem is resolved. For those suffering with secondary infertility, their pain is usually minimized by others who make comments such as "At least you have one child, you should be thankful."

Often, the infertile couple also experiences rejection when they perceive their siblings with children as being over-valued by their parents. For example, parents may spend more time at the homes of sons and daughters who have children; they may talk about how much pleasure they get from their grandchildren. The infertile couple may experience pain at family get-togethers around holiday times or celebrations such as a *brit* or bat mitzvah. These milestones, which traditionally serve to bring families together, end up leaving the couple feeling isolated, empty, and estranged.

For the many couples who are children or grandchildren of Holocaust survivors, feelings of strain or guilt may be exacerbated. They have grown up with the message embodied in that experience: that it is important to compensate for the losses of the Holocaust and ensure the continuity of the Jewish chain. This may add additional pressure or guilt for not being able to achieve this goal.

Couples and families can take steps to bring themselves closer together. Couples should be aware that their parents are also struggling with painful feelings. They need to assess what kind of emotional support they can realistically expect from their parents. Couples can educate and sensitize extended family members and let them know that they do not need to offer solutions or try to ease the pain with "helpful" advice. Just listening is often the most useful way to be supportive. Couples can also encourage family members to read literature on the emotional impact of infertility or to attend workshops that will make them more aware of these issues. It is not uncommon for family members to attend these workshops, even independent of the infertile couple. When couples are considering other options, like adoption, they can help other family members by introducing the idea gradually and not springing it on them. Family members do not need to wait for the couple to offer information, but can make independent efforts to educate themselves about infertility and adoption. The ability of couples and their families to feel more comfortable with each other around these issues of infertility is something that can take time to develop. When this process is worked on actively, it promotes connection, concern, and warmth that can be an anchor for the drifting, isolated couple.

Communal

Infertility also strikes out at social relationships and involvement with community events. Reminders of childlessness are built into the religious communal aspects of life. Where a synagogue used to be a place to relax and appreciate the joy of Shabbat, it now becomes a weekly reminder of how set apart the infertile members are from the rest of their peers. Synagogues are filled with children and pregnant women who enjoy discussing childbirth and child-rearing issues. The child-oriented festivals like Simhat Torah, Hanukah, Purim, and Passover make it painful for the infertile couple to participate, which leads to an increasing sense of isolation. One couple expressed their pain humorously: "We have no difficulty with the Jewish holidays—we just pack up and go to Florida!"

Other rituals present their own dilemmas. Among Ashkenazic Jews, a childless couple is frequently chosen to carry an infant to be circumcised at a *brit milah*. It is traditionally believed that the couple will merit children by virtue of their participation in this mitzvah. While some couples feel honored and privileged to be involved in the ritual, others may feel awkward and uncomfortable at being singled out so publicly. Couples should realize that they do not have to accept every invitation to, or honor at, social or religious events if doing so is painful for them. Alternatively, they may agree beforehand to attend but then leave as soon as it becomes too difficult for either one to handle. Couples might agree on a prearranged signal—a wink or gesture—and a prearranged excuse for leaving. Couples can also role-play with each other or prepare ways of responding to anticipated questions and comments about their situation. When a couple chooses to decline an invitation, it is important for them and their family to understand that this is a healthy choice; they are not "leaving" the family but just stepping back for a while. Families can help by accepting those decisions in a gracious way, recognizing the couple's need for "psychological space" and allowing them to preserve their dignity and self-respect.

In observant communities, where couples conceive soon after marriage, infertile couples soon become out of step with their peers. Close friends with whom they may have shared life-stage tasks and issues are now moving on and are consumed with discussions of a *brit*, diapers, child care, schools, and the like. Infertile couples find they have less and less in common with their friends. The turmoil of emotions they experience in social settings, such as embarrassment coupled with jealousy and resentment, may lead them to withdraw inward. The combination of having and sharing fewer common experiences, along with the difficult emotions evoked, places a strain on the continuity of meaningful relationships. Yet it is vital to avoid isolation and to receive appropriate social support. This does not mean having to share all the details of one's experience. Infertile couples have a hard enough time making sense and sorting through the issues they confront. However, people outside the experience can be more supportive as they become more aware, educated, and sensitized to these issues. It is helpful to choose a close friend who has shown sensitivity in the past and to educate this confidante. Let them know that rather than offering advice, listening is often the best they can do. Simply listening may seem like insufficient help, but a sensitive friend who can empathize is providing priceless support.

Interventions and Summary

As described above, infertility is an all-consuming crisis that pervades and disrupts multiple aspects of one's life. It is critical for infertile couples to develop coping skills and support systems to help deal with issues concerning themselves, their marriages, and their relationships with family, friends, and community.

It is easy to become absorbed by the emotional and medical aspects of infertility. Couples must actively develop and nurture other real and potential aspects of themselves and their relationships. Carving out time alone and with one another to pursue rewarding activities that have nothing to do with infertility provides a welcome and necessary safe haven. These "vacations" can vary from taking a weekend away to spending a half hour a day pursuing a relaxing activity. In addition, it is also important to remain mindful of small moments and experiences. For example, no matter how stressed one is by ongoing events, one may still appreciate the colors and scents of a spring day, cutting a beautiful vegetable salad, or the squeeze of a hand by an understanding friend. This helps promote living in the moment and a sense of gratitude.

Reaching out and connecting to others is probably the most significant action that the infertile couple can take to help themselves cope in more positive and productive ways. This includes connecting to family, friends, and other infertile couples. Specifically, connecting with others going through the infertility experience helps one feel strengthened and less alone. Connecting with the infertile community can be done in a number of ways, such as talking on an anonymous hotline with a volunteer or joining a peer group or support group and sharing the experience with others. Contrary to the popular conception, well-run support groups do not suggest that people sit around encouraging one another to drown in self-pity. Rather, they offer an opportunity for people to share their feelings and experiences, to learn from one another's coping skills, and to find strength. Support groups also provide the unique chance to offer strength to others. The goal is that people move forward in their lives in a more positive and productive way.

For those who need an extra boost to help them get through a rough period, individual or marital counseling with someone expert in this area can make a critical difference. These options are available through patient advocacy organizations. RESOLVE, Inc. and the American Fertility Association are non-profit, secular organizations that dispense medical information and support for couples with infertility. These self-help organizations provide information about the latest medical techniques as well as listings of qualified fertility specialists. ATIME (A Torah Infertility Medium of Exchange) is a non-profit organization founded for the specific purpose of providing information and support to infertile Jewish couples worldwide. Networking allows one to be more in control of one's self, one's situation, and one's medical treatment. Being more knowledgeable about treatments and treatment options allows couples to be more assertive with their physicians and to be able to pursue their treatments in a more proactive manner.

Infertility treatment can go on for years. It is important for couples to reevaluate their situation, not in order to forget their goal of becoming parents, but so that they can reserve their energy to pursue other credible options in parenting. Signs that will help a couple know that it is time to engage in this evaluation include: pursuing techniques over and over again despite low odds of a resulting successful pregnancy; ingesting large amounts of medication and ignoring potential side effects; depleting financial resources; and/or depleting emotional resources. It is not an easy decision to stop infertility treatments, especially in the light of tempting newly emerging high-technology treatments which seem to offer that one last hope. In reality, for many, these treatments offer low odds and are expensive and time consuming.

To posit that one must emotionally resolve one's infertility before pursuing other options would be erroneous. Resolving the emotional aspects of infertility is a life-long process that even the success of having biological children does not erase. Therefore, one can begin to explore other options even before one is ready to pursue them. This is especially true for couples who find that they are at different stages in looking at options. For many, foster-care, adoption, or volunteering with children is part of the resolution process. Couples can attend pre-adoption workshops even before they make a commitment. Some people pursue medical treatment following adoption with renewed energy; others feel ready to leave the treatments behind them. Couples can derive strength from looking at other families and learning how they have coped with infertility and how they have overcome their obstacles.

Judaism holds that events are not accidental or random. It becomes the challenge of those confronted with adversity to use these experiences as a catalyst for positive and meaningful development as a Jew. The Talmud explains that the patriarchs' and matriarchs' infertility was due to God's desire to bring them closer to Him. The struggles and suffering of infertility can lead to growth in one's self, one's marriage and one's sensitivity to others. It is up to the individual to translate this growth into an increased awareness and involvement in mitzvot. This is both on a personal level (between man and God) and an interpersonal level—reaching out to others in need (between man and man). It is in this way of viewing life events that we bring increased meaning and inspiration to our lives.

Endnotes

1. B.E. Menning. *Infertility: A Guide for the Childless Couple* (New York: Prentice Hall Press, 1988).

Allen Schwartz

A Rabbinic Response to Infertility

Procreation is the way a person acts in partnership with God to actually imitate His creation of man. It is the first commandment of the Torah, and, as the author of *Sefer Hahinukh* explains, "This is a great commandment by whose reason and means all other commandments are established." Yet some people are unable to become parents. How does Judaism teach such people to come to terms with their infertility? Is infertility God's will? If God commanded the human race to procreate, why does He make it impossible for some people?

Of course, this is a general question that religious people must face on a regular basis. God commands us to give charity, but suddenly our finances turn sour and we cannot fulfill God's will. Every fall, we prepare to fulfill God's will that we eat in a *sukkah*, and often He brings rain to frustrate our ability to fulfill this mitzvah. Somehow, we believe that the financial turn and the bad weather are part of God's plan for us and the world in which we live. We believe that only God knows why each event must take place and, in the course of life, we understand that fulfilling God's will takes a back seat to being part of God's plan.

God's will is that each and every human being be fruitful and multiply. Yet, in the scheme of God's plan there may be an external design in which a person's inability to procreate will produce something positive, such as bringing an adopted child into one's family, teaching others about sensitivity to the human condition, or being inspired to write these feelings for the public. This is the essence of Nahum Ish Gamzu's Talmudic dictum, "*Gam zu l'tova* (this too is for good)." Nahum, when faced with impending death, did not say "*Gam zu tova* (this too is good)," because death is not good. He said, rather, this too is *for* good, meaning, I feel confident that this event will have some positive outcome. One need not deny the negative aspect of a situation in order to see that it may have a positive result.

An infertile person must not see his or her condition as a punishment from God. We understand the Talmud's exhortation to "analyze ones deeds to determine the cause for suffering" to mean that one should analyze what one may learn from suffering. How can one improve his or her own life as well as the lives of others based on adverse circumstances? How can one get close to his or her spouse through this? When the rabbis of the Talmud and Midrash noted the infertility of the patriarchs and matriarchs, they explained that God wanted to elicit the prayers of the righteous, not that their suffering was due to some sin on their part. One thing is clear: One may not explain the suffering of another; to do so is to violate the Torah prohibition of verbal oppression. If a person suffers from tragedy or illness, no one may presume to attribute the suffering to sins. It is not for humans to undertake a direct correlation between someone's behavior and God's actions.

Let us return to the analogy of the *sukkah*. The Talmud relates that at the end of days, when the nations of the world ask for a mitzvah, God will grant them the mitzvah of *sukkah*. While sitting in their *sukkah*, the sun will beat down on them so strongly that they will be forced to leave. Upon leaving, they will knock down the *sukkah*. This aggression can be seen as anger over being unable to perform the mitzvah. The Talmud reflects that though they are halakhally justified in leaving the *sukkah*, they are wrong for expressing their anger thus and thereby forfeit their ability to perform the commandment again. One can draw a message from this story: If one is really interested in fulfilling God's will, one cannot be angry when God's plan interferes with one's ability to do so. Otherwise, we frustrate our ability to fulfill His will in the future.

In modern times, many options are open to couples with infertility that were not available to previous generations. The patriarchs and matriarchs had prayer and were successful at it. Today, medical advances can combine with prayer to serve as a powerful solution. The question we must answer is the extent of our *obligation* to do so. In other words, is an infertile couple halakhically *required* to seek medical help in assisting conception, or can they content themselves with prayer, as their forefathers did?

This question can perhaps also be approached through the same analogy of the *sukkah*. The Mishnah compares raining on the *sukkah* to a master pouring wine on his servant's face after the servant poured it for him. If the servant pours an additional cup, would not the master be incensed? In our situation, if God prevented a person from procreating—if it is part of God's plan that some *not* have children—who is that person to thwart God's plan? But the point is that we do not know God's plan. Perhaps the plan is that one should work *harder* to parent a child for a reason only God knows. When we *can* help ourselves, we ought to. In the case of rain in the *sukkah*, perhaps we can suggest that if there were some way for us to alter the rain on Sukkot, we also ought to. However, there is no reason to say that we would *have to* do so. Procreation is a positive commandment, and positive commandments must be observed only to the point of dispensing with up to 20% of one's assets. Putting oneself in harm's way would certainly be considered to be beyond a 20% dispensation of assets. However, if one wants to do so, one certainly may.

The fact that the Jewish community is family-centered can add to the emotional difficulties of the infertile couple. Rabbis are bound to deliver one or two sermons a year about the centrality of children in the synagogue and the community. Friends and family are bound to needle couples who remain childless after three or four years of marriage.

Talmudic and Midrashic sources refer directly to the relationship between the barren Hannah and her husband Elkanah's second wife Penina, who had children. Penina made Hannah's life miserable, taunting her that the Lord had closed her womb. Some rabbinic sources maintain that Penina had good intentions and only meant to push Hannah to action. Whatever the intentions, one source indicates that Penina would dress and wash her children and parade them before Hannah. She would take them to school and feed them in front of Hannah and gloat over her bounty. The Rabbis considered Penina's behavior so reprehensible as to warrant the death of all her own children. Indeed, a remarkable passage from *Sefer Hasidim* forbids parents from hugging and kissing their children in public, as one must be sensitive to both childless adults who might see this and long further for the child that they do not have to hug and kiss, and orphaned children, who would long for a parent to hug and kiss them.

The stories of the barrenness of the matriarchs teach that such circumstances can serve to increase love and sensitivity between husband and wife. The sensitivity is best expressed by Elkanah to his barren wife Hannah, when he told her, "Why are you crying, why won't you eat and why is you heart bitter? Am I not better for you than ten sons?" Perhaps Elkanah meant that he could not love Hannah more even if she had borne him ten sons. A couple's inability to have children can cause them to intensify their love for each other and to consider, if not giving life to an unborn child, then giving hope to a newborn child through adoption.

In his classic work, *The Kuzari*, Rabbi Yehuda HaLevi explains why God appears in the Decalogue as the "God who took you out of Egypt" and not the "God who created heaven and earth." While creation is a much greater event cosmologically, he says, the redemption from Egypt is more meaningful in our relationship. Creation implies a relationship between God and man; redemption proves that the relationship continues and intensifies.

If we can compare this to the process of adoption, the ones who raise the child are considered the redeemers and are on a higher level in the relationship than the creators. Rabbinic literature is replete with sources indicating that supporting or teaching a child is tantamount to actually parenting that child.

Midrash Devarim Rabbah refers to a man who has no garment yet makes *tzitzit* (ritual fringes) for others; one who has no house yet makes mezuzot for others; one who has no children yet teaches Torah to the children of others. These people will be rewarded, the Midrash says, as if they did the mitzvah themselves. An analysis of this Midrash leads to a startling conclusion. The Midrash refers to a man who cannot fulfill the mitzvot of *tzitzit* and mezuza yet helps others to do so. He also cannot fulfill the obligation of procreating, and yet teaches the children of others Torah! To be consistent, the Midrash should have had him somehow assisting in the process of birth as a doctor or supporter. This source teaches once again that the teaching of Torah to children is in some way a fulfillment of *peru u'revu* (be fruitful and multiply): "Whoever teaches his friend's son Torah *acquires him as a natural child*" (Sanhedrin 19b).

In his concluding Messianic prophecies, Isaiah addresses the strangers and childless, and teaches a powerful message on this topic.

> Thus said the Lord: And let not the eunuch say, "I am a withered tree." For thus said the Lord: As regards the eunuchs who keep My Sabbaths, who have chosen what I desire and hold fast to My covenant—I will give them, in My House and within My walls, a monument and a name, a *yad vashem*, better than sons and daughters. I will give them an everlasting name that shall not perish.

The childless, Isaiah says, will be given a *yad vashem*, a memorial better than sons and daughters, if they seek justice and specifically observe the Sabbath. The observance of the Sabbath is testimony to God's creation of the world and man. When the Jew observes the Sabbath, he or she is a partner in that creation. Every birth is a creation, but birth is not the only way we can be party to that first moment of this history of the universe. The observance of Sabbath, the teaching of Torah and the support of a child make one a party to creation as well. Once one can come to grips with one's destiny, one can derive and produce the joy and satisfaction that is available to all human beings. One can learn how to intensify the love of one's spouse. One can learn about a whole range of issues that may be plaguing others. And finally, one can come to grips with seeing how one fits in with God's plan, for nothing can change that, and it is always *l'tova*, for the good.

Rabbi Joseph B. Soloveitchik ל"זי

On Adoption

(*Editor's note: Despite the wonderful blessings brought by the assisted reproductive technologies, many couples find that their only possibility for parenthood involves raising children who are not their genetic offspring. It is valuable, therefore, to keep in mind the following thoughts on adoption by Rabbi Joseph B. Soloveitchik, excerpted from his* Family Redeemed: Essays on Family Relationships.[1])

Man's involvement with God is only realizable if he is ready to commit his offspring to God by imbuing them with Torah knowledge and Torah ideals. Maimonides writes "It is the duty of the father to teach his young son Torah as it is said: 'And ye shall teach them to your children to speak of them' (Deut. 6:7)…Just as it is a man's duty to teach his son, so it his duty to teach his grandson, as it is said: 'Make them known unto thy children and children's children' (Deuteronomy 4:9)." (*Mishneh Torah,* Hilkhot Talmud Torah [Laws of Torah Study] 1:1–2).

In the Aggadah, God Himself appears in the role of teacher. Every day God spends time instructing young children. Physical creation, sustenance of Being as such, are not enough. When one helps children find themselves by taking hold of their inherent aptitudes and acquainting them with the eternal verities which give man a sense of rootedness—only then is the creative gesture of God completed. Father and mother are not only a procreative natural community, but a creative teaching fellowship whose importance can hardly be overstressed and exaggerated.

At this point we may parenthetically mention the problem of the childless couple. Since existential completeness is possible only in a community of three personae—I, thou, and he—the married couple who was not blessed with a child never rids itself of the loneliness experience which is characteristic of a shattered and imperfect existence.

The answer to this problem is quite simple in light of what was said about the educational community which the parents and child form. Procreation is not creation. The latter is realized not in the fertilization of an ovum but in the formation of the child's spiritual personality, in fostering his or her good qualities and trying to sublimate the child's primitive desires and smooth out his rough edges. This can be accomplished not only by natural parents but by a couple to whom the happiness of natural childbirth was denied. They can become teachers and educators of children and by so doing fulfill their mission and find existential fulfillment in a creative act of education.

Judaism has advanced a new doctrine of teaching. Education is not just a technical activity. It is a soul-performance, an existential involvement of two strangers, an imparting not only of formal knowledge but of a total self-experience, of an ontic awareness. It expresses itself in the emergence of a new fellowship, within which master and disciple share one great adventure, that of creation. Therefore, the union of teacher and disciple does not terminate with the end of actual instruction. The community outlasts the physical nearness of these two individuals; it contains something of the covenantal community. The ideal of the rabbi is shining in the Jewish firmament. It outranks every other image, that of king, priest, and prophet. The role of the high priest was defined by Malakhi as consisting not of cultic but of educational duties: "The law of truth was in his mouth and iniquity was not found in his lips; he walked with me in peace and equity and did turn many away from iniquity. For the priest's lips should keep knowledge, and they should seek the law at his mouth for he is the messenger of the Lord of Hosts" (Malakhi 2:6). King David was depicted by the Aggadah as a scholar, devoting his time to the study of the law and the dissemination of knowledge. The prophets found their place among the *hakhmei haMasorah*, the sages of the transmission. "Moses received the Torah at Sinai and transmitted it…to the Elders who transmitted it to the Prophets" (*Avot* [Ethics of the Fathers] 1:1).

There is love for and identification with each other in this community of knowledge. Socrates spoke of the teacher as a midwife who merely helps the child to rediscover himself. This metaphor is in agreement with the Socratic-Platonic viewpoint that all learning is recollection (*anamnesis*), a reawakening of something which is dormant in the pupil. The teacher does not give anything of himself. All he does is bring out whatever the pupil possesses. The task of the teacher is not a creative one, and there is no intimate drawing toward each other involved in teaching. The existential embrace within which pupil and teacher find themselves ontically happy and enjoying a full life is missing in the Platonic philosophy. Judaism saw the teacher as the creator through love and commitment of the personality of the pupil. Both become *personae* because an I-Thou community is formed. That is why Judaism called disciples sons and masters fathers. As Maimonides writes:

> This obligation [of teaching Torah] is to be fulfilled not only toward one's son and grandson. A duty rests on every scholar in Israel to teach all disciples, even if they are not his children, as it is said, 'and you shall teach them to your children' (Deuteronomy. 6:7). The oral tradition teaches: "Your children" includes your disciples, for disciples are called children as it is said: "And the sons of the prophets came forth" (II Kings 2:3).
>
> *Mishneh Torah*, Hilkhot Talmud Torah 1:2

Our Talmudic sages stated, "Whoever teaches his friend's son Torah acquires him as a natural child" (Sanhedrin 19b). When the letter *hei* was added to Abram's name, he became Abraham, the father of many nations, the spiritual father of all he taught. Natural procreative Abramic parenthood was denied to the childless couple, yet the creative Abrahamic parenthood is a challenge which everyone is summoned to meet.

Judaism did not recognize the Roman institution of adoption since the Roman concept is directed toward substituting a legal fiction for a biological fact and thus creating the illusion of a natural relationship between the foster parents and the adopted son. Judaism stated its case in no uncertain terms: what the Creator granted one and the other should not be interfered with; the natural relationship must not be altered. Any intervention on the part of some legal authority would amount to interference with the omniscience and original plan of the Maker. The childless mother and father must reconcile themselves with the fact of natural barrenness and sterility. Yet they may attain the full covenantal experience of parenthood, exercise the fundamental right to have a child and be united within a community of I-thou-he.

There is no need to withhold from the adopted child information concerning his or her natural parents. The new form of parenthood does not conflict with the biological relation. It manifests itself in a new dimension which may be separated from the natural one. In order to become Abraham, one does not necessarily have to live through the stage of Abram. The irrevocable in human existence is not the natural but the spiritual child; the threefold community is based upon existential, not biological, unity. The existence of I and thou can be inseparably bound with a third existence even though the latter is, biologically speaking, a stranger to them.

Endnote

1.   David Shatz, Joel B. Wolowelsky, eds., *MeOtsar HoRav*, (New York: Ktav, 2001).

Part III

Diagnostic Evaluation of the Infertile Couple

Introduction

Infertility is never a problem that is solely male or solely female. It affects a couple, together, profoundly. Inevitably, however, medical techniques identify the physical source of infertility as residing in one or both of the partners. When the male is involved, special problems arise that pose formidable halakhic challenges.

Within the framework of halakha, it is the man and not the woman who bears the special commandment to "be fruitful and multiply."[1] The Talmud, in *Yevamot* 65b, explains that the biblical verse ties the obligation to "be fruitful and multiply" with the obligation to "fill the earth and conquer it." As "conquest" is intrinsically tied to warfare, which is taken to be a characteristic of men, the Talmud concludes that it is only men who are obligated to fulfill the commandment. Why women are exempt is a matter of conjecture. It is possible, on the one hand, that the Torah viewed motherhood as so natural a tendency in women that a specific commandment was not necessary. On the other hand, it is noted that in the past, the very act of pregnancy could be a life-threatening experience, and perhaps the Torah did not wish to obligate an action that would put one's life in danger. In any event, the commandment to the man does not imply free reign to spread his seed. On the contrary, the halakhic requirement for a man to reproduce comes with an accompanying set of halakhic restrictions on sexual activity that is elaborate in detail. In general, these guidelines serve to strengthen the bonds between husband and wife and to ensure the continuity of the Jewish people. Unfortunately, in situations where the cause of infertility resides in the male, those same guidelines may frustrate all attempts at proper diagnosis and treatment.

As a rule, men do not respond as well as women to the need for diagnostic testing, especially physical examinations. Even today, when the value of preventive care is widely accepted, men are more reluctant than women to have annual physical exams. The idea of establishing contact with a physician may be a strange and threatening one, and few regard it as a purely clinical, emotionally neutral exercise. This fear and anxiety which many men feel is understandably compounded for the halakhically committed man. He may perceive that, should he be found infertile, the solution to his problem will require him to tread on thin halakhic ice.

These considerations, together with some legitimate halakhic concerns, lead many Orthodox couples to delay the evaluation of the husband entirely until every imaginable test has been performed on the wife. Inevitably, for some couples this only delays proper diagnosis. Still when a male factor is suspected of impeding fertility, it must be properly evaluated.

As a practical matter, investigating the cause of infertility gen-erally begins with the woman. Here, the halakhically problematic issues mainly concern timing; issues that often require rabbinical input involve the appropriate time to initiate the evaluation and also how to perform testing to interfere as little as possible with *taharat hamishpa'ha.*

The following chapters will explore the basic principles that govern the evaluation of reproductive failure in both the male and female. Rabbi Weiss addresses the halakhic issues pertinent to the work-up of the female. Because most issues in this regard involve the problem of the *niddah* status of the woman, he precedes his discussion with an outline of the basic principles of *niddah.* Dr.

Jakobovits outlines the halakhic issues pertinent to the diagnosis of male factor problems. Modern testing of the male is centered mainly around the examination of sperm. It is likely that future tests will also concentrate on methods, albeit more reliable ones, of sperm evaluation. Therefore, the bulk of this chapter is devoted to the issue of the procurement of sperm for evaluation.

Before getting to the halakhic issues, it is essential to understand some basic elements about the infertile Jewish couple. Although generalizations are hard to stand by, all involved must understand the traditional Jewish approach to seeking medical care and the specific religious guidelines in which fertility treatments can be given. This section begins, therefore, with a general description of the setting in which fertility care is rendered. Following that, I present an introduction to the physiology of conception and a description of how practicing physicians currently approach the evaluation of infertility. With that as a foundation, we then explore those elements of the reproductive process where problems might occur and how to go about uncovering those problems. A discussion of the interventions aimed at solving those problems will follow in the next section.

Endnote

1. Yevamot 65b; *Mishneh Torah*, Hilkhot Ishut 15:2; *Shulhan Arukh*, Even HaEzer, 1:1.

Richard V. Grazi

The Couple, the Physician and the Rabbi: A Triumvirate Partnership

Before we delve into the intricacies of caring for traditional Jewish infertile couples, it is useful to understand the decision-making process that typically occurs behind the scenes of their care. This is because the couples involved differ, at least in some respects, from others who may request treatment for infertility. Surely, their situation is different from the outset in that they bring to the process a third party—their rabbi—who will eventually become an inextricable part of solving the problem. Although all involved are motivated to achieve the same ultimate outcome—a healthy pregnancy—their immediate agendas may be different.

The Couple

In a certain sense, it is not proper to speak of a couple as a unified entity, for no matter how aligned a husband and wife may be in their desire for a child, infertility affects each of them differently. To a certain extent, this is because infertility affects every individual differently. But on a broader level there is a difference between how men and women each react to the appearance of a fertility problem in their marital life. Although there are no rules that govern these differences, years of caring for couples bring to the fore certain generalities. For example, one partner almost always leads the quest for medical therapy. Whether this is the husband or wife depends on the particular dynamic of the couple. Rarely will both participate at the same level. Instead, one is usually the "designated driver," researching the problem, finding the physician, scheduling the appointments, arranging the necessary post-visit feedback, and making sure that adequate records are kept. Who assumes this responsibility may be a practical matter, assumed by the partner who has the most time for it, or a matter of personality, assumed by the partner with the more aggressive, and usually more organized, personality type. However, often the cause of designation is more amorphous, and it is impossible to define why a particular partner has shouldered the bulk of the responsibility.

THE WOMAN

Women are more commonly the designated drivers of the infertility management process. This is almost never a reflection of their having more time to engage in the work that the process demands. In modern Jewish households, women are just as likely as their husbands are to be engaged in paid work outside the home, especially where there are no children. If not professionally engaged, they may be equally busy with community works of *hesed*, volunteering their time for charitable causes. In many traditional and *haredi* households, the young wife is often the main breadwinner, her husband spending the bulk of his days and nights learning in yeshiva.

No formal studies have been done to discern why one partner

is chosen to lead the effort to solve infertility, or why the woman will more commonly take on this burden. However, it seems intuitive that women *feel* more directly affected by infertility, at least in its earliest stage, than men. Once the couple begins trying to conceive—often, but not always, just after marriage—it is she who has the monthly reminder that conception has not occurred. Orthodox women, in particular, are keenly attuned to their monthly cycle, as much of marital life—even outside the sexual relationship—is affected by her cycle and her *niddah* status. Over time, her physical perception of "failure" may motivate her to initiate the quest for a medical solution.

Women may also become aware much sooner than men that a fertility problem is likely. In the course of a healthy marital relationship, a man has no way of knowing that he has compromised fertility potential other than by trying to initiate a pregnancy and awaiting the result. A woman, however, may anticipate that she has a reproductive disorder on the basis of menstrual cycle abnormalities or other physical manifestations. It is not uncommon for women to raise this issue with their intended *shiddukh* even before they are married, so that the matter may be dealt with promptly. Men have no such telltale signs of infertility.

For halakhic reasons, the investigation of infertility almost always begins with the female. The Orthodox Jewish woman is aware that, no matter what the ultimate source of the fertility problem, the preliminary investigation is going to focus on her. Unless a significant male factor is discovered, it will ultimately be her physician who directs the care of the couple. Knowing this, she may be motivated to make the first decisions regarding which physician to consult and when that consultation will take place.

Women also have more resources at their immediate disposal than men. By the time that infertility is apparent, a woman will likely have already established a relationship with a gynecologist. She may have already expressed a concern about fertility at an annual check-up, and may feel comfortable scheduling an early revisit just to make sure that nothing obvious is awry. She is also more apt to have seen literature on the subject, either at her physician's office or in a women's magazine. In general, women are more open with each other than men about health issues. A woman who finds herself in an infertile marriage is more likely than her husband to know a friend or family member who has already been through this experience and from whom she can seek advice. Unfortunately, for cultural reasons, unsolicited advice will also more commonly be directed toward the childless wife than to the husband. These unpleasant comments may serve to further motivate her to seek professional help.

It is not uncommon, for all of these reasons, for a woman to arrive at her initial consultation alone but well-armed with information. She may already have researched general facts about infertility, fertility therapies that have been given to other women she knows, a presumptive self-diagnosis that she has made, and even the physician's practice. An educated patient is always easier to deal with than those who must be taught the basics. As such, her physician will usually welcome all such preliminary information. Nevertheless, it is important for even the most educated patient understand that no amount of research, on the internet or even in textbooks, will supercede the judgment of a highly trained and experienced caregiver.

THE MAN

In his best-selling thesis, *Men are from Mars, Women are from Venus*, Dr. John Gray explains the numerous ways in which men and women differ in their approach to life. Men are by nature more focused on direct problem-solving, and in that focused mode they often overlook the many and varied consequences of the problem itself. Thus, in the initial stages, they may experience infertility as a straightforward physical problem to be dealt with and not sense the overwhelming ramifications that it may have on their marital life. Other than when a sexual problem is perceived as the cause of infertility, a man may believe that the problem lies with his wife and feel comfortable ceding the leadership role to her.

But other issues may come to play. Men are physically more separated from their fertility potential. Other than sexual competence, they have no physical clues to alert them about any problem that may be brewing. While a man may be aware of his wife's monthly cycle, and keeping *taharat hamishpaha* may indeed rule his physical needs, he does not directly experience the same physical reminder. He is not focused on counting days, checking for bleeding, and figuring out when immersion in the *mikvah* will occur. In addition, he is less likely to have visited a physician for a general, routine examination, let alone a urological examination.

The possibility of needing to visit a physician to probe into the cause of infertility may be daunting to the Orthodox man. Sitting in the gynecologist's waiting room is not something that he has been prepared for. It is unlikely that he will have shared his anxiety with a friend or family member. He may see the interviews and examination of his wife as an invasion into their highly guarded privacy. He might be wary of the potential halakhic conflicts, which he may have learned about as part of his yeshiva studies. In *haredi* communities, boys often grow up without a comfortable working knowledge of the vernacular language. As grown men, the expectation that they will need to communicate effectively with a physician can be intimidating. Indeed, his level of education aside, this may be the man's first-ever need to have a meaningful conversation with someone who is not a co-religionist. Against this background, it is not surprising that men will often absent themselves, not only from the initial physician encounter, but also from all others until the time that an absolute need becomes evident or pregnancy is established.

Of course, these are generalizations, and specific couples differ in many ways. There are many circumstances when men practically drag their wives to the consultation, and spend a lot of energy keeping them focused on what needs to be done. Some men seem to be more aware of their wives' cycles than the wives themselves. And some women defer completely to their husbands when it comes to choosing a physician and arranging for all of the follow up. How this works for each couple is not necessarily dependent on who is diagnosed with the "problem." What is clear is that there is almost never an equal degree of awareness, motivation and activity among partners in the marriage. Sometimes, this can lead to resentment and a breakdown in the problem-solving process. What is useful to remember is that women and men are different creatures, not only physically but also psychologically.[1] It is virtually impossible for a man to completely feel what his wife is feeling, and to think what she is thinking, and vice versa. Effectively wading through the process of fertility diagnosis and treatment requires that they acknowledge this and respect their innate differences.

The Physician

It is not possible to practice as a reproductive specialist without being moved by the plight of couples who come to the consultation room, or rejoicing with them when one's well-designed practices have played a role in the miracle of their new child. Deep professional satisfaction results from properly understanding the science and changing rules of clinical practice. Personal satisfaction is also profound, a result of successfully applying with one's patients—who all too often are also neighbors and friends—the art of medicine. Yet with all of the wonderful moments, the actual day to day interaction with patients is an endless flow of clinical conundrums and distractions, side by side with a constant struggle to rein in patient anxieties.

Reproductive medicine is a field that continues to change at a feverish pace. Much of the training of the reproductive specialist—in the United States this is typically a seven-year process that begins after graduation from medical school—is designed to prepare him or her to respond to those changes in a careful and thoughtful way. While innovation is encouraged and welcomed, not all treatments that are touted as "new" or "better" are immediately incorporated into actual practice. Good medicine is grounded in scientific evidence and evolves over time. While certain achievements may seem newsworthy to a couple grappling with infertility, it does not make them relevant, applicable, or even desirable from the standpoint of clinical management. Physicians expend a lot of energy explaining why treatment X that has just worked for one patient in Rome may not be appropriate for all infertile women in Miami, or why treatment Y that was successful with Rachel is not relevant to the care of Leah. These discussions may be very frustrating when the couple has done exhaustive research into their new-found cure and is convinced that, by insisting on adhering to the "tried and true," the physician is denying them success.

At other times it may be the couple who is unwilling to undergo a change of direction in their clinical care. But new information may prompt the physician to make unanticipated recommendations. For example, couples with male factor infertility may be "fast tracked" to assisted conception. Medically, the clinician may see this as their shortest, least invasive and least expensive way to have a baby. He is focused on efficiency. The couple, on the other hand, may perceive this treatment plan as halakhically problematic. (They may be surprised to hear that, depending on their circumstances, this may not be so.) They might decide to instead focus on the male factor directly and to use hormonal therapy or surgery with the hope of improvement. Though it may take them another year or two to achieve the same percentage chance of pregnancy, such a course of action might be preferable to them. They are focused, foremost, in living as Torah Jews. Needless to say, these paradigms are not static. The same couple might make a different decision if it happened that a specific course of action offered a better chance.

There are, of course, other avenues of frustration that can develop during the treatment process. Astute clinicians are aware of the many psychological, logistical, and financial pressures that are brought to bear during treatment of all infertile couples. But specific problems that may arise during the treatment of Orthodox couples should be mentioned. First is the physician's perception that halakhic restraints conflict with his ability to help his patients meet their goal. For the secular Jewish or non-Jewish physician in particular, it may seem strange that a couple is heartbroken by their infertility, yet may refuse a straightforward solution on technical halakhic grounds. Second is the need to tailor diagnosis and treatment in ways that circumvent the usual pattern or chronology. In standard practice, semen analysis is done at the outset of diagnosis. In keeping with halakhic concerns, this is usually delayed. Medical protocols may also need redesigning in order to conform to the rules of *taharat hamishpa'ha*, and procedures may need to be advanced or delayed by the occurrence of the Sabbath. Sometimes these changes conflict with what the physician feels is medically prudent. At such times, trust between patient and physician is paramount.

It is important for all caregivers to understand that Orthodox couples function within a strict set of guidelines. Fertility therapy is almost never a matter of life or death. Any violation of the Sabbath that can be avoided must therefore be avoided, even if it might result in an unsuccessful treatment cycle. The rules of *niddah* are fairly clear. Even slight modification requires input from an authoritative halakhic source. For one unfamiliar with the demands of the halakhic process, the involvement of a third party in personal decisions seems strange. The rabbi may be perceived as intrusive or even inappropriate. But ultimately the couple depends on him for something even more important than resolving their infertility.

Of course, there are many physicians who have much more familiarity with halakha, either because they themselves are observant or because they work with large numbers of observant patients. They, especially, must be careful not to assume what the correct halakhic solution might be, or to extrapolate from the halakhic decision for one couple to the circumstances of another. The spectrum of opinions and approaches within the halakha varies widely. The halakhic decisions of rabbis may differ, and the same rabbi may give different decisions regarding the same clinical matter if, as he understands them, the circumstances of the couple differ.

Traditional Jewish couples who seek modern medical care see the abilities of their physicians as God-given. Physicians who practice with respect for this system of beliefs enable their patients to stay focused on the medical issues and overcome them. In so doing they also build the trust that underlies their success.

The Rabbi

The role of the rabbi is to teach and to counsel. The subjects about which he teaches and counsels go beyond the law and the spirit. It is not uncommon that the rabbi's role extends to the personal and psychological well-being of his congregants. In some communities he meets the physical needs as well, at times even prescribing medicine or folk-remedies (a practice that would be better avoided). In many cases, it is he who makes appropriate referrals to professionals. Some rabbis have a special interest in medicine and halakha; some are particularly well-versed in reproductive halakha.

When infertility is prolonged or resistant to easy solutions, there is no substitute for a rabbi who is willing to consult with the couple and their physician and to offer reasoned halakhic decisions. Occasionally, the couple may confront their *posek* with a situation or recommendation that sounds wrong to him, giving the impression that the couple is not getting sound medical advice. In such cases direct communication between the rabbi and the physician will clarify the issues. A sophisticated physician looks forward to the rabbi's call and will use that opportunity to make him conversant with the clinical picture and medical logic that are the bases for treatment.

The ethical standards of medicine demand that physicians closely guard the confidentiality of their patients. Couples are often so close to their rabbi that they ask his advice before they agree to any kind of medical care. They do not see conversations on their behalf by their doctor and rabbi as breaches of that confidentiality. Indeed, it is they who usually initiate such conversations. However, all involved must bear in mind that consent to discuss their care must be written or specifically implied. A physician may refuse to carry on a discussion when he or she believes that the patient does not countenance doing so.[2]

The effort on the part of the rabbinate to become familiar with halakhic dilemmas in reproductive care is a very positive recent development. In numerous communities there are rabbis who can speak authoritatively on these issues, many of whom are familiar with the specialists who care for their congregants, and have consulted with them before arriving at their *pesakei halakha* (halakhic verdicts). The views expressed in these verdicts are multifarious. For example, while all agree that the halakhic obligation to "be fruitful and multiply" does not include an obligation to undertake assisted conception, there is general agreement that, as a practical matter, the child relates to his genetic parents just as he would if he were conceived naturally. Some, however, oppose any artificial interruption of natural marital life. Others are willing to allow it for only one child. Others limit their objections to overcoming some of the technical halakhic problems.

For the committed Jewish couple there is a requirement to involve one's halakhic authority when difficult discussions arise. The Talmud tells us that three partners are involved in the creation of a child: mother, father, and God. Modern reproductive medicine has brought in the doctor as a fourth partner; God remains represented by His Torah authorities.

Endnotes

1. For interesting insights into this subject, see Deborah Blum, *Sex on the Brain,* (New York: Viking Press, 1997).
2. The Health Information Privacy and Portability Act, HIPPA, was enacted by the United States in April 2003. HIPPA governs all communications between physicians and outside parties about private medical matters. By law, all such communications now require a signed, HIPPA-compliant consent form.

Richard V. Grazi

The Physiology of Conception

The average person has a general understanding of "how babies are made." A somewhat more sophisticated knowledge of the reproductive process is necessary, however, for one wishing to appreciate the demands of fertility diagnosis and therapy on the couple and how they interface with halakhic concerns. While the language in the following short discussion is at times technical, the concepts are straightforward and easily absorbed.

Sperm

Sperm cells are produced in the testis and carry half the genetic information necessary for the creation of a new human being. (The other half is contained in the egg.) This tightly packaged genetic material, consisting mostly of DNA, is protected within the sperm head. The tail, in turn, endows the sperm with motion, or motility, which is necessary for its migration through the female genital

tract and final union with the egg. Sperm are unique in their ability to propel themselves. Unlike eggs, which are produced in the
ovary only during fetal life and never again, sperm are continually
produced in large numbers during the reproductive life of every
normal man.

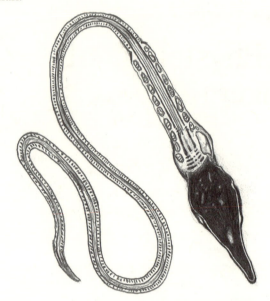

A sperm cell: A cross section of the sperm show three
distinct portions: the head, midpiece and tail

Once ejaculated into the vagina, the sperm must undergo
a long and complex journey before they are capable of fertilizing
an egg. Most die before they traverse the cervical canal, which is
the entrance to the womb. Of the relatively few that do manage to
survive, only a small number will actually be able to enter into the
fallopian tubes. Fewer still will swim successfully to the end of the
tube, where fertilization of the egg occurs. Even then, the journey is
incomplete. Once the egg is encountered, the sperm must disperse
the surrounding layers of cells, penetrate through the hardened
shell of the egg, pierce the egg membrane and, finally, fuse with
the genetic material contained in its nucleus. Because the process is
so complex and, to a certain extent, inefficient, it is necessary that

a critical number of normal sperm be present in the ejaculate to ensure that at least one will successfully fertilize the egg.

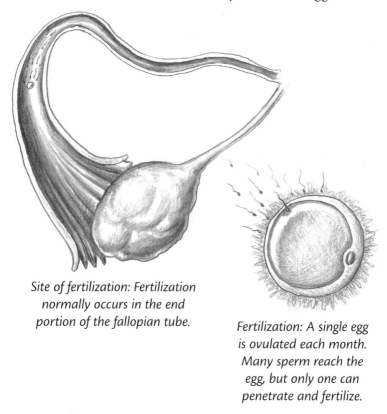

Site of fertilization: Fertilization normally occurs in the end portion of the fallopian tube.

Fertilization: A single egg is ovulated each month. Many sperm reach the egg, but only one can penetrate and fertilize.

Cervical Mucus

Most women, upon arising after intercourse during which male orgasm and ejaculation has taken place, sense that the seminal fluid "falls out." This is normal and cannot be considered a cause of infertility. Seminal fluid, the liquid medium in which the sperm are delivered to the female, is always discharged after intercourse. What is more, during most of the menstrual cycle, which averages 28 days in reproductive-age women, the sperm within the semen is discharged as well. There is only one interval during the cycle when this expulsion does not occur. At or near the time of ovulation, the mature egg sends a signal to the cervix (in the form of the hormone estrogen), stimulating it to produce copious amounts of a watery substance called cervical mucus. This mucus acts as a reservoir for motile sperm, which penetrate into it upon contact. It can harbor live sperm for up to 72 hours. Thus, during the fertile period leading up to ovulation, even though the semen is expelled, healthy sperm are retained within a woman's genital tract. In fact, many women can determine their "fertile time" by the appearance of this watery mucus discharge. It is a reliable sign that a fully ripened egg is about to be released.[1]

Several conditions may render the cervical environment hostile to sperm. These include infections, antibody production and inadequate mucus production, whether due to previous surgery or to abnormal hormonal stimulation. In these cases, the cervix may act as a physical barrier to the progression of sperm through the reproductive tract. The impact of fertility treatments on cervical

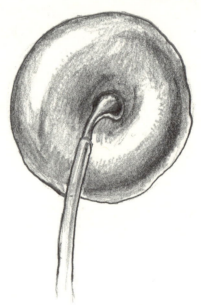

Cervical mucus: The cervix is easily visualized during a speculum exam. Cervical mucus can be aspirated and examined for the presence of sperm.

mucus production is discussed in "Halakhic Considerations in the Treatment of Female Infertility."

Fallopian Tubes

After the sperm traverse the cervix, they are propelled upward through the uterine cavity and the fallopian tubes toward the ovary. But it is not enough for the tubes to simply be open; they are not merely conduits for sperm and eggs. In fact, they participate in the reproductive process in ways which, when disrupted, are difficult to overcome.

The inner channel of the fallopian tube is lined by cilia, hair-like structures that help propel the sperm toward the far end of the tube, where the egg is fertilized. Somewhat paradoxically, and in ways that are not completely understood, these same cilia propel the egg in the opposite direction, from the ovary toward the uterus. Using fimbriae, small, finger-like projections at its very end, the tube sweeps over the ovary and captures it within its inner lining. If motile sperm are present in this area, the egg may be fertilized. However, for a normal pregnancy to be initiated, the tubal muscle must undergo rhythmic contractions which, in concert with the

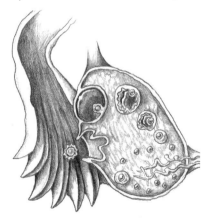

Fallopian tube: As the egg emerges from its
follicle, it is captured by the tube

motion of the cilia, bring the fertilized egg to the uterus, where it may implant. This process takes approximately three days, during which time the tubal secretions must be sufficient to maintain the enormous nutritional and energy requirements of the rapidly dividing embryo.

Unfortunately, the very specialized functions of the fallopian tubes are exquisitely sensitive to even the smallest degrees of damage, in particular by infection. When blockage occurs in both tubes, this results in sterility. It is important to understand that, although a variety of surgical procedures may be used to open blocked tubes, any underlying damage to the propulsive and nutritional functions of the tube may result in permanent infertility or, in some cases, tubal pregnancy. In the latter case, the fertilized embryo actually implants within the tubal wall. As the tube cannot accommodate a growing fetus, however, the situation poses a potentially grave hazard to the woman and necessitates the removal of the pregnancy by either chemical or surgical means.

Ovulation

There are certain fundamental differences between egg and sperm production. Unlike sperm, which are continuously produced in vast numbers, the human ovary generally produces only one mature egg during each fertile cycle. Also, eggs have no innate propulsion system. As they are released through the ovarian capsule, they rely on the fallopian tube to transport them to proximity with sperm. Finally, egg production, in contrast to sperm production, is a non-renewable process. The human female is born with all the eggs she will ever have (and 99% of them die before they even have a chance to be fertilized). Ovulation is the process by which an egg that has lain dormant—sometimes for three or four decades!—is activated, matured, and released from the ovary.

Normal ovulation depends on a complex interplay between the developing egg and centers in the brain called the hypothalamus and pituitary gland. The pituitary gland is responsible for the release of two hormones (follicle stimulating hormone, or FSH, and luteinizing hormone, or LH) that stimulate the growth, maturation and

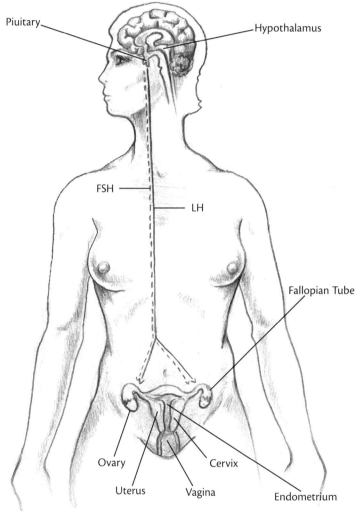

Ovulation: Hormones secreted from the pituitary gland control the ovarian cycle

release of the eggs within the ovary. The hypothalamus plays a role by releasing a hormone (gonadotropin releasing hormone, or GnRH) which is necessary for normal pituitary functioning. The developing egg, mainly through its release of estrogen, interacts with the hypothalamus and pituitary in ways that control its own development and that ensure that one egg is ovulated each month.

Following ovulation, the supporting cells of the egg that are left behind in the ovary become the corpus luteum (sometimes called the "ovulation cyst") and produce progesterone. Progesterone prepares the uterine lining for implantation of the fertilized egg. In the absence of pregnancy, the corpus luteum has a defined lifespan of fourteen days. As it dies, hormonal production wanes and uterine bleeding follows. During this menstrual period, another egg is recruited for the following ovulation, a process that takes approximately 14 days. It is this continual replenishment of mature eggs and limited functioning of the corpus luteum that is responsible for the 28-day, cyclic menstrual pattern of most women.

Because cyclic bleeding is the end result of a process that depends on the proper integration of so many hormonal signals, it is a phenomenon that can be disrupted at numerous points. Excessive physical stress, anxiety, malnutrition, and obesity are among the more common conditions that can prevent ovulation and, therefore, cyclic menstruation. "Fertility drugs" are all designed to manipulate the hypothalamus, pituitary, or ovaries and thereby stimulate ovulation.

Uterus

The goal of all reproductive processes is to produce a healthy, growing fetus within the uterus, or womb. Although anatomical obstructions within the uterus may occur, the more common problems relate to the uterine lining itself. This lining sheds and regenerates itself each month under the influence of hormonal stimuli from the ovary and its developing egg. Any disturbances in egg recruitment, development, ovulation, corpus luteum formation, or hormonal secretion will translate into a disordered development of the uterine lining. In such situations, if a fertilized embryo were to enter the uterine cavity, it would likely not implant. Even if implantation were to occur, the embryo would not properly develop. Thus, a disordered uterine lining is commonly associated with infertility or repeated miscarriages. It is worth noting, however, that this usually reflects a problem elsewhere in the hormonal system, and not primarily with the uterus itself.

Other Factors

Listed above are only the main events in human reproduction: (A) Sperm need to be ejaculated into the vagina; (B) They need to penetrate into the cervical mucus and (C) they must find an open passageway to the egg. (D) In addition, an egg must be released from the ovary and, after fertilization, (E) it must be able to grow within a normal uterine environment. While these are all neces-

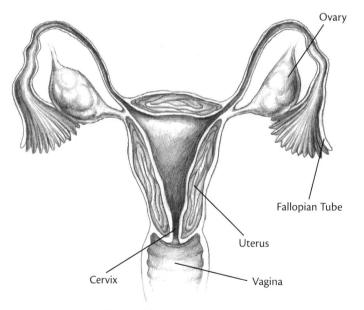

Normal female anatomy

sary for conception, clearly they are not in themselves sufficient. Indeed, reproductive science is constantly shedding new light on the complexity of these processes. As our knowledge of genetics, immunology and molecular biology continues to increase, our sophistication with respect to reproductive physiology and the correction of infertility will also grow.

Endnotes

1. Pregnancy may occur with intercourse occurring as many as six days prior to ovulation, indicating that cervical mucus may begin to appear even longer than seventy-two hours prior to ovulation. However, the chances of pregnancy increase as intercourse approaches the day of ovulation. See A.J. Wilcox, C.R. Weinberg, D.D. Baird, "Timing of sexual intercourse in relation to ovulation—effects on the probability of conception, survival of the pregnancy, and sex of the baby," *New England Journal of Medicine*, 333:1517–21, (1995).

Richard V. Grazi

General Aspects of Female Infertility

Defining Infertility

Infertility affects approximately 1 in 6 couples during some part of their reproductive lifetime.[1] A couple is infertile if they have failed to conceive after having unprotected intercourse for more than 12 months. This 12-month standard is based on the statistical probability of pregnancy occurring in a couple with *normal* fertility. On average, couples with normal fertility will take six months to conceive. This means that an equal percentage of couples takes more than six months as takes less. Although it may seem to infertile couples that pregnancy occurs almost at whim for everyone else, this is not the case. Some couples do in fact conceive the very first month they try, but an approximately equal number do not conceive until the twelfth month of trying.

     To help understand the cumulative chances of pregnancy, it is sometimes helpful to think in terms of 100 couples with normal fertility. If all 100 begin trying to conceive on the same month, 50 will be pregnant after six months. After nine months, 85 will be pregnant; after twelve months, 95 will be pregnant. It is worth noting that the last five couples will not conceive until well into the second year of trying despite their having normal fertility. Nevertheless, because 95% of normal couples conceive within the first twelve months, this is used as the medical defining point for couples with infertility. Putting that same statistic a little differently: if a couple has not conceived after twelve months, there is only a 5% chance that they can expect a pregnancy to occur naturally. The chance that such a couple is truly infertile is, on the other hand, 95%.

Cumulative pregnancy rates are best viewed visually on a "life table." Researchers in the field of infertility commonly use such tables to measure the effect of a given therapy. An example is shown in the figure below, which depicts monthly pregnancy rates in women treated for endometriosis.[2]

Life Table: Conception rates are shown as a function of time

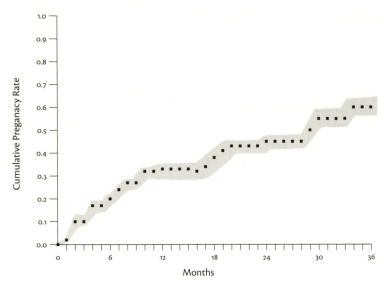

Graphic representation of a table based on the conception rate of 88 women undergoing conservative surgery for endometriosis-associated infertility. The shaded area indicates variance at each time point.

Couples undergoing medical intervention for infertility should absorb the significance of such statistics. They remind us that, even under normal circumstances, human reproduction is a highly inefficient process. For most couples, repeated exposure is required for conception to occur. This means that even in the case where the source of infertility is clearly defined, correction of the problem cannot be expected to result in instant success. Success rates after the surgical correction of fertility disorders are typically reported for intervals of one to two *years* following surgery.

As with natural conception, all fertility interventions that are targeted to a specific reproductive cycle have a success rate that is cumulative with time. No particular intervention can ever reliably produce a pregnancy on the first time, every time. This is the reason why physicians will often tell couples to repeat a treatment cycle that has failed. For many couples and many different types of treatment, the statistical likelihood of success is not diminished until three failures have occurred. Pregnancies can still occur even on the fourth or fifth try of the same therapy.

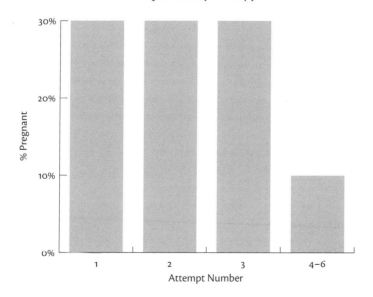

Successful Fertility Therapy

Realistically speaking, most couples begin to feel some anxiety after one failed treatment cycle; after two, the disappointment is even greater and anxiety is heightened; after three, most are convinced that there is no further chance of success. Although this is technically incorrect, most medical intervention protocols call for the changing of therapy after three successive failures.

It is often difficult for couples in therapy to understand how it is possible that conception might *not* occur. For example, couples with infertility who have no anatomical abnormalities and no functional abnormalities of sperm or eggs are often treated in ways that maximize the woman's exposure to sperm at exactly the time of ovulation. (This is described in more detail in the next chapter.) Depending on the medications used and the woman's age, such intervention has a 30–45% chance of success over three cycles of treatment. This translates into a 10–15% pregnancy rate per treatment cycle. Still, couples undergoing such treatment are typically astounded if pregnancy does not occur on the first attempt. How can it be, they ask, that sperm and eggs can meet yet pregnancy not result? And, if pregnancy has not resulted, what possible utility can there be of repeating the same treatment?

The obvious answer to both questions is that infertile couples are no different than fertile couples in their need for repeated exposure before pregnancy occurs. Just as normally fertile couples may take a long time to conceive, so may infertile couples undergoing treatment. The reason is the same for both: Pregnancy is not just about combining sperm and eggs. The egg and sperm must both be genetically normal; the resulting embryo needs also to be genetically normal, so it can divide and develop; it then needs to make its way through the fallopian tubes to the uterus; the uterine lining needs to be perfectly developed to allow implantation, and the woman's hormonal secretions need to support the developing pregnancy. Malfunction in any of these areas poses an obstacle to pregnancy. And this is just the short list. There are, of course, thousands of processes, most still hidden to us, which need to occur perfectly in order to start growing a healthy human being.

The complexity of making a healthy baby can also be seen in

the vast embryonic wastage that occurs as part of natural human reproduction. It has been estimated that only 30% of all conceptions are even noticed by women. Studies of large groups of women using daily sensitive pregnancy tests show that most eggs that are fertilized never implant, and many that do are lost without significantly disturbing the normal menstrual cycle.[3] Of the 30% that are recognized as pregnancies, a further 20–50% will miscarry. Miscarriage rates rise with age, regardless of the circumstances of conception.[4] In other words, women who conceive with treatment are no more likely to miscarry than those who conceive naturally. On the other hand, nothing about treatment conveys any protection against miscarriage, either.

The inefficiencies of reproduction are likely founded in the genetic complexity of human beings. The ovary is the storage site for hundreds of thousands of eggs, all of which lie dormant in a suspended state of development from the time of birth until decades later, when they are activated to mature. During this period of dormancy, eggs are susceptible to genetic damage. The later in life they are activated to mature and ovulate, the higher the probability that some genetic damage will have occurred. This explains why miscarriage rates rise with age. Still, even in younger women, genetically abnormal eggs can and do ovulate. Likewise, normal men produce sperm by the millions on a continual basis. Such voluminous and incessant sperm production allows ample opportunities for the transfer of genetic information to go awry. Studies of conceptuses from spontaneously miscarried pregnancies show genetic abnormalities in 60–70%. These abnormalities may have their origin in abnormal eggs, abnormal sperm or both. In either case, such miscarriages must be viewed as nature's way of assuring that most babies that are born are healthy. Indeed, it is only a tiny minority of genetically abnormal embryos that escape this process and ultimately survive to birth.

For all of these reasons, reproductive specialists usually recommend that "older couples"—meaning those where the woman is age 35 or older—seek medical attention if pregnancy has not occurred after six months of trying. After a woman reaches the age of 40, her window of potential success is very small. In such instances, the case for an expedited evaluation and medical intervention is especially compelling.

Origins of Infertility

Studies examining the origins of infertility generally follow a 40–40–20 rule. A predominant male factor is identified in 40% of cases, a predominant female factor in 40% of cases, and combined male and female factors in 20%. Male causes are discussed in Part IV. Female factors break down into the following categories: disorders of ovulation, 40%; tubal abnormalities, including blockage or scar tissue, 20%; endometriosis, 20%; and cervical or uterine factors, 10%; At least 10% of women with infertility will have no identifiable cause, or so-called unexplained infertility.

It is interesting to note that these commonly accepted figures may not hold true in the observant Jewish community. The epidemiology of infertility among observant Jewish couples may be different because behavioral patterns differ. Endometriosis, for example, is a progressive disease associated with infertility that tends to become more clinically apparent and significant in women as they age. Endometriosis is also known to improve or disappear with the occurrence of pregnancy. Thus, endometriosis is typically found in women who have reached their thirties with no previous successful pregnancies. Early marriage and pregnancy, typical in many Jewish communities, makes the occurrence of endometriosis less likely. Disease of the fallopian tube, which largely (but not always!) occurs as a result of sexually transmitted diseases, is uncommon for obvious reasons. On the other hand, ovulatory disorders are very common, and make up for the relative paucity of anatomical problems. Disorders of ovulation are directly linked to a woman's weight and physical activity. Eating disorders are common in Jewish communities. In some, a great focus on weight motivates women to eat less and exercise incessantly, which can result in low body weight, cessation of ovulation and the disappearance of menstrual cyclicity. In other communities the problem is the opposite—opportunities for physical activity are limited, and women may instead be confined to the home for extensive periods of time, resulting in high rates of obesity. Polycystic Ovary Syndrome, which is often associated with obesity, is probably the most common cause of infertility in observant women.

Male factor infertility may also be disproportionately high among Orthodox couples. There are two explanations for this. The first, as already described, is the relative scarcity of tubal factor infertility and endometriosis in this group. From a purely statistical point of view, this means that when infertility occurs in an Orthodox couple, it is more likely to be due to a male factor. Secondly, lifestyle differences, particularly among certain sects, may predispose men to conditions that can cause infertility. It is well known that a sedentary lifestyle, sitting for prolonged periods of time and lack of exercise are associated with the development of varicoceles (see Part IV "Evaluation and Treatment of the Male") and low sperm counts. This accurately describes the life of many yeshiva and *kollel* students.

There is one more type of infertility that is seldom discussed but nevertheless demands attention. This infertility results from sexual dysfunction. Why it may disproportionately affect Jewish couples is a subject that is difficult to broach. In general, it is problematic to equate infertility in any way with sexual dysfunction. Among physicians, it is well known that infertility is almost always the result of discrete and identifiable malfunctions in physical systems, and almost never a result of anything psychological. Infertility resulting from sexual dysfunction is therefore quite rare. Still, in popular lore, infertility is linked with psychological and/or sexual disturbances. The oft-repeated advice from well-meaning friends and family that infertile couples should "relax," "take a vacation" or try having "better sex," is a result of this misconception and can be a source of great frustration and emotional pain for the infertile couple. Giving any legitimacy to this concept has the potential of inflicting on them greater psychological stress. Moreover, the traditional Jewish perspective on sexuality within the context of marriage is a very positive one, with an emphasis on fostering healthy sexual relations between husband and wife. To discuss sexual pathology in observant couples is, in a sense, to expose weaknesses that should not exist. Finally, *tzini'ut*, or sexual modesty, is one of the pillars of Judaism. Addressing sexual problems requires a frankness that can easily violate the principles of *tzini'ut.*

These reservations notwithstanding, there is compelling reason to include sexual dysfunction as a cause of infertility, and that is to reassure couples affected in this way that they are not alone and that a solution exists for them, too. It is not difficult to imagine the turmoil that visits the couple with sexual dysfunction. Not only is their infertility obvious and open to all, they must also live with the disappointment and guilt over the failure of their intimate life. Personal embarrassment, as well as the sense that any discussion of sexual matters might violate the laws of *tzini'ut,* may make them reluctant to seek help for many years.

To be sure, sexual dysfunction resulting in infertility is not a particularly Jewish problem. No studies have identified it as occurring more often among certain ethnic or demographic groups. However, when such problems occur in observant Jewish couples, it bears reflecting on the probable origins. Rigorously Orthodox boys and girls are forbidden any physical contact with someone of the opposite sex. In some communities, social contact is also severely restricted. Boys and girls are schooled separately and intentionally segregated in non-school activities, sometimes even within their own families. Yet they are expected to marry young and then to build families right away. In many Orthodox communities, dating proceeds at a furiously determined pace. Once the right match is found, the wedding quickly follows. In Hasidic communities, the concept of dating is anathema; it is still common for marriages to be arranged. Bride and groom commonly enter the bridal canopy with little knowledge of each other and no previous experience of physical intimacy. Still, they are expected to have sexual intercourse that very first night!

That this system works for the vast majority of couples is a tribute to the generally healthy attitudes that Judaism fosters about sexual relations within the framework of marriage. Although there is no *actual* experience prior to marriage, there certainly is preparation. But for some couples the transition from no contact to normal marital relations cannot be bridged in so short a time. For them, the marriage will not be consummated right away. In some cases, the couple makes a conscious pact not to have sexual relations for the first few months, preferring first to "date" and then to allow their relationship to progress gradually, in a manner typical of unmarried secular couples. Of course, there is nothing at all surprising or wrong with such decisions. But for other couples the solutions may not come so easily, and they may have trouble consummating their marriage month after month. Fear, anxiety, and confusion are only some of the emotions that can interfere with proper sexual relations, and husband, wife, or both may be equally affected.

Sexual dysfunction may occasionally result from technical naivete. More commonly it is associated with low libido, vaginismus, erectile dysfunction, or inability to ejaculate (anejaculation). All such situations require a highly patient and sensitive approach on the part of the treating professional. The operative word is *professional*. Sexual dysfunction is a serious problem that should be addressed by someone with special expertise in this area. There is no place here for "dabbling," either by rabbis, physicians, or interested laypersons. A trained sex therapist or psychologist should be sought when such situations are encountered.

Basic Evaluation

HISTORY

The standard approach to evaluating any medical complaint is to take a thorough history, and this is especially true of infertility. This history includes the identification of any medical illnesses in either partner, including medications taken, review of any previous surgical procedures, and a review of any social habits that may interfere with a healthy pregnancy, such as smoking, alcohol, and substance abuse. Family and genetic histories are also useful. A detailed menstrual history often will provide a clue to the etiology of infertility, especially if there is significant irregularity or absence of menstrual cycles. For the woman who observes the laws of *taharat hamishpa'ha*, or family purity, it is especially important to ascertain that ovulation does not occur during the time of *niddah*. A sexual history should also be taken, as it too may play a role in infertility.

Coital frequency is a lifestyle issue that must be explored. The Talmud sets forth guidelines for women's conjugal privileges. These are the minimum levels of sexual relations that should occur between couples, and they are dependent on the stature and work obligations of the husband. Sometimes a couple may take upon themselves the habit of having sexual relations only on Shabbat, which is a stringency that more properly belongs only to the greatest of sages.[5] They may take on this extra measure of observance specifically to demonstrate their piety and to exact the reward of children. Ironically, such low levels of coital frequency may yield the opposite result. Overcoming barrenness in such couples is merely a matter of convincing them that sexual relations may properly occur more frequently.

Timing of intercourse is another important historical detail that should not be overlooked. Observant couples commonly are taught that the peak fertility potential of a woman exists around the time of her immersion in the *mikvah*. But that is so only in the average woman who has a recurring 28-day cycle with a 5–7 day menstrual period. These intervals translate into immersion on day 12–14 and then ovulation on day 14. Longer cycles, shorter cycles and longer periods of bleeding may all result in dysynchrony between immersion, sexual relations, and ovulation. In general, it is useful for couples to understand their particular cyclic patterns of fertility to make sure that sexual relations occur during those times. (The specific problem of ovulation prior to *mikvah* is addressed in "Halakhic Considerations in the Treatment of Female Infertility")

The initial visit is the proper time for the couple and their physician to review any other lifestyle habits that may be interfering with conception. Eating disorders and smoking are examples

of problems that can be corrected without specific medical intervention.

OBESITY—A SPECIAL CONSIDERATION

The task of the reproductive specialist is not only to help a woman
conceive, but also to assure that the pregnancy has an optimum
chance of being successfully completed—i.e. that delivery of a
healthy infant at term will occur.[6] Maintenance of body weight
that is close to ideal is important for assuring this result. Obesity,
a problem that is prevalent among American women, has not
spared Jewish women. Because obesity poses a particular obstacle
to pregnancy, addressing this problem bears special consideration
during the initial evaluation of infertility.

An overweight or obese person has excess body fat. Women
store most of their body fat in the midsection that includes the
abdomen, hips, and thighs. The measurement of overall body fat
is determined by calculation of Body Mass Index (BMI) and waist
measurement. BMI measures body weight relative to height and
is used by clinicians to determine total body fat content in adults,
being a better indicator than weight alone. Waist measurement
indicates body fat stored specifically in the abdominal area. Women
with fat concentrated in their abdominal region are more likely to
develop health problems associated with obesity. Total body fat
and concentration are factors of greater importance in determining
health risks than weight alone. In non-pregnant women, a BMI of
18.5–24.9 represents a healthy weight. A BMI of 25–29.9 is considered
overweight, and a BMI exceeding 30 is considered obese.[7]

More than 50% of women in America are overweight or
obese. Many of these women feel that their weight is out of propor-
tion to their food consumption. However, in the absence of specific
medical conditions, which are rare, most obesity is the result of
eating too much and/or exercising too little. If one consumes too
many calories that are not needed for immediate energy, most of
the extra calories are stored as fat. Total weight and fat distribu-
tion—especially abdominal fat—are factors that contribute to
health risks.

BMI (kg/m2)	19	20	21	22	23	24	25	26	27	28	29	30	35	40
Height (in.)	Weight (lb.)													
58	91	96	100	105	110	115	119	124	129	134	138	143	167	191
59	94	99	104	109	114	119	124	128	133	138	143	148	173	198
60	97	102	107	112	118	123	128	133	138	143	148	153	179	204
61	100	106	111	116	122	127	132	137	143	148	153	158	185	211
62	104	109	115	120	126	131	136	142	147	153	158	164	191	218
63	107	113	118	124	130	135	141	146	152	158	163	169	197	225
64	110	116	122	128	134	140	145	151	157	163	169	174	204	232
65	114	120	126	132	138	144	150	156	162	168	174	180	210	240
66	118	124	130	136	142	148	155	161	167	173	179	186	216	247
67	121	127	134	140	146	153	159	166	172	178	185	191	223	255
68	125	131	138	144	151	158	164	171	177	184	190	197	230	262
69	128	135	142	149	155	162	169	176	182	189	196	203	236	270
70	132	139	146	153	160	167	174	181	188	195	202	207	243	278
71	136	143	150	157	165	172	179	186	193	200	208	215	250	286
72	140	147	154	162	169	177	184	191	199	206	213	221	258	294
73	144	151	159	166	174	182	189	197	204	212	219	227	265	302
74	148	155	163	171	179	186	194	202	210	218	225	233	272	311
75	152	160	168	176	184	192	200	208	216	224	232	240	279	319
76	156	164	172	180	189	197	205	213	221	230	238	246	287	328

A Typical BMI Table

Obesity has been directly linked to serious diseases, including cardiovascular disease, high blood pressure, and stroke. The livers of obese women produce increased amounts of cholesterol and triglycerides, both of which are known risk factors for heart disease. An increased strain on the back and legs from increased weight can lead to osteoarthritis. Increased insulin resistance can lead to Type II Diabetes and Polycystic Ovary Syndrome (PCOS). Aside from the physical and physiological consequences of obesity, there are also emotional and social consequences.

Weight problems, and especially obesity, have a major impact on a women's reproductive performance. Although there are many overweight women who are fertile and have children, studies have shown that the overall prevalence of reproductive disorders increases with increasing BMI. These disorders include amenorrhea (absent periods), oligomenorrhea (irregular periods), anovulation (lack of ovulation), infertility, and poor response to fertility drugs. Women with a high BMI who do conceive, whether naturally or with fertility treatment, are at increased risk for spontaneous miscarriage[8] as well as pregnancy-related complications such as diabetes, pregnancy induced hypertension (PIH), pre-eclampsia (toxemia), and delivery of larger babies, which increases the risk of cesarean delivery. Recent studies have also identified obesity with increased risks of stillbirth, neonatal death, and even birth defects.[9]

Obese women are also at increased risk for the most common reproductive disorder associated with infertility, PCOS. PCOS is a metabolic disorder that affects 5–10% of all women. It is the most common female cause of infertility. In this syndrome, there is an accumulation of many incompletely developed egg follicles in the ovaries, which is a result of, as well as a cause of, anovulation. These follicles fail to mature and ovulate and they appear in the ovary as small "cysts," hence the term "polycystic" to characterize a PCOS-affected ovary.[10]

The polycystic ovary produces too much androgen and estrogen, both of which interfere with follicle stimulating hormone (FSH).

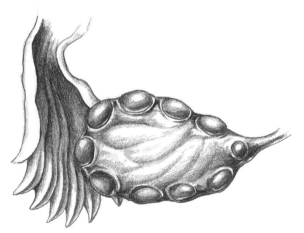

Polycystic Ovary: The ovary is filled with immature follicles

The result is failure to ovulate. Without ovulation, the ovary does not produce enough progesterone necessary to bring on normal menstruation. High androgen levels and failed ovulation contribute to the typical characteristics of PCOS. These include irregular periods, hirsutism (excessive growth of facial and body hair), acne, weight gain and/or infertility.

Normal ovarian function is dependent on the proper secretion of several different hormones, including insulin. Failure of one or more of these hormones to be produced at the right time interferes with normal function. Insulin is thought to play a major role in how PCOS develops. Many, though not all, obese women are resistant to the effects of insulin, which causes their insulin levels to rise. High levels of insulin (hyperinsulinemia), in turn, may cause further weight gain due to insulin's role in promoting fat storage. The result is a vicious cycle of weight gain, further insulin resistance resulting from weight gain, then insulin resistance causing further weight gain. The body's attempts to compensate for insulin resistance further results in higher levels of circulating insulin. These high insulin levels cause the ovaries to become polycystic.[11] The primary modality of treatment is to lower insulin levels. Although there are medications that can be used for this purpose, the best way to do so is to restrict food intake and increase exercise, both of which will inevitably result in weight loss, decreased insulin resistance, and the normalization of ovarian function.

Overweight and obese women whose failure to conceive is not related to anovulation, but to other factors such as tubal blockage or male factors, also benefit from weight loss. This is because the success rates of other fertility treatments increases as body weight approaches normal. Behavioral interventions to improve diet and physical activity are the primary methods used to promote and maintain weight loss and reduce infertility. Insulin sensitizing medications are used along with lifestyle modification only in patients who are at a significantly elevated risk because of obesity, and where lifestyle modification has not resulted in sufficient weight loss.

INFECTIOUS DISEASES TESTING

All couples presenting for infertility evaluation must undergo standard preconception testing, which includes testing for infectious diseases. Although it may seem odd to test even monogamous couples for HIV infection, physicians cannot discriminate in testing on the basis of assumptions about religious people. In addition, other infectious diseases, such as hepatitis, must also be tested for. Active infection may have serious consequences, including transmission between partners or between mother and infant.

Couples should also be tested for immunity to certain viral infections that have been associated with fetal damage. Rubella (German measles) and varicella (chicken pox) infections are in this category and are absolutely preventable. Women who wish to conceive and who have not previously been exposed to these infections should be vaccinated. In addition, the presence of certain antibodies, such as the easily measurable antibodies to chlamydia, has potential clinical significance. Infection with chlamydia, a sexually transmitted bacteria, can cause tubal damage and pelvic adhesions. Women who are antibody positive have been exposed to chlamydia and are therefore at higher risk of having tubal infertility than women who are antibody negative.

SCREENING FOR GENETIC DISEASES

Many women begin their relationship with their obstetrician/gynecologist after they are pregnant. By that time, testing for genetic diseases in the prospective parents is too late. Infertile women, on the other hand, seek medical attention before they conceive, enabling them to be educated about and tested for genetic diseases during the evaluation process.

Ashkenazic Jews have been carefully studied and are now known to be frequent carriers of some potentially devastating genetic diseases. Most these genetic diseases are recessive. This means that in order for a child to be affected, both parents need to be carriers for the disease. Carriers, like non-carriers, generally enjoy perfect health. There is no way to detect the carrier state other than to undergo testing. If one spouse is a carrier and the other is not, their children cannot be affected by the disease. If both are carriers, there is a 25% chance that a child will be affected. Examples of these recessive diseases include the following:

Bloom Syndrome is a DNA repair disorder. Clinical features include growth deficiency, sun-sensitive facial erythema (redness), other pigmentation abnormalities of the skin, immunodeficiency and predisposition to cancer. Death from cancer usually occurs before the age of 30 years. Intelligence is normal. A single mutation in the BLM gene is responsible for 97% of Bloom Syndrome in affected Ashkenazi Jewish individuals. The carrier frequency of this mutation among Ashkenazi Jewish individuals with no family history of Bloom Syndrome is approximately 1 in 100.

Cystic fibrosis is the most common recessive lethal genetic disorder among Caucasians, with an incidence of approximately 1 in 3,300 live births. It is characterized by pulmonary and gastrointestinal manifestations of varying severity. Although there is some variability of clinical expression, most individuals with cystic fibrosis require lifelong medical care and experience reduced life expectancy. Intelligence is normal. The carrier rate among Ashkenazi Jews, as in all Caucasians is 1 in 26.

Canavan's Disease (also known as Spongy Degenerative Disease) is a severe, progressive neurological disease caused by a deficiency of the enzyme aspartoacylase, which leads to an elevated level of N-acetylaspartic acid. This results in demyelination and spongy degeneration of the brain. Clinical characteristics include developmental delay, hypotonia (poor muscle tone), macrocephaly (large head) and poor head control. The first clinical symptoms usually appear between 3–6 months of age. Spasticity, seizures, optic atrophy, gastrointestinal reflux, and feeding difficulties develop as the child gets older. Currently there is no effective treatment and most children with Canavan's disease die within the first decade of life. The carrier frequency among Ashkenazi Jews is 1 in 40.

Familial dysautonomia is a disorder affecting the autonomic nervous system. Affected individuals suffer from various symptoms including insensitivity to pain and temperature, cardiovascular instability and labile blood pressure, aspiration pneumonia and recurrent crises which consist of paroxysms of vomiting, cramping and emotional lability. Intelligence is normal. Approximately half of all affected individuals die before the age of 30. The carrier frequency among Ashkenazi Jews is 1 in 30.

Fanconi anemia is a condition that leads to bone marrow failure (pancytopenia). It is also associated with congenital malformations, chromosomal instability, and an increased risk of cancer. While there is variability in physical manifestations, affected individuals frequently exhibit short stature, bony abnormalities of the upper extremities, and genital abnormalities. Learning disabilities or mental retardation may occur. Fanconi anemia is associated with a very high risk of early onset leukemia and an elevated risk of gynecological and head/neck cancer in adulthood. Death from cancer usually occurs before the age of 30 years. The carrier frequency among Ashkenazi Jews is 1 in 89.

Gaucher's Disease is a disease with variable severity. It is caused by a deficiency of glucocerebrosidase, the enzyme required for the degradation of glycolipids in the liver. Gaucher's Disease has a wide range of clinical manifestations, ranging from significant disease to no symptoms at all. Virtually all Ashkenazi Jewish individuals affected with Gaucher's Disease have Type 1, the mildest type of Gaucher's Disease. Type 1 is associated with liver enlargement, blood abnormalities and skeletal problems, including deformity of the femur (thigh bone), aseptic necrosis of the femoral heads (hip bones), bone infarcts and fractures. Type 1 Gaucher's can be readily treated with enzyme replacement therapy. The carrier frequency among Ashkenazi Jews is 1 in 15.

Mucolipidosis Type IV is a progressive neurological disease caused by liver enzyme abnormalities. It is characterized by psychomotor retardation and a variety of eye diseases such as corneal clouding, retinal degeneration, and strabismus (cross eye). Motor and mental retardation ranges from mild to severe. Onset is usually within the first year of life, with a maximal developmental age of 1 to 2 years. No effective treatment is currently available. Patients currently range from 1 to 45 years of age. The carrier frequency among Ashkenazi Jews is 1 in 22.

Niemann-Pick Disease is caused by a deficiency of acid sphingomyelinase, the enzyme required for the degradation of sphingomyelin in specialized liver cell components called lysosomes. It can occur in all ethnic groups, but has the highest prevalence in the Ashkenazi Jewish population. Individuals with type A disease have a clinical course characterized by failure to thrive, liver enlargement and a progressive neurodegeneration which leads to death by 2–3 years of age. Currently there is no therapy for Niemann-Pick Disease. The carrier frequency among Ashkenazi Jews is 1 in 90.

Tay-Sachs Disease is a disorder caused by a deficiency of the enzyme hexosaminidase A, which results in the build-up of certain lipids in the liver that cause progressive neurological degeneration. Development is typically normal during the first several months of life. Progressive deterioration then causes blindness, deafness, seizures, and paralysis. Children do not usually live beyond the age of five. There is currently no treatment or cure for this disease. Tay-Sachs Disease occurs most frequently in populations of Ashkenazi Jewish descent and French Canadian descent. The carrier frequency among Ashkenazi Jews is 1 in 30.

Dor Yesharim is a Jewish communal organization whose mission is to prevent the occurrence of recessive genetic diseases in the Ashkenazic Jewish community. It offers anonymous testing for high school students in the anticipation that some day they all will marry. Each individual is given an identifying code. When a potential mate is found, Dor Yesharim is given the couple's codes. Unless both partners are carriers of the same genetic disease, the union is blessed and left to develop. But in the rare instances that both are carriers, the couple is informed, the relationship usually comes to an abrupt end and the partners seek other opportunities elsewhere. No one is ever actually told of his or her results, preventing the stigma that might accompany a known carrier of a lethal genetic disease.

Couples who have undergone testing with Dor Yesharim are often reluctant to subject themselves to further genetic testing. At first glance, it seems repetitious. It is worth noting, however, that Dor Yesharim can only test for those genetic diseases which are known to be prevalent and problematic at the time the test is done. It cannot make up for an evolving science. It cannot anticipate the discovery of new genetic illnesses. The longer in the past the testing was performed, the less complete it therefore will be. There is good reason to update testing to reflect the gamut of diseases currently known.

Many couples, having the sense that there is no point in screening once they have already married, still opt to defer. They assume that, even if it turns out that they both are carriers, there is no option available to them other than to take a chance and try. Once they conceive, they often will also not avail themselves of prenatal diagnosis, thinking that the abortion of a genetically impaired fetus is against halakha. However, there is no uniform Jewish viewpoint on abortion. Rabbi Waldenberg allows abortion of a fetus with Tay-Sachs Disease until the seventh month.[12] Moreover, recent developments, such as preimplantation genetic diagnosis, make it possible not only to prevent the transmission of genetic disease but also to avoid the religiously problematic act of aborting a genetically defective fetus.

ENDOCRINE TESTING

For the ovary to function properly, it must be able to signal and respond to the pituitary gland. But the pituitary controls endocrine glands other than the ovary. These include the thyroid, breast and adrenal glands. Physical examination of the thyroid gland and breasts is therefore a routine procedure in evaluating infertility. The adrenal glands are not accessible to physical examination. In rare circumstances, they may need to be imaged using special x-ray techniques.

Reproductive endocrinologists will generally measure thyroid function and prolactin levels on all women who present with infertility. The thyroid gland is important for general metabolic processes. Control of thyroid hormone secretion from this gland is exerted by thyroid stimulating hormone (TSH, or thyroxine), which is secreted from the pituitary gland. Abnormally low secretion of thyroid hormone is one of the most common disorders in women, and can be detected by elevated levels of TSH. Prolactin is a hormone secreted by the pituitary gland, typically in pregnant or nursing women. Although its major function is to stimulate milk production, low levels of prolactin are found in all women and are necessary for normal fertility. Abnormally high levels of prolactin can cause menstrual disturbances that result in infertility. On occasion, high prolactin levels will cause infertility or recurrent miscarriage in the absence of any noticeable change in menstrual function. Galactorhea, the inappropriate secretion of breast milk may, however, be present. Increased prolactin levels may or may not be associated with small tumors, called microadenomas, of the pituitary gland.

Approximately 5% of women with infertility will be hypothyroid and another 5% will have above normal prolactin levels. Although cause and effect is not always provable, these hormonal disorders should be corrected prior to instituting any other fertility therapy. Hypothyroidism is corrected by administering thyroid supplements in dosages sufficient to normalize the thyroid function tests. Prolactin disorders are usually correctable with the administration of either bromocriptine (Parlodel®) or carbergoline (Dostinex®) in doses sufficient to normalize the prolactin level. It is not uncommon for these simple corrections to restore normal fertility.

Women with menstrual cycle abnormalities, especially those who are at risk for having PCOS, are generally tested for levels of the pituitary hormones LH (luteinizing hormone) and FSH; the adrenal hormones DHEAS (dihydroepiandosterone sulfate) and 17-hydroxyprogesterone; as well as for testosterone, which is produced in both the ovary and the adrenal gland. These tests are necessary to pinpoint the area of the body that is not functioning properly, and then to tailor treatment accordingly.

Physical Examination[13]

PELVIC EXAM

Assessment of the infertile woman should always include a standard pelvic ("internal") examination, consisting of both visual inspection and feeling (palpation) of the pelvic organs, also known as a bimanual exam. Visual inspection of the vagina and cervix is possible with a speculum and, in experienced hands, usually involves no or minimal discomfort. This inspection is necessary to rule out abnormalities that might interfere with pregnancy occurring or with treatment being given. When the history is consistent with

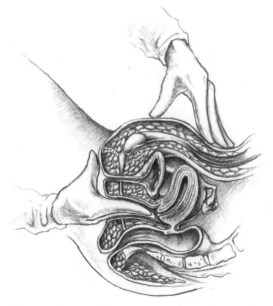

Bimanual exam: The uterus and ovaries can be palpated between the two examining hands

sexual dysfunction, the vaginal exam can confirm whether or not intercourse has taken place.

During a bimanual exam, the physician feels the pelvic organs in between two fingers inserted in the vagina and a separate hand placed over the lower abdomen. This examination is useful to detect uterine or ovarian enlargement, which would indicate myomas or cysts. In addition, the position of the uterus and its mobility can alert the skilled physician to the existence of adhesions or other conditions such as endometriosis. Pain on bimanual exam is not usual and may indicate the possibility of internal anatomical abnormalities.

PELVIC ULTRASOUND

Ultrasound (sonogram) examination of the pelvis has become increasingly useful for revealing the soft tissues of the pelvis. The development of transvaginal ultrasound has changed the practice of gynecology in general and the assessment of infertility in particular. When utilized properly, the ultrasound probe can be an extension of the gynecologist's hand, essentially allowing him or her to "see" with the fingers. Especially desirable features of transvaginal ultrasound are that, unlike ultrasound examinations that are done over the abdominal wall, the resulting picture is sharp and not limited by the amount of body fat. A full bladder is not required in order to do the exam, which also makes it more comfortable to perform.

In the context of the infertility investigation, ultrasound is used to assess the uterine anatomy and to detect abnormalities of the ovaries. Small cysts are easily detectable and may point to conditions that require further assessment by laparoscopy. Egg follicles within the ovary are also easily seen. Many specialists use the assessment of these follicles as an adjunctive test to determine whether ovulation is taking place and what the woman's egg supply might be. The "antral follicle count," which is determined by using ultrasound to count the number of resting egg follicles during a woman's menstrual period, is a good predictor of a how she might respond to stimulation with fertility drugs.

Generally speaking, the fallopian tubes are not detectable on

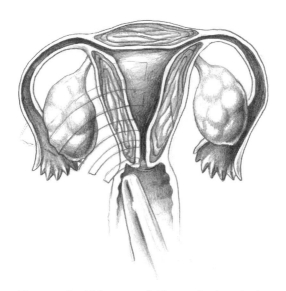

Transvaginal Ultrasound: The vaginal probe is used to visualize the uterus and ovaries

an ultrasound examination. In conditions of tubal blockage, when the tubes are filled with fluid (hydrosalpinx), the tubes may show up as masses near the ovaries. The management of hydrosalpinx is complex and requires consultation with a reproductive endocrinologist skilled in surgery and in vitro fertilization.

Neither the routine pelvic examination nor a transvaginal ultrasound examination can render a woman *niddah*. This is because direct touching is limited to the vagina and cervix. There is no dilation of the cervix and no trauma to the uterine lining during either of these exams. Thus, any bleeding that occurs following such exams may be assumed to be vaginal or cervical in origin.

Specific Fertility Tests

OVARIAN RESERVE SCREENING

While infertility can be due to a variety of causes, the age of the woman is often a significant factor. Many couples delay childbearing until their later reproductive years, with 20% of American women having their first child after age 35. After age 30, monthly pregnancy rates decline; this decline is even more pronounced after age 35. Although it is commonly believed that infertility affects 10–15% of couples, the rate of infertility approximately doubles after the age of 35, and nearly half of women over the age of 40 experience infertility.[14] Furthermore, advancing age is associated with an increase in miscarriage rates as well as chromosomal defects. As a result, couples in this age range require an efficient and timely approach to infertility diagnosis and management.

All infertile women, regardless of age, are routinely asked about the regularity and length of their menstrual cycles. While menses ceases at menopause, in the years preceding menopause menstrual cycles may change significantly. Skipped or shortened cycles may occur over time. Even when a woman's cycles does not change appreciably, the natural aging process brings with it a depletion of healthy eggs, i.e. eggs that can be fertilized and produce a normal pregnancy. The ability of the ovaries to produce healthy eggs, either naturally or in response to fertility medications, is called "ovarian reserve." A decrease in ovarian reserve is most commonly seen with aging. However, compromise of the ovarian reserve may also cause infertility in younger women.

Reproductive specialists separate chronological aging from biological aging. Some women, especially those who have borne many children, appear to retain a healthy ovarian reserve well into their late forties. On the other hand, the ovaries of some younger women appear to undergo a rapid aging process, so ovarian reserve may be compromised in their early thirties or even during their twenties.[15] It is therefore imperative to evaluate the ovarian reserve in women with infertility prior to beginning treatment, especially with fertility medications. Accurate assessment helps the physician to determine the likelihood of pregnancy and to discuss these matters prior to treatment.

Ovarian reserve is usually reflected in the levels of FSH and estradiol circulating in a woman's body during her menses. The physiology behind this is as follows: Ovarian follicles—the structures from which ova, or eggs, are released—are stimulated to develop by FSH, a hormone that is secreted by the pituitary gland, which sits at the base of the brain. Cells that compose the ovarian follicle produce their own hormones; two of the most important are estradiol (an active form of estrogen) and inhibin. Among their many roles, these two hormones suppress pituitary FSH secretion, allowing one follicle to develop without competition from other follicles. With advancing age, ovarian follicles become less functional and secrete less inhibin. As a result, FSH levels rise with age, providing a useful marker for ovarian reserve. In fact, an age-related rise in FSH may precede menopause by as much as a decade. The rise in FSH initially causes a rise in estradiol. Therefore, estradiol levels are used as another marker of ovarian reserve. (As follicles deplete, however, estradiol levels will eventually fall and are low in postmenopausal women.)

Typically, screening for ovarian reserve is performed early in the menstrual cycle (days 2, 3, or 4). Serum FSH and estradiol levels are drawn and analyzed. FSH levels in excess of 10–20 IU/L (depending on the laboratory test used) are associated with poor egg supplies—both qualitatively and quantitatively—and therefore with lower pregnancy rates. Similarly, elevated estradiol levels have negative prognostic implications.[16]

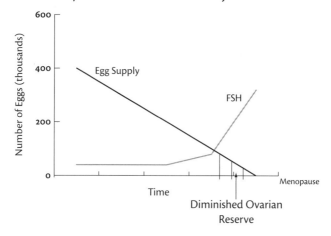

Time and Fertility Potential: The rate at which egg depletion occurs varies in every woman

Many physicians perform additional clomiphene citrate challenge tests (CCCT) on selected patients. In this test, FSH and estradiol levels are drawn on day 2, 3, or 4 of the menstrual cycle and 100 mg of clomiphene citrate is taken on days 5–9 of the menstrual cycle. The woman then returns on day 10 for another FSH level. The pattern of these laboratory values provides an even more sensitive marker of the individual woman's ability to respond to fertility medications and to conceive.

The value of these tests in terms of their ability to separate those women who will eventually conceive from those who will not is not perfect. Problems include significant variations between what physicians consider a "normal" FSH level. Furthermore, FSH levels may vary between laboratories and even between cycles in the same patient. Therefore, while highly predictive, a small percentage of patients with elevated FSH and estradiol levels may still conceive. Similarly, woman with normal ovarian reserve may respond poorly to fertility therapy. This is especially true of women in their mid- to late-forties, whose innate fertility is not well measured by the occurrence of regular menstrual cycles and the finding of normal ovarian reserve.

Ovarian reserve screening is very helpful to physicians who must make recommendations to couples regarding their best chances for success. In couples being evaluated for in vitro fertilization, for example, poor test results may elicit a discussion of special stimulation protocols, the use of donor eggs or, alternatively, adoption.

EVALUATION OF THE MALE

Although it may at first seem odd to include the testing of the male as a component in the evaluation of the female, this is in fact a necessary step. Because most cases of infertility are not clearly male or clearly female, as a practical matter it is important that both partners be tested before any conclusions are reached as to the source of the problem. Assigning infertility solely to a "female factor" necessitates exclusion of a "male factor."

Testing for male fertility is simple, noninvasive and inexpensive, which is why nearly all reproductive specialists, including gynecologists, will generally ask for the male to be tested as the first step in their evaluation of infertility.

EVALUATION OF SPERM

Although it is difficult to precisely define the determinants of male fertility, most doctors accept certain criteria to determine if a man is fertile, subfertile, or sterile. Mostly, these relate to the examination of sperm, or semen analysis. In general, fertile males have greater than 20 million sperm in each milliliter of ejaculated semen. Men with no sperm in the ejaculate (due to failed production or blocked ducts) are considered to be sterile.[17] Sperm counts anywhere in between define a male as subfertile. In addition to the standard sperm count, semen analysis includes examination of other sperm characteristics, such as motility or morphology. At least 50% of the sperm must be motile, or moving, and preferably in a straight and progressive way in order for a male to be considered fertile.

In addition, for many years reproductive specialists have relied heavily on sperm morphology characteristics to predict male

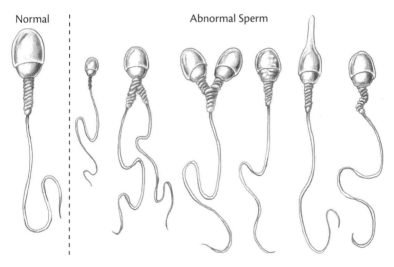

Sperm morphology: Sperm are found in many different shapes, but only the one at left is considered normal

fertility. The standard evaluation of sperm morphology, as classified by the World Health Organization, requires that 30% of the sperm be normal in shape in order for the test results to be normal. In 1986, Tineas Kruger described more exacting criteria for classifying sperm as normal or abnormal.[18] Subsequent data bear out his original findings, which were that very few morphologically normal sperm are needed for normal fertility, and that fertilization rates are proportional to the percentage of normal sperm, as measured by his strict criteria (now also called Kruger criteria). In many laboratories, the finding of as little as 4% normally shaped sperm is sufficient to classify as a normal test. As laboratories may differ in the way that sperm are assessed, the limits of normal will vary between laboratories.

Clearly, measurements of sperm count, motility, and morphology are not the only ways to assess male fertility. Scientists continue to investigate different tests as predictors of male fertility. Computer assisted semen analysis (CASA) has been a welcome addition to most fertility laboratories. CASA allows for more objective assessment of sperm counts and movement, and can also measure characteristics of sperm not apparent to the human eye. Other tests are being developed that may allow clinicians to assess the fertilizing capacity of sperm. Biochemical testing, as well as testing for antibodies attached to sperm, are sometimes useful. Although all of these add to the time-honored semen analysis, none has proven to be entirely accurate in distinguishing male fertility from subfertility. Research in this area is active and ongoing.

It should be noted that, with all the limitations of testing, the semen analysis is still the only way for a man to tell if he is fertile or not. The ejaculation of semen during orgasm does not indicate anything about fertility potential, because even men who have no sperm at all have semen. Also, some men who produce no semen because of anatomical abnormalities may have perfectly normal sperm production. The advent of assisted reproductive technologies (See Part IV, "Assisted Reproduction") has certainly changed the way doctors think about male fertility and infertility. Still, the semen analysis has remained a mainstay of diagnosis since its introduction at the beginning of the twentieth century.

POSTCOITAL TEST

Because male factors are so prevalent a cause of infertility, it is self evident that semen analysis should be done early on in the investigation of the infertile couple. However, halakhic concerns often move observant patients to defer the semen analysis. Depending on the clinical circumstances, a postcoital test (PCT) may be performed instead.

The PCT is a simple, painless procedure that evaluates both the cervical mucus for receptivity to sperm and the sperm for its ability to survive once in the vaginal environment. The test involves the examination of the woman's cervical mucus shortly after intercourse. It must be performed just prior to the time of ovulation. Correct timing is usually assured by the woman using an ovulation predictor kit (OPK) to detect her "LH surge." (LH is released by the pituitary gland prior to ovulation. When detected in the urine, the LH surge indicates that ovulation will occur within 24 to 36 hours.)

The PCT is performed much like a routine pelvic exam. A sample of cervical mucus is obtained and is immediately examined

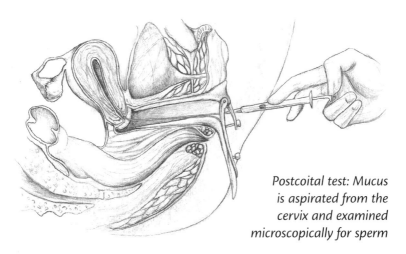

Postcoital test: Mucus is aspirated from the cervix and examined microscopically for sperm

under a microscope for quality and also the number of live sperm. Results are available right away. A good result shows that the female partner secretes adequate mucus around the time of ovulation, and that her partner's sperm can survive in this mucus. When highly active sperm are found in the cervical mucus, it is reasonable to presume that some sperm will make their way through the uterus to the fallopian tubes.

There are several different causes for a poor PCT. The most common of these is poor timing. Proper timing is crucial, as sperm can only live inside a woman's body around the time of ovulation, when cervical mucus protects them.[19] Cervical mucus is produced in response to estrogen, which is secreted as the egg approaches maturity, and reaches its peak just at ovulation.[20] In the days of the menstrual cycle that precede egg maturation, there is insufficient cervical mucus to protect sperm from the acidic environment of the vagina. Once ovulation occurs, progesterone secretion from the ovary renders the cervical mucus thick and impenetrable to sperm. The window of time during which sperm can actually survive in a woman's body is therefore relatively small. This underscores the need for LH testing to time the PCT. If LH testing is performed improperly, or if the time of ovulation is estimated instead of doing LH testing, the actual time of ovulation may be missed, and the PCT result will be poor. Infection, disease of the cervix, and poor sperm are other causes of poor results.

Though a good number of live sperm suggests normal male fertility, the PCT cannot replace a semen analysis. The latter is necessary when a fuller evaluation of the male factor is needed. If repeated, well-timed postcoital testing fails to reveal sperm or suggests a sperm problem, formal semen analysis should be performed. Under these circumstances, if rabbinical permission for semen analysis is not given, the couple should request that their rabbi conference directly with their physician so that the urgency for further testing can be discussed directly.

Couples often feel a great deal of pressure when they need to have intercourse "on schedule" for the PCT, which at times renders them unable to do so. Often they assume that intercourse needs to occur just before their visit to the doctor. It should be understood that the PCT must be done *close* to the time of intercourse, but it need not be done immediately afterward. Anywhere from 2–24 hours may elapse from the time of intercourse to the performance of the PCT.

ENDOMETRIAL BIOPSY

Sampling of the uterine lining, or endometrium, is sometimes useful in the diagnostic evaluation of infertility. When properly timed, the test may provide clues about a woman's ovulatory cycle that might otherwise go undetected. This is because the uterine lining is exquisitely responsive to the hormonal output from the ovary, both before and after ovulation. A biopsy of the uterine lining will reveal not only if a woman has ovulated, but also precisely when and whether or not the ovary has sent the proper signals to prepare for implantation of the embryo.

Endometrial biopsy is generally simple to perform. The actual biopsy takes approximately 5–10 seconds and, in experienced hands, the pain from the biopsy is minimal. Newly developed instruments facilitate biopsy without any trauma to the cervix and with virtually no dilation of the cervical canal.

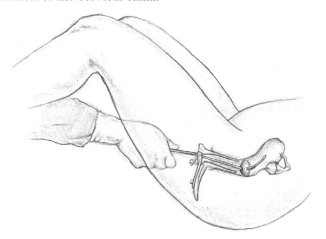

Endometrial biopsy, side view: A metal or plastic tube is inserted through the cervix into the uterus

There is still significant debate among practitioners about the usefulness of the endometrial biopsy. This is because the biopsy may detect abnormalities that are not recurrent, thus suggesting problems where there are none. The standard recommendation is to repeat the biopsy if the initial result is abnormal in order to eliminate a "false positive" result. However, the need for repeat biopsies makes the test unattractive. The widespread use of fertility drugs, which tend to improve endometrial development, renders the test extraneous in many clinical circumstances. In some situations, however, the endometrial biopsy is extremely useful. Women with abnormal bleeding that is suspected of having a hormonal basis as well as women with recurrent miscarriages will often undergo endometrial biopsy.

HYSTEROSALPINGOGRAM

The hysterosalpingogram, or HSG, is a special type of x-ray that has become a time-honored tool in the evaluation of tubal and uterine anatomy. The results of the HSG are often crucial in determining the most appropriate treatment for infertility.

HSG is generally performed by a radiologist or a gynecologist in conjunction with a radiologist. The test is done under fluoroscopy, a type of x-ray equipment that allows the physician to peer inside the body in real time. Unfortunately, a simple x-ray cannot outline the soft tissues of the reproductive tract. It is therefore necessary to fill them with a liquid known as contrast dye (usually a clear liquid containing iodine)[21] that is opaque to the x-ray. This outlines the anatomy on standard x-ray film. Using a device inserted near or through the cervical canal, the contrast is injected into the uterus and, if the tubes are open, it will traverse the entire length of the tubes and spill into the pelvic cavity. Movement of the contrast is seen immediately by the radiologist. The contours of the uterine cavity, the anatomical detail of the insides of the fallopian tubes, and the spillage pattern of dye from the tubes into the pelvis are all important markers. Many abnormalities of the uterine cavity and fallopian tubes may be diagnosed in this way.

Although the test is simple to perform and takes only a few

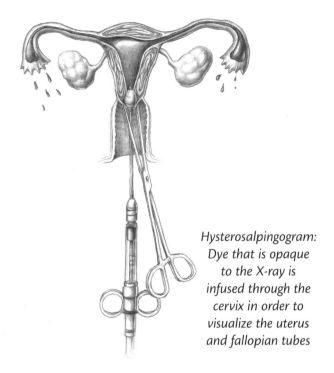

Hysterosalpingogram: Dye that is opaque to the X-ray is infused through the cervix in order to visualize the uterus and fallopian tubes

minutes, some women experience significant discomfort during and after the injection of dye. The perception of pain is somewhat related to the previous occurrence of a vaginal birth: women with primary infertility tend to feel the most pain while those with several previous births tend to feel very little or no pain. The pain from HSG is generally described as menstrual-like cramping. It can be minimized by the ingestion of an anti-inflammatory agent such as ibuprofen prior to testing. Antibiotics are also often given in order to minimize the possibility of infection.

The HSG assesses first and foremost whether or not the fallopian tubes are open, or patent. If they are patent, then an assumption may be made that conception can occur *in vivo*, i.e. within the fallopian tube. The finding of tubal occlusion, or blockage, would indicate that conception can only occur *in vitro*, unless the occlusion can be repaired. There are certain caveats that should be kept in mind regarding the HSG results. Firstly, the test has a 20% false positive rate, meaning that when the tubes are read as occluded there is a 20% chance that they are actually patent. Such a misreading is more likely when the tubes are found to be blocked at their beginning (or proximal part) than when they are found to be blocked at their end (distal part). Technique is an important aspect of this procedure, so it is important that it be performed by an experienced radiologist. Secondly, tubal patency as assessed by HSG is not the last word on a woman's anatomy. While it is obvious that tubal occlusion is a barrier to pregnancy, the finding on the HSG that both tubes are open does not necessarily establish that they are normal. Scar tissue around the tubes, such as that which results from endometriosis or pelvic surgery, can severely damage the fallopian tubes without blocking them. When, on the basis of clinical factors, the physician believes that such intrapelvic pathology exists, laparoscopy may be done following the HSG, or the HSG may be dispensed with altogether. Finally, the HSG will often detect blockage on one side and patency on the other. The precise interpretation of this finding and how it is handled must be left to the skilled reproductive specialist.

In addition to testing the fallopian tubes, the HSG is also an accurate way of assessing the anatomy of the uterine cavity. Its greatest utility is in the assessment of women with recurrent miscarriages, since it can detect congenital abnormalities of the uterus that can cause miscarriage. Examples include bicornuate uterus and septate uterus. However, there are also instances when the uterine anatomy as determined by HSG is helpful in managing infertility. The HSG can detect abnormalities within the uterine cavity, such as scar tissue, myomas, and polyps that may cause infertility or interfere with fertility interventions. Correction of such uterine problems should usually precede other fertility interventions.

Much has been said and written about the occurrence of pregnancy as a result of HSG. This is a known phenomenon, likely due to a flushing out of obstructing debris from within the tubes during the instillation of contrast dye. However, as there is no way

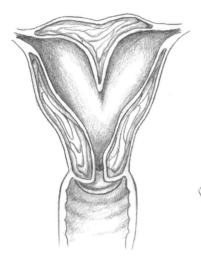

UTERINE
ANOMALIES

*Septate uterus: The external
contours of the uterus are normal,
but the interior is divided*

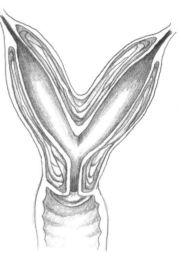

*Bicornuate uterus: The precursors
of the uterus have not fused,
leaving two separate cavities*

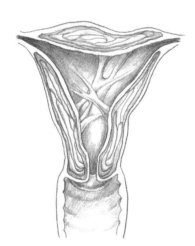

*Uterine adhesions: Scarring
within the uterus is diagnostic
of Asherman's Syndrome*

to predict when a woman might conceive after HSG is performed, the test is best thought of as diagnostic and not therapeutic.

SONOHYSTEROGRAM

There are some occasions when an evaluation of only the uterine cavity, without reference to tubal anatomy, is required. Examples might include assessment of abnormal bleeding associated with infertility, or preparation for specific therapy such as in vitro fertilization. In such cases, the HSG exam may be replaced by a simpler sonohysterogram. This exam is a hybrid test that involves injection of fluid into the uterus, as with the HSG, but the use of ultrasound instead of x-ray.

Standard ultrasound exams of the pelvis are an excellent way to examine the uterine anatomy. However, the actual cavity of the uterus is usually not visualized because the walls of the uterus are in contact with each other, sealing off the potential space between them. When a better and more detailed view of the uterine cavity is required, sonohysterogram is done. This is performed by the reproductive specialist in the office exam room. Using a speculum to visualize the cervix, a thin catheter is placed through the cervix into the uterus and connected to an instillation device through which saline can be injected. After the catheter is in place, the speculum is removed and a transvaginal ultrasound probe is inserted into the vagina. Under ultrasound guidance, saline is then gently instilled into the uterine cavity through the catheter. The dark appearance of saline on the ultrasound picture helps to clearly outline the inner contours of the uterus. In this manner, polyps, fibroids, and other abnormalities of the uterine cavity may be detected. Unlike the HSG, the sonohysterogram does not help visualize the fallopian tubes. The test is also less painful, rarely inducing even mild pain.

HYSTEROSCOPY

Although the sonohysterogram is a very simple and accurate way to peer inside the uterine cavity, the ultimate assessment of this structure is accomplished by direct inspection. This is done using the hysteroscope, a very thin telescopic lens that can be inserted

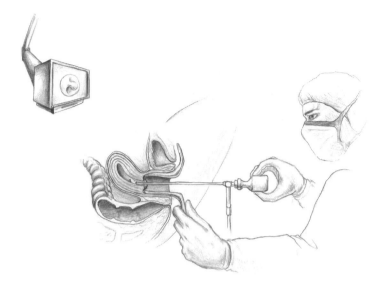

Hysteroscopy: A thin telescope is placed through the cervix in order to assess the uterine cavity

through the cervix and into the uterine cavity, facilitating direct examination. In order to perform hysteroscopy, special fluids are used to distend, or open up, the uterine cavity during the inspection. Often the hysteroscope is connected to a small video camera, which magnifies the picture and increases physician and patient comfort.

Hysteroscopy is the gold standard for assessing the intrauterine anatomy. Its greatest utility, however, is its ability to facilitate surgical procedures from within the uterus. This is called operative hysteroscopy. Fibroids, polyps, and scar tissue may be removed in this way. Certain congenital abnormalities of the uterus are also repairable by hysteroscopy.

LAPAROSCOPY

Physical evaluation of the infertile woman includes a complete pelvic examination, which provides some information about the size and mobility of her pelvic organs, especially the uterus and ovaries. When a woman's previous history and/or physical examination are suggestive of pelvic disorders such as endometriosis, ovarian cysts, scar tissue, uterine fibroids, or other masses, it is often necessary to visualize her pelvic anatomy directly. In the past, such visualization would require admitting a patient to the hospital and performing an incision to open up the abdominal cavity. Such operations required many days of pre- and postoperative hospitalization, missed work days, and several weeks for complete recuperation. Physicians today perform laparoscopy, a much less invasive procedure, to either diagnose (diagnostic laparoscopy) and/or treat (operative laparoscopy) pelvic abnormalities.

Laparoscopy is generally performed on an outpatient basis. As general anesthesia is used, leaving the patient completely unconscious during the operation, there is no pain. A thin needle is inserted through the navel and carbon dioxide gas is used to distend the pelvic and abdominal cavities. The surgeon then removes the

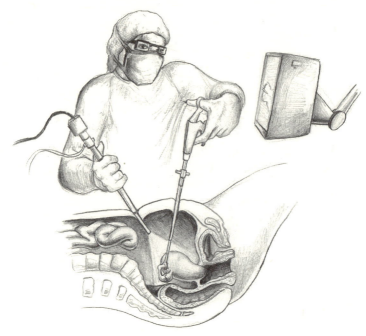

Laparoscopy: A thin telescope is placed throught the abdominal wall to assess the pelvic cavity

needle and introduces a laparoscope with an attached video camera through the incision. This allows good visualization of the pelvic organs. If better visualization is needed, thin metal instruments which allow the pelvic contents to be manipulated are inserted through additional tiny incisions that are made lower down on the abdominal wall. Postoperative pain is usually minimal to moderate. Generally, it results from residual carbon dioxide distending the abdomen, which is usually resorbed in three to four days, after which the pain typically resolves. Complete cosmetic healing of these incisions generally follows.

Laparoscopic instruments may be used not only to visualize pelvic organs but also to treat pelvic disorders. This is called operative laparoscopy. Operative procedures may involve cutting or excising scar tissue, dissecting out cysts or masses, removing fibroids or other diseased tissues, or coagulating lesions using electrocautery or lasers. Many of these operative techniques can be implemented at the time of the initial diagnostic evaluation, making the laparoscopic evaluation not only diagnostic but also therapeutic.

A physician may choose to do laparoscopy if he or she suspects pelvic disease or, more commonly, as part of a complete infertility evaluation. Pelvic disorders may be found even when not previously elicited by physical examination. Therefore, diagnostic laparoscopy is frequently done prior to initiating ovulation induction. It is also commonly performed in couples with unexplained infertility.

OTHER TESTING

As is evident from the above, the variety of tests to determine the cause of infertility currently available is small. Usually the diagnostic evaluation can be completed within the course of a month or two. However, many couples are found to have completely normal test results, even despite many years of infertility. Of course, this does not mean that there is no reason for their infertility; rather, the diagnosis of "unexplained infertility" simply means that our current testing methodologies are insufficiently sensitive to detect the actual cause.

In order to further elucidate more subtle causes of infertility, physicians and scientists working in the field of reproduction are constantly trying to improve the diagnostic accuracy of testing. Examples include biological testing of sperm for their capacity to fertilize the egg, detection of uterine substances that may be involved in the implantation process, and the measurement of antibodies circulating in the body that may interfere with both fertilization and implantation. Although couples with uncertain diagnoses may understandably chase such testing, it is important to note that newly developed tests must undergo extensive experimental investigation before they are deemed to be of any usefulness. Many tests that were once thought to add great insight to the diagnostic evaluation have proven to be of limited value. Therefore, great caution should be exercised in interpreting and valuing the results of tests that have not yet been accepted by the medical community as part of the standard evaluation.

It should be emphasized that, despite our limited ability to assess the cause of infertility in many cases, treatment for most cases of infertility is available and generally successful, even for couples with unexplained infertility.

Treatment Strategies

An obvious principle of medical treatment is that it should follow diagnosis and identification of the problem whenever possible. In other words, treatment should be directed toward correcting a specific disorder. However sensible this notion, it is nonetheless true that many women are given hormonal treatments to treat their infertility despite inadequate evaluation. The reasons for this are complex, and call into play the pressures that infertility puts on women and their caregivers. Every woman with infertility has heard of "fertility pills." They often think of them as a simple, almost magical solution for infertility, no matter what the cause. In actuality, the term refers to clomiphene, a stimulant of egg development in the ovaries (see next section) that is useful for the correction of only certain types of infertility. This view of clomiphene therapy as a benign intervention may compel them to request, and to be given, prescriptions for clomiphene by their gynecologists. It is never appropriate, however, to use clomiphene as the first response to infertility. In recent years, prolonged exposure (more than twelve months) to clomiphene has been associated with the occurrence of certain types of ovarian tumors.[22] For this medication to be used safely, therefore, other causes of infertility must first be ruled out and the therapy monitored to assure that maximum benefit is being achieved.

Assuming that a thorough evaluation as defined above has been completed and that the source of infertility is pinpointed, treatment should then be directed toward correcting the specific cause of infertility. Examples would include the following:

SURGICAL REPAIR

The most straightforward correction of infertility occurs when a specific anatomical disorder has been identified and it is surgically correctible. Most structural damage to the reproductive organs is acquired, resulting from prior pelvic surgery, infection, or endometriosis. Any of these conditions may cause scarring or closure of the fallopian tubes and thereby block the key passageway for conception. Surgical repair may be accomplished by laparoscopy or open surgery (laparotomy). When successful, surgery is followed by the occurrence of pregnancy in the natural manner and within an acceptable time frame. The extent of the underlying damage is as important as the skill of the surgeon in determining the chances for postoperative success.

It should be noted that the time frame for success with surgery is the same as for any couple beginning to attempt conception. Assuming that the surgery is successful, it is expected that conception may take up to a year to occur. Many women who undergo surgical correction become impatient with this time interval. Expectations for pregnancy are best reviewed with the reproductive surgeon prior to undergoing surgery. In women who are in their later reproductive years, and particularly those who are past the age of 40, surgical correction of anatomic disease may not be appropriate because of the anticipated long time frame for success.

OVULATION INDUCTION

Ovulation induction (OI) is used to treat myriad disorders that interfere with the regularity of ovulation or prevent ovulation altogether. Indirectly, ovulation may be induced by administering thyroid hormone to a hypothyroid woman, bromocriptine to a woman who has hyperpolactinemia, or steroids to a woman with an overly active adrenal gland (most commonly a result of congenital adrenal hyperplasia). In recent years, women who fail to ovulate because they have polycystic ovary syndrome (PCOS) have been treated with Metformin. Metformin is an insulin sensitizing agent that can correct insulin resistance in women with PCOS, causing the ovary to ovulate spontaneously. These are all forms of OI. However, ovulation induction is more commonly thought of as the intentional and direct stimulation of the ovaries to ovulate.

Clomiphene

The most commonly used medication for OI is clomiphene citrate (Clomid®, Serophene®). Clomiphene works by blocking receptors for estrogen in the pituitary gland, causing it to sense a low estrogen environment. The pituitary gland responds by releasing more FSH. In response to the higher FSH levels, the ovary begins the process of egg maturation. If the dosage of clomiphene is appropriate, normal ovulation will ensue.

Clomiphene has been used for ovulation induction since the late 1960s. It is safe, relatively inexpensive and has relatively few side effects. The expected twinning rate with clomiphene is 5–8%, and only 0.5% of women who conceive with clomiphene have more than two fetuses. It is commonly taken for five days at the beginning of a menstrual cycle, with little or no monitoring of response required. The ease with which this drug can be administered has enhanced the prevalence of its use for appropriate as well as inappropriate indications.

Gonadotropins

Gonadotropins are a class of medications identical to the natural pituitary hormones FSH and LH which control egg development in the ovary. These medications are used as alternatives to clomiphene when it fails to induce ovulation or pregnancy, or when certain clinical circumstances make the use of gonadotropins preferable. Nearly all in vitro fertilization cycles require preparation with gonadotropins.

Gonadotropins are commonly given over a period of seven to ten days in order to stimulate growth and maturation of eggs. The dose used to produce the desired effect is individualized for each patient and may vary from day to day and from one cycle to the next. The response to therapy must be monitored by frequent measurements of blood estrogen levels and ultrasound examinations of the ovaries. When egg follicles are of the appropriate size and the appropriate estrogen level is achieved, ovulation is triggered with the use of hCG (human chorionic gonadotropin). Intercourse, insemination or egg retrieval for in vitro fertilization is then planned.

The cost of gonadotropin therapy is high, often running in the thousands of dollars for each treatment cycle. Approximately 25% of pregnancies induced with gonadotropins are multifetal, most being twins. The triplet rate is approximately 5%. Another problem with gonadotropin use is the risk of Ovarian Hyperstimulation Syndrome, a condition that in its severest form may result in ovarian enlargement, abdominal bloating, dehydration and clot formation. Rare complications of severe ovarian hyperstimulation can be fatal. Proper monitoring can prevent complications and also maximize the efficacy of therapy. Unlike clomiphene use, gonadotropin therapy is generally restricted to the domain of the reproductive endocrinologist.

GnRH analogs

Gonadotropin releasing hormone, or GnRH, is produced in a central area of the brain called the hypothalamus and is, reproductively speaking, the master hormone. It controls the pituitary production and release of LH and FSH, which in turn control ovarian function. In recent years, a new class of medication has been developed by modification of the natural GnRH molecule. These GnRH analogs selectively bind to the gonadotropin-producing cells of the pituitary gland and exert the opposite effect of GnRH; that is, they *turn off* the secretion of LH and FSH. Without these two hormones, natural egg maturation in the ovary essentially shuts down, allowing the reproductive specialist complete control over ovarian function. Two classes of GnRH analogs are currently available. One is a class of *agonist* hormones (Lupron®, Synarel®), which temporarily stimulate and then suppress pituitary function. The other, *antagonist* hormones (Antagon®, Cetrotide®), result in immediate suppression of pituitary function. GnRH analogs are generally used in conjunction with gonadotropins when complete control is necessary. This includes many cases of ovulation induction and almost all cases when the ovaries are being stimulated in preparation for in vitro fertilization.

Safety of Ovulation Induction

Intense media interest in assisted reproductive technologies has focused the attention of the general public, as well as couples with infertility, on a possible link between fertility drugs and cancer, in particular ovarian cancer. Because the use of ovulation-inducing agents to treat infertility is so common, with more than two million women using these drugs worldwide every year, it is important to put this issue into proper perspective.

Ovarian cancer is the fourth most common cause of cancer-related death in women, although it accounts for a mere 4% of all female cancers. The high degree of mortality is due to the fact that there are no reliable screening methods for ovarian cancer, and therefore most women diagnosed with ovarian cancer are already at an advanced stage. Most studies of ovarian cancer in previous users of fertility drugs are limited by one or more methodological biases. Women who have been studied for an increased risk of ovarian cancer due to fertility drugs are infertile and have been compared in most cases to women who are not infertile. But studies reveal that there is a general increased risk of ovarian cancer in infertile women, regardless of treatment. This makes it hard to isolate any specific effect of treatment as the cause for increased risk. Additionally, the observation in many of these studies of cancers arising within two years of the start of fertility treatments begs the question of whether the fertility drugs are *stimulating growth* of already preexisting malignancies, as opposed to actually *causing* cancer.

Controversy surrounding this issue remains intense despite much reassuring data. What bears reiterating is the fact that infertility is itself a risk factor for ovarian cancer. This has been shown in virtually every study, with increased risk estimates ranging from two to six-fold. Many of these studies also suggest that the risk of ovarian cancer in infertile women is greatest when the infertility is due to ovulatory problems. This suggests that women who are successful with their treatment *lower* their risk of ovarian cancer. Nearly every study of risk factors for ovarian cancer has demonstrated that childbirth is protective. It has been estimated that each birth reduces a woman's lifetime risk of ovarian cancer by 20%. Nursing further reduces this risk. These facts together make a compelling case for the correction of ovulatory infertility.

It is also important to note that the actual underlying risk that any woman will develop ovarian cancer in her lifetime is approximately 1.5%. A *doubling* of that risk would raise the actual risk for an individual woman to only 3%. While most studies show *no* increased risk, the small actual risks identified by some studies would likely not deter most women from treatment, providing that treatment with "fertility drugs" were the only reasonable way they could start a family.

If studies concerning a link between ovarian cancer and infertility treatment are inconclusive, studies regarding a link to breast cancer are negative—i.e., fertility treatment does not seem to increase the risk of a woman incurring breast cancer. Breast cancer is the most common cause of malignancy among women and the second most common cause of death due to cancer. The lifetime risk for a woman approaches 12.5%. It is thought that bearing fewer children and the use of the female ovarian hormones estrogen and progesterone increase the risk of succumbing to this tumor. The role of ovarian hormones was supported by the observation that removal of both ovaries before the age of 35 decreased the risk of breast cancer by 60 to 70%.

Large studies have found no statistical elevation in breast cancer in treated infertile women as compared to fertile women, which negates the possibility of a causal relationship between infertility, fertility drug use, and breast cancer. Several studies have found no statistical difference in the occurrence of breast cancer in infertile women exposed to fertility treatments, as opposed to those who were not. Other studies have separated women with breast cancer and a history of infertility according to the causes of their infertility, and found no significant elevation in the risk among those with hormonal dysfunction as the cause.

Further research regarding the safety of fertility drugs is ongoing. Currently, the American Society of Reproductive Medicine recommends limiting the use of clomiphene to no more than six months. At the current time, there is no data to support specific restrictions on the use of injectable gonadotropins.[23] While all patients need to be aware of the potential risks of fertility drugs, current information about the safety of these medications should be reassuring to women who require their use.

Another concern commonly expressed by women contemplating or undergoing ovulation induction relates to their mistaken impression that ovulation induction uses up their egg supply more rapidly and, therefore, will bring about an earlier menopause. This is not correct. During a normal menstrual cycle, eggs are constantly activated to go through the cycle of maturation and atresia, essentially growth and death. Approximately 1,000 egg follicles are lost to this process each month, with only one escaping and ovulating. This accounts for the loss of approximately 400,000 egg follicles, the normal complement at the onset of puberty, through the completion of approximately 400 ovulatory cycles during the average woman's reproductive life-span. When their effect is optimal, ovulation agents rescue a few follicles that would otherwise have succumbed to atresia, allowing them to achieve maturity and ovulation. These medications cannot, however, accelerate the rate of egg loss.

INSEMINATION

Artificial insemination is often, but not exclusively, used to treat couples who are infertile as a result of male factors. Semen abnormalities involving mild abnormalities in sperm count, motility, or morphology are often overcome by insemination. Less commonly, but with good success, artificial insemination is used in cases where the sperm do not naturally come into contact with the female reproductive tract. One example is retrograde ejaculation, a condition resulting in the ejaculate flowing backward into the bladder. This is most often found in men with a history of diabetes or trauma to the neck of the bladder. It can also be a side effect of certain

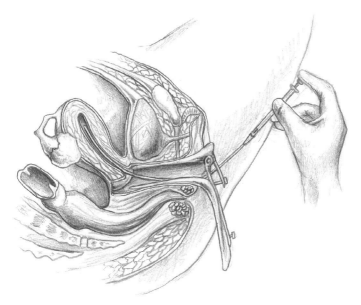

Intrauterine insemination: Sperm is injected through a soft catheter into the upper reaches of the uterine cavity

medications. Other examples include anatomical abnormalities and sexual dysfunction, or cases when sperm have been frozen for storage prior to chemotherapy or testicular surgery. Artificial insemination may also be used to overcome female factors, such as disorders that prevent sperm from traversing the cervix to the uterus.

The most commonly used technique is intrauterine insemination (IUI), in which sperm are placed past the cervix directly into the uterus. This allows large numbers of sperm to reach the fallopian tubes, where fertilization occurs. The procedure requires that the semen specimen first be processed, or "washed," in order to separate the seminal fluid and dead sperm from the most active sperm. The result is usually a concentrated suspension of the most highly potent sperm. The sperm suspension is subsequently inserted into the uterus using a very thin, soft plastic catheter.

OVULATION INDUCTION WITH INSEMINATION

Although OI and IUI are distinct treatment modalities, they are commonly used in combination, especially in instances of unexplained infertility. This type of infertility is common for two reasons. Firstly, complete evaluation will fail to reveal the cause of infertility in at least 10% of infertile couples. Secondly, many couples who are treated, either for male or female causes, fail to conceive. When correcting the known cause of infertility fails to produce a pregnancy, such a couple may also be said to have unexplained infertility.

It is important to point out that, in cases of unexplained infertility, OI and IUI must be used in conjunction with each other in order for them to be successful. IUI alone or OI alone have not been shown to be efficacious.[24] The same is true in the treatment of mild male factor infertility. In both cases, per cycle success rates for OI and IUI in combination are better with gonadotropins than with clomiphene.

Couples undergoing treatment cycles with any modality should be careful to distinguish between the expected pregnancy rate and the expected pregnancy rate *per cycle* of treatment. In the example cited above, couples treated with OI+IUI had a 33%

	Pregnancy rate per couple	Pregnancy rate per cycle
Cervical insemination alone	10%	2%
IUI alone	18%	5%
OI + cervical insemination	19%	4%
OI + IUI	33%	9%

Typical Results of OI and IUI

chance of conceiving during the duration of the study. However, their chance of conceiving on any one cycle was 9%. The per cycle pregnancy rates are cumulative, accounting for the discrepancy. As already noted earlier in this chapter, fertility treatment is a process that has a certain chance of succeeding over time. Couples are best served by adjusting their expectations prior to the onset of therapy, so that frustration with that process does not interfere with its completion.

ASSISTED REPRODUCTION

Assisted reproduction refers to harvesting gametes (sperm and eggs), processing them in the laboratory, and implanting them in a woman with the expectation that pregnancy will occur. It includes a variety of procedures that are and have been used in order to alleviate infertility. These are discussed in further detail in Part IV, "Assisted Reproduction."

Original indications for the use of assisted reproduction were limited to diseases of the fallopian tube requiring in vitro fertilization (IVF). With the improvement of the assisted reproductive technologies (ART) and the limited usefulness of other modalities for certain conditions, the use of ART has become widespread for many indications. In addition to its use in the treatment of common causes of infertility, ART is used in all cases where egg donation is needed (as in the case of premature ovarian failure); whenever a gestational surrogate is required; and when a history of genetic disease indicates that preimplantation genetic diagnosis is required to assure the delivery of a healthy baby.

Assisted reproduction was once thought of as a last resort therapy. This was due to the low success rate, high cost, and invasiveness of the procedures. Many of these difficulties no longer hold true. IVF as currently practiced is minimally invasive, has high success rates especially in younger women and, increasingly, insurance companies have agreed to cover its cost.[25] Because of these changes, assisted reproduction has assumed its natural, medically-driven position as just one of many possibilities in the treatment armamentarium of the reproductive specialist. Exactly when and how it is used depends on the treatment strategy that is worked out with each individual couple.

Indications for IVF

Anatomical disease
    Endometriosis
    Adhesions
    Tubal blockage
Unexplained infertility
    Failure to concieve with other treatments
Severe male factor

Treatment Algorithms

A variety of factors has led physicians to develop standardized treatment strategies for certain diseases. These directives for treatment have been organized into flow charts called algorithms. The algorithms take into account the statistical probability of success with each intervention and are based on best practices as identified by experts in the field. Many algorithms also take into account the cost of each intervention.

MANAGEMENT OF INFERTILITY IN
PATIENTS WITH ENDOMETRIOSIS

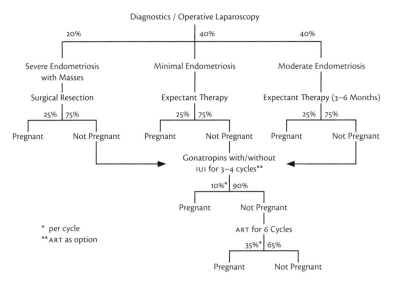

Example of Treatment Algorithm[27]

Infertility in particular lends itself to treatment algorithms,[26] as the treatment has a clearly defined end point—pregnancy. Also, regimens and protocols used for treating infertile couples have predictable outcomes that make it possible to develop statistical tables for the probability of success. Some insurance companies "manage" infertility care by requiring that physicians follow strict treatment algorithms. Alternatively, physicians who are paid fixed fees for managing infertility may follow algorithms in their attempt to provide the most cost-efficient care.

Many treatment algorithms are based on the supposition that repeated exposure is necessary for success to occur, but that the probability of success with repeated exposure declines after three attempts. For example, it is well known that 90% of pregnancies that occur in response to ovulation induction with clomiphene will occur within the first three ovulatory cycles. Each of these three months carries with it an approximate 30% chance of success, so failure on the first cycle does not affect the chance of success on the second cycle, and failure on the second cycle also does not affect the chance of success in the third cycle. The remaining 10% of pregnancies that occur with clomiphene are spread out over the fourth through the sixth cycles. This means that if three ovulatory cycles have failed to produce a pregnancy, the statistical likelihood of success in subsequent cycles diminishes considerably. A more aggressive intervention is subsequently introduced.

In couples being treated for ovulatory dysfunction, mild sperm abnormalities, or unexplained infertility, it is common to begin therapy with clomiphene and intrauterine insemination. When a treatment cycle does not result in pregnancy, the physician will review the ovulatory response and the results of sperm washing for insemination. If the parameters are normal, then a repeated attempt is made. Sometimes the ovulation induction protocol is modified in order to elicit a better response. Overall, approximately 30% of women so treated will conceive. If three cycles of treatment with a reasonably normal response do not result in pregnancy, treatment with gonadotropins and intrauterine insemination is usually instituted. Again, therapy is limited to three cycles. Overall, approximately 40% of women so treated will conceive. The remainder are generally put into a program of in vitro fertilization. It is helpful for patients and their physicians to review these treatment strategies prior to their onset. Knowing what their fallback options are is often reassuring to patients embarking on a treatment plan. Also, it is helpful for couples to understand from the outset that having one or two failed cycles does not necessarily indicate that the treatment strategy is faulty.

Many factors will determine how strictly the treatment algorithm is followed. Fertility treatment centers with well-established programs for assisted reproduction may view in vitro fertilization as the surest and quickest route to pregnancy, and tend to fast-track patients to IVF. This is justifiable for younger patients because their expected success rates are so high. It is equally justifiable for older patients, because their expected success rates are low enough with conventional therapies that there seems to be a compelling need for them to get to aggressive therapy quickly. Cost factors may also play a role. Couples facing the prospect of having to pay the high price of gonadotropins may look to assisted reproduction as a more efficient use of their financial resources, especially if their insurance covers them for parts of their treatment.

Algorithms may also be side-stepped for purely medical reasons. Among the most common is the desire to avoid multifetal pregnancy. It has been suggested that IVF, when used judiciously, can decrease the risk of high order multifetal pregnancies (more than twins).[28] Younger women, women with PCOS and women who hyper-respond to ovarian stimulants are all at risk for developing complex multifetal pregnancy. Although multifetal pregnancy reduction is feasible in most circumstances (see Part VI "New Ethical Issues"), the procedure is psychologically traumatic and occasionally results in complete loss of the pregnancy. On the other hand, multifetal pregnancy is a serious complication of fertility therapy, with many significant costs to both the couple and to society, and solving it has been identified by reproductive endo-crinologists as one of their highest priorities.[29] IVF can be used to limit the number of embryos that reach the uterus and therefore the risk of multifetal pregnancy.

A problem often encountered by observant Jewish couples with infertility is that they will not fit neatly into established treat-ment algorithms used by their physicians. As already noted, the chronology of diagnostic testing is often reversed because of the requirement that semen analysis come toward the end, rather than the beginning, of the evaluation. In addition, treatment itself is also subject to the demands of halakha. Thus, many couples with unexplained infertility are reluctant to undergo IUI in conjunc-tion with their ovulation induction due to halakhic considerations. Some may be averse to using gonadotropins because of their fear of multifetal pregnancy. In vitro fertilization, while accepted among most rabbinic authorities, is nevertheless viewed as a last resort. It is not uncommon for couples undergoing ovulation induction and IUI for male factor to persist with this treatment even after multiple failed cycles because of their reluctance to move on to

IVF. In any situation where the couple requests that their physician deviate significantly from accepted medical practice, it is crucial for the physician to ascertain if the reason for the departure is the expressed unwillingness of the couple's rabbi to permit the needed therapy or the couple's *assumption* that permission would not be granted. If the latter is the case, then it is helpful to include the rabbi in the consultative process. Couples are often surprised that, when there is clear medical rationale, the halakha allows great latitude for their rabbinical authority to issue instructions that will facilitate success.

Summary

Most cases of infertility are treatable. When possible, it is desirable to accurately determine the cause of infertility and to direct therapy specifically to solving that problem. However, accurate diagnosis is not always possible. In such cases, and also in cases where correction of the known problem is not successful, empirical therapies using ovulation induction, insemination, or assisted reproduction are indicated. The exact progression and time frames for these interventions depends on the particular clinical circumstances, including the woman's age, the length of their infertility, the results of specific fertility testing, and the couple's emotional readiness to move forward to the next step. Until pregnancy is reached, most couples will not have complete confidence in the steps they are taking. Proper counseling prior to treatment, including the rationale for therapy as well as the expected time frame for success, is essential in order to keep the couple focused on the imperatives of their care. While it is true that halakhic concerns may pose obstacles to following through with standard, medically accepted treatment options, the halakha does allow great latitude in fertility care. When problems arise, the inclusion of the couple's rabbinical authority in the decision-making process is essential. Proper communication between the couple, the physician and their rabbi facilitates expert caregiving and also gives the couple the psychological comfort they may require in order to persist in the sometimes long road to pregnancy.

Endnotes

1. J. Abma, A. Chandra, W. Mosher, et al. "Fertility, family planning, and women's health: New data from the 1995 National Survey of Family Growth," National Center for Health Statistics, Vital Health Statistics 23:19, (1997).
2. D.L. Olive, "Analysis of clinical fertility trials: a methodological review," in E.E. Wallach, R.D. Kempers, eds. *Modern Trends in Infertility and Conception Control* (Chicago: Year Book Medical Publishers, Inc., 1988).
3. J.D. Biggers, "In vitro fertilization and embryo transfer in human beings," *New England Journal of Medicine*, 304:336–42, (1981). X. Wang, C. Chen, L. Wang, et al. "Conception, early pregnancy loss, and time to clinical pregnancy: A population-based prospective study," *Fertility and Sterility*, 79:577–584, (2003).
4. K. Pezeshki, D.E. Stein, S.M. Lobel, J. Feldman, R.V. Grazi, "Bleeding and spontaneous abortion following therapy for infertility," *Fertility and Sterility*, 74:504, (2000).
5. *Yalkut Shimoni*, Tehillim 247:617.
6. The expected length of a normal human pregnancy is 40 weeks from the last menstrual period prior to conception. Any pregnancy that progresses beyond 37 completed weeks is considered to have reached "term." It is worth noting that obstetricians, by convention, date pregnancy from the last period, even though, in the average situation, conception does not occur until 14 days later. This is why the gestational age as computed by the obstetrician is never the same as embryologic age. The difference is occasionally important halakhically, as when determining if a miscarriage has caused *peter rehem*.
7. BMI can be used as a means of standardization across cultural or time period variations. From these evaluations, multiple conclusions may be drawn. Depending on which scale is used, it can either be measured using inches and pounds, or meters and kilograms.

$$\mathrm{BMI} = \frac{Weight\ in\ Pounds}{(\text{height in inches}) \times (\text{height in inches})} \times 703$$

or

$$\mathrm{BMI} = \frac{Weight\ in\ Kilograms}{(\text{height in meters}) \times (\text{height in meters})}$$

For adults, the use of body mass index or BMI to define overweight does not depend on age or gender. For the purposes of this equation, people 20 years or older are considered adults.

8. J. Bellver, L.P. Rossal, E. Bosch, et al., "Obesity and the risk of spontaneous abortion after oocyte donation," *Fertility and Sterility* 79:1136–40, (2003).

9. M.I. Cedergren, "Maternal morbid obesity and the risk of adverse pregnancy outcome," *Obstetrics and Gynecology* 103:219–24, (2004) M.L. Watkins, S.A. Rasmussen, M.A. Honein. "Maternal obesity and risk of birth defects," *Pediatrics* 111:1152–1158, (2003).

10. The "cystic" in the term "polycystic" ovary should be distinguished from other ovarian cysts, which are benign or malignant tumors of the ovary and require removal. The "cysts" in PCOS are just tiny egg follicles that do not mature properly. They represent physiologic structures and almost never require surgical removal.

11. B. Haas, R. Carr, G.C. Attia, "Effects of metformin on body mass index, menstrual cyclicity and ovulation induction in women with polycystic ovary syndrome," *Fertility and Sterility,* 79:469–481, (2003).

12. *Tzitz Eliezer,* vol. 9 #51:3 (1968); *Tzitz Eliezer,* vol. 12 #102, (1979).

13. The halakhic issues involved in the various physical examinations described are discussed in further detail in the following chapter, "Diagnostic Procedures in the Female Patient."

14. L. Speroff, R.H. Glass, N.G. Kase. *Clinical Gynecologic Endocrinology and Infertility,* 5th ed. (William and Wilkins, 1994).

15. Some women are frankly menopausal—having exhausted their entire egg supply—even in their teens. This is most often, but not always, due to a genetic abnormality.

16. A.J. Levi, M.F. Raynault, P.A. Bergh, et al., "Reproductive outcome in patients with diminished ovarian reserve," *Fertility and Sterility,* 76:666–669, (2001).

17. Men who produce any sperm at all, even if only in very small numbers and only in the testes itself, can still father children using in vitro fertilization and intracytoplasmic sperm injection. Traditional distinctions between fertility and sterility therefore may not hold true in today's clinical setting.

18. T.F. Kruger, R. Menkveld, F.S.H. Stander, et al., "Sperm morphological features as a prognostic factor in in vitro fertilization," *Fertility and Sterility,* 46:1118–1123, (1986).

19. See cervival mucus illustration, figure 6

20. A common perception of women with infertility is that they do not conceive because they lose semen after intercourse. Folklore abounds in sexual techniques and positions that minimize semen leakage from the vagina. It is important to note that this phenomenon is normal and occurs in fertile women also. The importance of cervical mucus is that it acts as a reservoir for normally motile sperm, even if the seminal fluid is lost in the normal postcoital discharge.

21. Women who have known histories of allergy to iodine generally should not undergo hysterosalpingogram.

22. M.A. Rossing, J.R. Daling, et al., "Ovarian tumors in a cohort of infertile women," *New England Journal of Medicine,* 331:771–776, (1994).

23. S. Kashyap, O.K. Davis, "Ovarian cancer and fertility medications: A critical appraisal," *Seminars in Reproductive Medicine.* 21:65–71, (2003).

R.T. Burkman, C.T. Mei-Tzu, K.E. Malone, et al., "Infertility drugs and the risk of breast cancer: Findings from the National Institute of Child Health and Human Development Women's Contraceptive and Reproductive Experiences Study," *Fertility and Sterility*, 79:844–851, (2003).

24. D.S. Guzick, S.A. Carson, C. Coutifaris, et al., "Efficacy of superovulation and intrauterine insemination in the treatment of infertility," *New England Journal of Medicine*, 340:177–183, (1999).

25. The rationale for the shift in the policies of insurers ranges from a reaction to coercion from state legislatures (which have passed mandated coverage laws in several states) to voluntary expansion of benefits as a means of controlling the cost of care.

26. See G.W. Bates, S.R. Bates, "The economics of infertility: Developing an infertility managed care plan," *American Journal of Obstetrics and Gynecology* 174:1200–7, (1996).

27. R.E. Blackwell. "Algorithm for evaluation and treatment of infertility." Update in *Infertility and Reproductive Endocrinology*, vol. 7, no. 3, (July, 1995).

28. T. Jain, B.L. Harlow, M.D. Hornstein, "Insurance coverage and outcomes of in vitro fertilization," *New England Journal of Medicine*, 347:661–666, (2002).

29. Proceedings of an expert meeting: "Infertility therapy-associated multiple pregnancies (births): An ongoing epidemic," *Reproductive Biology Online*, vol. 7, suppl. 2, (2003).

Richard Weiss

Diagnostic Procedures in the Female Patient

Introduction to the Laws of *Niddah*

The halakhot (religious laws) surrounding a woman's menstrual cycle form the basic backdrop of our discussion as they govern the normal sexual life of a religiously committed Jewish couple. An understanding of these basic concepts is indispensable to the professional managing fertility therapy for an observant couple. In general, this is a very complicated area of halakha and requires a particular expertise to be able to render proper judgments. There exists a core of biblical law surrounded by a host of rabbinic legislation. On a practical level, individuals do not differentiate between biblical and rabbinic prohibitions. However, when a rabbi is faced with a difficult set of social circumstances, the fact that a particular prohibition might be rabbinic rather that biblical gives him legitimate leeway in addressing the problem.

　　Biblically, a distinction exists between a *niddah*, a woman who experiences vaginal bleeding derived from the uterus during her expected menstrual period, and a *zavah*, a woman who experiences bleeding at times other than during her expected period.[1] A woman is a *niddah* for seven days from the onset of normal menstrual bleeding, regardless of the duration of bleeding, provided that all bleeding has stopped prior to sunset of the seventh day.[2] Shortly before sunset of the seventh day, the woman performs an internal examination to be certain that the bleeding has actually stopped.[3] A *zavah*, as more precisely defined by the Talmud, is a woman who experiences bleeding during the eleven days immediately after completing a seven day sequence of *niddah*.[4] If bleeding occurs on three consecutive days during the eleven day period, the woman begins a sequence of seven clean days, but only after all bleeding has ceased. To ascertain this fact she performs an internal examination prior to sunset of the last day of bleeding. (For bleeding of less than three consecutive days, a status of *zavah* is created but of a lesser form, without the need for a full sequence of seven clean days.) Both a *niddah* and a *zavah* immerse themselves in a *mikvah* at the conclusion of their respective seven day periods.[5] From the onset of bleeding until the conclusion of the seven days, all sexual intercourse and other physical modes of affection are prohibited between a woman and her husband.[6] It is only after immersion in the *mikvah* that these restrictions are lifted.[7]

Biblically, an important precondition for a woman to become either a *niddah* or a *zavah* is that she experience an awareness or sensation of the bleeding occurring.[8] Three forms of sensation are described in rabbinic literature.[9] They are: 1) the sensation of an internal flow of fluid (blood) exiting the uterus; 2) the sensation of the opening of the entrance to the uterus, or cervix, (to allow for the egress of blood); 3) physical sequelae associated with the discharge of blood or the opening of the uterus, such as a tremor of the body. We will return to the issue of sensation later in the discussion.

The laws of *niddah* have developed through various stages. The most influential development was the undertaking of additional stringencies in the time of the Talmud, which caused the distinction between a *niddah* and a *zavah* to become less relevant.[10] In practice, any minute amount of bleeding—with or without any associated

Richard Weiss

sensation and regardless of the timing of such bleeding—invokes the stringencies of both a *niddah* and a *zavah*.[11] In addition, all bleeding must cease before observing a required interval of seven clean days.[12] The woman goes to the *mikvah* on the evening following the conclusion of the seventh clean day and is then permitted to have intimate relations with her husband.[13] These halakhot fundamentally apply to spotting as well.[14] Furthermore, any amount of bleeding or spotting during the seven clean days cancels this sequence retroactively, thus requiring a new seven-day series.[15]

The Rama, Rabbi Moses Isserles (c. 1520–1572), records the additionally accepted practice that a woman does not begin the seven day sequence until at least five days after the onset of menstrual bleeding or spotting.[16] The first day of bleeding is included in these five additional days.[17] (The reason for this rabbinical amendment is related to the impurity that the semen deposited in the woman's reproductive tract can cause.[18] The halakha, however, applies regardless of any actual intercourse having taken place.)[19] Thus, a woman committed to following the halakha is unable to have sexual relations with her husband for a minimum of twelve days, regardless of the length of her menstrual bleeding or spotting. For example, if a woman's first day of menstruation occurs between Saturday night and Sunday evening, she must wait until Thursday when, if the flow ceased, she performs an internal examination before sunset to verify this fact and begins the seven day sequence that night. During the seven days, she must continue to perform internal examinations with a cloth or pad.[20] Assuming that no further bleeding occurs during the seven clean days, the sequence ends on the following Thursday evening, at which time she immerses herself in a *mikvah*.

In the course of our discussion, we will mention the positions of classic and contemporary rabbinic authorities whose opinions have wide currency in the halakhic community. While the names may be irrelevant for the medical professional, they are important for the rabbinic authorities who address these issues. (Dates are not given for contemporary authorities.)

191

Basic Principles

The diagnostic procedures used in the evaluation of the infertile woman are closely related to four major issues within the laws of *niddah*: anatomy, physiologic effects on menstrual flow, cervical dilation, and injury, or *makkah*. First and formost are the issues of anatomy. We begin, therefore, with a brief description of the female reproductive tract.[21]

ANATOMY

The female anatomy is divided into "external" and "internal" organs. The external organs include the labia majora and minora, clitoris, vestibule, urethral opening and hymen. The labia (lips) majora are two rounded folds of adipose tissue, or fat, covered with skin and hair. They cover the labia minora, which are two flat folds of skin which are reddish in color. The labia minora converge superiorly, or above, to form the clitoris, a small cylinder-like body similar in some respects to the male penis. The area enclosed by the labia minora is termed the vestibule. The urethra (from the urinary bladder) opens into the vestibule as does the vagina. The vagina opens into the lower portion of the vestibule and the urethra above that. The hymen is a skin like membrane, or covering, that surrounds the vaginal opening more or less completely. It has a small opening which allows for blood to flow out. Because it contains many blood vessels, tearing of the hymen during the first intercourse usually results in bleeding. On occasion the hymen is resistant to penetration by the penis and a surgical procedure is required to open it.

The vagina, the first of the internal organs, is an elastic, muscular tube that extends to the uterus. It sits between the urinary bladder anteriorly (toward the front of the body) and rectum posteriorly (toward the back of the body). It functions in the act of intercourse and as the birth canal. The lower end of the cervix, or neck of the uterus, projects into the upper end of the vagina at a 45°–90° angle. It has two oses, or openings: the external os (mouth) that opens into the vagina and the internal os that opens into the uterus. They are separated by the cervical canal, which measures

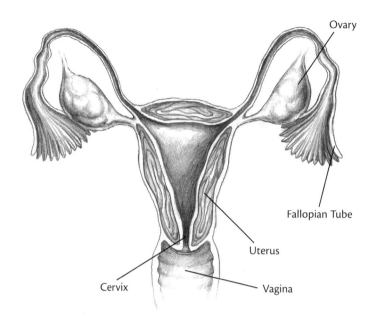

Normal female anatomy

about three to four centimeters in length. The external os is usually open about three millimeters in diameter.

The uterus is a flattened, pear shaped, muscular organ lined with a tissue called the endometrium. It, too, sits between the bladder and rectum and is continuous with the cervix below. The fallopian tubes are connected to the uterus. At their other (lateral) ends, they lie in close proximity to the ovaries. Sperm are transmitted to this region of the tube via the vagina, cervix, and uterus. Mature eggs are captured in this area of the tube during the process of ovulation, when an egg is released directly through the surface of the ovary. If the egg is fertilized, the resulting preembryo is then propelled toward the uterus, where it implants and develops into an embryo and fetus.

The menstrual cycle is a series of regular cyclic changes that occur in preparation for pregnancy, the most prominent being the development of the endometrial lining. If implantation does not take place, the endometrium is shed. This spontaneous shedding is associated with bleeding, primarily from arteries supplying the uterine lining. The menstrual flow contains dead cells of the endometrium mixed with blood. It generally lasts 2–6 days and results in 20–65 milliliters (⅔–2 ounces) of bloody discharge. The blood flows from the uterus through the cervical canal, into the vagina and out of the body.

According to Talmudic law, a woman is not considered a *niddah* unless the bleeding originates from the uterine lining and then flows out of the uterus.[22] A significant discussion exists among the commentators regarding the anatomy of the reproductive tract. Beside the historical interest, the discussion as it relates to the anatomical landmarks that define a state of *niddah* is very significant.

The Mishnah states that the blood must flow from the "inner compartment" into the "outer compartment" but need not flow out of the body to create a state of *niddah*.[23] The simple understanding of commentary is that the blood must flow just past the external os of the cervix.[24] This understanding is adopted by Rabbi Moses Sofer (1762–1839) and is accepted as conclusive by several other authorities.[25]

Based on this approach, one may conclude that the point of demarcation is the external os and any source of bleeding internal to that point is considered "inner" according to the Talmud. Bleeding from the cervical canal could therefore also create a state of *niddah*. (Blood from the cervix outside the external os would be of no significance.) However, no explicit reference to cervical blood is made by Rabbi Sofer, in contrast to Rabbi Avrohom Blumenkrantz, who does state that cervical bleeding creates a state of *niddah,* though he records no specific source for this.[26] On the other hand, Rabbi Shimon Eider refers only to uterine bleeding,[27] and Rabbi Aharon Pfoifer concludes unequivocally that cervical bleeding due to any cause does not create a state of *niddah*, and that only uterine bleeding is significant. As he points out, this is because cyclic shedding and bleeding occur only from the uterus, not the cervix.[28]

A second understanding of the anatomical boundaries is based on the commentary of Rashi, Rabbi Shlomo Yitzhaki (1040–1105).[29] This opinion, quoted by Rabbi Abraham Karelitz

(1878–1953), places the point of demarcation somewhere in the vagina itself, in front of the cervix.[30] Rabbi Shlomo Zalman Auerbach also adopts this view and even interprets Maimonides' commentary in this way, dissenting with Rabbi Sofer's interpretation.[31] Vaginal bleeding from inside this point would be of no significance, as the uterus is the only source of bleeding with halakhic import. The only question is whether cervical bleeding is of importance, as it can be viewed as part of the uterus, and hence included in the "inner compartment" according to this approach as well.

A third approach places the point of demarcation at the internal os. According to this view the woman is a *niddah* as soon as blood enters the cervical canal from the uterus and, obviously, any bleeding from the cervix would be of no significance. This opinion is quoted by Rabbi Auerbach, who rejects it. As a practical matter, this author feels that cervical bleeding, due to any cause, does not create a state of *niddah*, regardless of which approach is adopted. Rabbi Pfoifer's opinion and reasoning quoted above seem most authoritative and logical, though some authors do present evidence to support the notion that cervical bleeding would be halakhically equivalent to that of uterine bleeding.[32] Lastly, blood found anywhere in the vagina during an internal examination imposes a state of *niddah* unless the source of blood is known to be outside the uterus. The same applies to the spotting of undergarments.[33]

PHYSIOLOGIC AND NORMAL FLOW

A second important issue in halakha is what constitutes a normal menstrual flow, and how much import to give the distinction between natural physiologic factors and other factors. The Talmud discusses a "tube" as an exception to the principle that uterine bleeding creates a state of *niddah*. It bases itself on a deduction that in order to impose a state of *niddah*, the blood must flow directly through the reproductive tract and not through some other medium or tube.[34] Thus, if a tube was inserted into the uterus and blood was withdrawn without leaking, the woman would not be a *niddah*.[35] The reason for this exemption, according to some authorities, is that *niddah* blood must be in physical contact with the reproductive tract. The tube functions as an interruption, or barrier, between the flow of the blood and the tract.[36] Accordingly, even if the tube was not inserted completely into the uterine cavity but just beyond the point of demarcation (at the external os) so that the flow of blood never made contact with the "outer compartment," the woman would not be a *niddah*.[37] If the blood is on the external surface of the tube, the woman would be a *niddah*, as there is no physical barrier between the blood and the tract.[38]

Another rationale for the exception of the tube is that the blood must flow naturally and in a normal fashion in order to create a state of *niddah*.[39] From Rabbi Auerbach's writings it would appear that the bleeding must occur as a result of natural causes and not be initiated by other factors. Secondly, the actual flow must also proceed normally and not, for example, assisted by some other means (such as a tube). Even a naturally induced flow which in any manner proceeds abnormally is incorporated into this exemption. Therefore, a natural flow from the uterus that travels in a tube inserted just past the external os would not create a state of *niddah*. (It is not normal for the blood to flow in a tube, regardless of whether or not its egress from the uterus is part of a natural and spontaneous process.)[40] The general concept of a normal physiologic flow has also been developed independently by Rabbi Eliezer Waldenberg. He discusses bleeding resulting from the presence of uterine fibroids, and maintains that a woman becomes a *niddah* only if the flow of blood is part of a natural and normal physiologic process that occurs spontaneously.[41]

According to the analysis suggested above, two of the essential criteria for uterine bleeding to create a state of *niddah* are: 1) The bleeding must be physiologic and spontaneous, i.e. not caused by other factors; 2) The actual flow of the blood must occur in a normal fashion through the reproductive tract. It is this second requirement which is adopted by the *Shulhan Arukh*, the definitive *Code of Jewish Law*, as the explanation for the "tube" exemption discussed above.[42]

It is significant to note that the argument could be made that the nature of the cause of bleeding is irrelevant. As long as the anatomical source is the endometrium, or uterine lining, it is considered *niddah* bleeding by definition. However, there would still be a requirement that the actual flow occur normally and unassisted—not through a tube, for example. This second requirement is the only one explicitly expressed in the Talmud; the first one is not. This is perhaps the most fundamental issue at the heart of the practical matters discussed in this chapter. This author feels that the issue is at present inconclusive and in need of further analysis.

A third rationale which explains the exemption of the tube is that some form of sensation by the woman is required.[43] Flow in a tube occurs without the sensation of something flowing, and is therefore exempt from the biblical laws of *niddah*, which require some kind of sensation associated with the bleeding. Still, such a woman should be a *niddah* based on rabbinic legislation. All authorities agree, however, that with the tube scenario, the woman is not a *niddah* on either a biblical or a rabbinic level.[44] Therefore, this approach has been rejected.

CERVICAL DILATION

A third important issue is that of technical halkhic bleeding—i.e. the creation of a state of *niddah* based on an assumption that bleeding has occurred, regardless of whether actual physical blood has been observed. The Talmud discusses the case of a woman who experiences a miscarriage without any associated bleeding.[45] This phenomenon, as described in the Talmud, is referred to as a "dry birth." Two questions arise. The first is whether such an event is equated with normal delivery, which imposes ritual impurity similar to that of *niddah* upon the woman. The second is, even if it is acceded that such a birth does not constitute a delivery, is the woman still considered a *niddah*, as there might have been unobserved bleeding.[46]

In the discussion regarding the latter possibility, a disagreement emerges as to whether the opening of the cervix is always assumed to be associated with bleeding.[47] Maimonides explains the authoritative view, which is that it is impossible for something to be discharged from the uterus without accompanying bleeding, though the amount of blood may be so minute as to have gone unnoticed.[48] Other commentators explain that the mere probability that bleeding is occurring is sufficient to render the woman a definite *niddah*.[49] Alternatively, the Talmud offers an opinion that it is possible for the cervix to be opened without bleeding and, therefore, such a woman is not definitely classified as a *niddah*.[50] The *Shulhan Arukh* rules that the opening of the cervix is associated with bleeding. Therefore, a woman who experiences a miscarriage even within 40 days of conception (which is not considered a delivery) is assumed to be a *niddah*.[51]

Rabbi Ezekiel Landau (1713–1793) carries this further and maintains that any opening of the cervix, whether internally or externally induced, qualifies as an opening.[52] This would include not only a miscarriage, but also a procedure or examination by a physician which involves the opening of the cervix. This ruling introduced for the first time the possibility of a physician inducing a state of *niddah* in the course of a medical procedure.

Rabbi Abraham Danzig (1748–1820) disagrees with Rabbi Landau.[53] However, it is not clear if he disagrees in principle or only with regard to the reality of a manual pelvic examination causing such an opening.[54] Some authorities question Rabbi Landau's view because he lacks a source.[55] The Talmudic examples all involve an obviously internal delivery or labor process. The birthing process was generally assumed to be associated with bleeding, as due to its nature, the discharge of the uterine contents drags blood along. Therefore, even if the "dry birth" was premature and not labeled technically as a delivery, it was assumed that it was accompanied by bleeding. However, the simple external opening of the cervix does not necessarily result in bleeding.[56]

It is clear from the Talmudic and halakhic discussion that uterine bleeding does not have to occur in the context of menstruation in order to render a woman a *niddah*. Any bleeding, even if it occurs in response to some external stimulus (such as physical activity) imposes a state of *niddah*, provided it is still a physiologic and normal event.[57] It remains questionable whether the opening of the cervix induces a state of *niddah*. While the issue remains incompletely resolved and in need of further analysis, Rabbi Landau's view is adopted in practice by many authorities, including Rabbi Moshe Feinstein.[58]

A further controversy exists over which portion of the cervix, if opened, causes a suspicion of uterine bleeding and, therefore, a state of *niddah*. Some maintain the view that the internal os must be dilated for any concern to arise, while others maintain that dilation of even the external os causes such concern.[59] In support of the first opinion is the anatomical fact that the external os has no real connection with the uterus and, therefore, opening it cannot truly cause uterine bleeding. If the internal os remains closed, the uterus cannot be affected by the pressure generated by the external os being opened.[60] However, Rabbi Auerbach discusses this issue and concludes that the dilation need only occur at the external os to cause concern for uterine bleeding and thereby induce a state of *niddah*.[61]

Another question associated with the dilation of the cervix is the minimum diameter of the opening necessary to create a concern for bleeding. Rabbi Yosef Karo, author of the *Shulhan Arukh*, rules that a very narrow tube does not dilate the cervix sufficiently to stimulate bleeding.[62] Some accept this leniency with the condition that the woman performs an internal examination and that no blood is found.[63] Rabbi Feinstein accepts this view without any such condition and defines the diameter of the opening to be three quarters of an inch, or approximately 19 millimeters.[64] Others record diameters of 15 or 13 millimeters.[65]

MAKKAH

The last issue we will consider is that of a *makkah* (wound). The Talmud and *Shulhan Arukh* rule that bleeding from a wound or lesion does not render the woman a *niddah*, even if the wound is in the uterine lining itself.[66] The exemption of *makkah* does not always require absolute knowledge that the source of bleeding is the wound. As long as it is known that the woman has a wound or lesion, and that this type of wound normally bleeds, the bleeding may be attributed to that wound, and she does not become a *niddah.*[67] However, this rule does not apply at the time that normal menstrual bleeding is expected.[68] The leniency at other times of the menstrual cycle is still appropriate for most women today, though they may experience some degree of irregularity in the timing of their periods.[69] Examples of wounds include fibroids, lacerations, ulcerations, and inflammation.[70] The question is whether a simple abrasion or cut resulting in transient bleeding is considered a *makkah.* In this case, no physical wound existed prior to the bleeding, nor does any gross healing process ensue that might constitute an observable wound. Some authorities seem to consider this a *makkah.* It would appear from the halakha of hymenal bleeding discussed next that any bleeding induced by physical trauma constitutes a *makkah.*

A woman does become a *niddah* on a rabbinic level as a result of the tearing of the hymen during the first intercourse, and the normal laws of *niddah* follow.[71] On occasion, the hymen can be resistant to penetration and a surgical procedure may be required to incise it. Rabbi Feinstein rules that hymenal bleeding following such a procedure does not make a woman a *niddah.* He points out that, in all cases, hymenal bleeding is really only that of *makkah.* While the rabbis nevertheless ruled that hymenal bleeding creates a state of *niddah,* they imposed this injunction only in cases of bleeding resulting from normal intercourse. In cases of instrumentation, the normal law of *makkah* takes over.[72] Even those who disagree with Rabbi Feinstein's conclusion concede that fundamentally this is a case of *makkah.*[73] Therefore, any instrumentation that causes bleeding falls under the category of *makkah.*[74]

Rabbi Feinstein elsewhere seems to be of the opinion that bleeding from the uterus caused by instrumentation renders the woman a *niddah.* He discusses the use of some kind of an electrical instrument, perhaps a laser, in the treatment of fibroids that have become enlarged because of a pregnancy. He claims that if the instrument itself causes bleeding from the uterus not at the site of the wound or lesion, the woman is a *niddah.*[75] The specific case involved the seven clean days, and therefore, they would be cancelled as a result. Although the cause was clearly traumatic,

Rabbi Feinstein did not consider it a *makkah* because the bleeding was not from an actual lesion. However, in yet another case, he implies that instrumentation by the physician *is* considered a *makkah*.[76] Prof. Abraham S. Abraham understands Rabbi Feinstein's view in this way as well.[77] The issue discussed there was that of cervical dilation. Rabbi Feinstein is not concerned if the diameter of the opening is less than three quarters of an inch, as previously discussed. Therefore, if there is bleeding and the physician claims it is due to the instrument, Rabbi Feinstein seems to consider it wound-bleeding, or *makkah*.

It would appear that bleeding caused by any physical trauma should not create a state of *niddah*. As mentioned previously, both Rabbis Auerbach and Waldenberg seem to define *niddah* bleeding as being a natural and spontaneous physiologic process. Any traumatic bleeding is, by its very nature, not a naturally occurring process. For this reason, Rabbi Auerbach claims that even if the same arteries that bleed during menstruation are bleeding as a result of *makkah*, the woman is not a *niddah*.[78] In other words, wound-bleeding falls under the principle derived from the "tube." Such bleeding is not considered the normal mode of bleeding. Furthermore, Rabbi Karelitz, in a response to Dr. Moshe Taub, delineates the various categories of uterine bleeding. He states that bleeding resulting from a cut in the uterine lining is a *makkah*. His argument is that only bleeding from the uterus that is unique to the uterus creates a state of *niddah*. This includes menstruation and the birthing process. However, bleeding that results from other causes that may similarly affect other organs of the body—such as abrasions and lacerations—does not create a state of *niddah*.[79] A woman with this type of bleeding is considered to have a *makkah* and is therefore not to be considered a *niddah*. Elsewhere, Rabbi Karelitz also explains the exemption of *makkah* to be that such bleeding is not considered the normal mode of bleeding from the uterus. Rabbi Pfoifer quotes this latter notion from Rabbi Karelitz as he explains the exemption of *makkah*.[80] Both concepts presented here should be applicable to any traumatic bleeding.[81]

While traumatic bleeding may not create a state of *niddah*, it is still significant for a woman beginning the sequence of seven clean days. All bleeding must cease prior to the seven clean days to enable a woman to realistically and accurately perform internal examinations. Even bleeding due to a *makkah* prevents a woman from discerning whether she is independently still bleeding due to her regular period. This condition applies to the first of the seven days as well, for if bleeding occurs then, the seven day sequence must be reinitiated. The examination prior to beginning the seven clean days (*hefsek taharah*) together with that of day one confer upon a woman a halakhically presumptive state of purity (*hezkat taharah*). Therefore, these two internal examinations must be accurate. If wound bleeding occurs any time after the first day, that bleeding is insignificant and may be disregarded. Rabbi Feinstein makes note of these qualifications in regard to the general exemption of *makkah*.[82] It should be noted that if the trauma was induced by a physician during an examination or procedure, he or she may be relied upon to categorically claim that all the bleeding that was observed was traumatic in origin. Bleeding that occurs sometime after the physician has completed the procedure cannot be categorically assumed to be entirely traumatic in origin, even if the physician claims it to be. In such a case, all bleeding must stop prior to beginning the seven clean days.[83]

The Gynecological Exam

We now turn to various gynecological examinations and their possible impact on a patient's *niddah* status. A preliminary word, however, is necessary on the issue of modesty.

Women who observe the laws of *niddah* maintain a commitment to laws of modesty that run counter to contemporary norms. Thus, for example, a male doctor should be aware that a religious woman would be very uncomfortable being left alone with a man—even her doctor—in a closed room, even before the physical examination has begun. Some patients may feel uncomfortable in asking for a nurse to be present, thinking that the doctor might take offense. Here, the doctor should take the initiative in guaranteeing that a third person is present in the room, or that the door to an adjacent occupied room is left open.

Based on the preceding presentation, it is possible to analyze the implications of the four halakhic principles discussed for specific diagnostic procedures in the female patient. The diagnostic procedures used during the fertility investigation are designed to follow a logical order and are generally performed beginning with the least invasive procedure and ending with the most invasive. Each procedure is designed to examine one or more possible causes of infertility.

I. PELVIC EXAM

The pelvic exam, incorporating speculum and bimanual exams, is designed to assess abnormalities of the external genitalia as well as internal structures such as the vagina, cervix, uterus, fallopian tubes, and ovaries. Infections, tumors, lacerations, and structural abnormalities can be diagnosed. The speculum exam allows for visualization of the cervix, at which time a Papanicolaou (Pap) smear is often performed. The Pap smear involves collecting samples of cells from the area around the external os and cervical canal and observing them under a microscope. A spatula of plastic or wood is used to abrade or scrape the external cervical surface for cells. A thin cotton swab or bristle tipped brush is often used to obtain cells from the cervical canal. Information regarding infections and tumors can be gleaned from a Pap smear. The bimanual exam involves the insertion of one to two of the physician's fingers into the vagina until the cervix is felt. A second hand is used externally to feel, or palpate, the uterus, and adjacent structures.[84]

The pelvic exam (including the Pap smear) poses absolutely no problem with respect to the laws of *niddah*. The bimanual and speculum exams do not involve dilation of the cervix and do not, in general, cause any bleeding. If perchance they do, the bleeding does not anatomically involve the uterine lining in any way. If the physician makes contact with the cervix manually or with the speculum, no penetration of the cervical canal occurs. Bleeding from the cervix

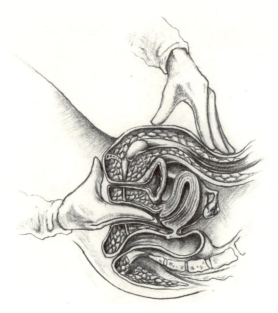

Bimanual exam

outside the external os is certainly not of significance. This basic view is the conclusion of many authorities.[85]

A Pap smear that involves inserting a cotton swab or brush into the cervical canal is also of no concern. The cervix is not dilated to any significant extent, if at all. Rabbi Feinstein's minimum measure of dilation is approximately 19 millimeters. The external os is normally open approximately three millimeters in diameter.[86] Therefore, the concern of somehow stimulating bleeding from the uterus by dilating the external os is not a realistic one. Also, according to many authorities, it is the dilation of the internal os that is of significance. If the scraping of cells from the cervical canal produces bleeding, it is not bleeding that creates a state of *niddah* because, as already discussed, only bleeding from the uterine lining constitutes bleeding of a *niddah*. Although Rabbi Blumenkrantz seems to be concerned about cervical bleeding, this does not represent the predominant view.[87] Dr. Abraham also dismisses the Pap smear as a reason for concern, based purely on anatomy. [88] Furthermore, cervical bleeding caused by a Pap smear might be equivalent to a *makkah*, or wound. As was already discussed, bleeding from a *makkah* does not render a woman a *niddah*.[89]

II. POSTCOITAL TESTING (PCT)

This test involves the collection of a specimen of mucus from the cervical canal. The mucus is examined for quality and quantity as well as for signs of infection. Cervical mucus is important for sperm motility and penetration. The test is an indication of the function of the ovaries, as hormones produced by the ovaries affect the nature of the mucus. The examination is performed at the time of ovulation, which is approximately two weeks after menstruation. The patient should have had intercourse within 12 to 24 hours before, hence the name "postcoital." As a result, the PCT also allows for an initial evaluation of the sperm in terms of motility and other qualitative and quantitative analyses.

A syringe attached to a soft catheter is used to aspirate mucus from the canal. The exam can be performed in conjunction with the pelvic exam and Pap smear.[90] No significant dilation of the external os occurs. No bleeding should occur and any that does is not uterine. Due to the required timing of the test, the PCT normally does not occur immediately before or during the seven day period. If it does, some qualifications apply, as will be discussed later.

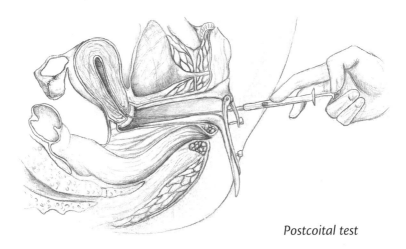

Postcoital test

III. CERVICAL DILATION AND ENDOMETRIAL BIOPSY

The dilation of the cervical canal at both the external os and internal os is performed to gain access to the uterine cavity. This allows an endometrial biopsy to be performed. The biopsy is aimed at obtaining tissue, or cells, from the uterine lining. This provides information about both ovarian function and uterine capacity for implantation. It can, for example, diagnose endometritis, or inflammation of the uterine lining. It is best performed one or two days before the onset of menstruation.[91]

The biopsy is performed by visualizing the cervix through a speculum placed into the vagina, then grasping its anterior (upper) lip (around the external os) with a wire hook, or tenaculum, in such a way as to avoid the blood supply to the cervix. (However, superficial bleeding from the cervix can occur.) On occasion, the cervix must first be dilated with a thin probe, or dilator, which can measure 7–11 mm in diameter. A curette, or scraping device, is then

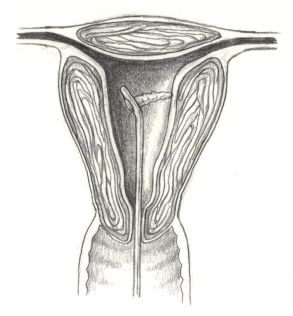

Endometrial biopsy, front view

inserted into the uterus to scrape off cells from the lining. The dilators and curettes can be hollow, thus allowing for blood to egress. Bleeding is a normal occurrence after any type of endometrial biopsy and can last a couple of hours to one or two days. Newer instruments have recently been developed that allow a biopsy to be taken without grasping the cervix and without forcefully dilating the cervical canal. Thus, a tenaculum may not be needed and dilating the cervix is usually not necessary. Flexible, disposable cannulas, for example, have replaced metal curettes and involve very little dilation of the cervix (less than 7 mm, if any).

Any bleeding from the cervix at the area of the external os or the cervical canal is anatomically not *niddah* bleeding. Cervical dilation does not create a state of *niddah*, as the dilation of the internal os is insufficient to render the woman a *niddah*. While the consensus of rabbinic authorities is that the opening of the internal os, even in the absence of observable bleeding, causes a woman to become a *niddah*, Rabbi Feinstein has established the minimum diameter for such dilation as 19 mm. Clearly, the dilation performed during biopsy is comfortably less than this minimum diameter. It is also less than Rabbi Blumenkrantz's 12.7 mm cutoff. The bleeding that results from the actual biopsy may be problematic. The blood that flows from the uterus through a hollow curette out of the cervical canal does not, according to most opinions, impose a state of *niddah*, as we have seen with the principle of the tube. The blood that exits around the curette, as well as bleeding that ensues sometime after the procedure is completed, may or may not create a state of *niddah*. This depends on the discussion earlier regarding the requirement of a natural and spontaneous flow and whether instrumentation-induced bleeding is exempted based on the principle of *makkah*. This author feels that the issue remains inconclusive.[92]

Since the biopsy is performed very near to the expected date of menstruation, the practicality of intimate relations with one's spouse may not exist. The laws of *niddah* proscribe intercourse for a period of time immediately prior to the anticipated onset of bleeding as a safeguard against having relations once the menstrual period has begun.[93] Depending on the woman's natural cycle, there may still exist one or two nights during which intercourse would be permissible.

Another issue to consider is the onset of the five initial menstrual days prior to the beginning of the seven clean days. They do not begin with the uterine bleeding from the biopsy. Since biopsies are sometimes performed just at the onset of menstruation, attention should be directed at discerning when the menstrual bleeding begins.

IV. HYSTEROSALPINGOGRAM (HSG)

This HSG test is considered to be the gold standard in assessing fallopian tube architecture and function. In order to visualize the uterus and fallopian tubes by x-ray (fluoroscopy), a dye must first be injected into the uterine cavity and fallopian tubes. If the dye is observed to spill out of the tubes and into the pelvis, this verifies that the tubes are patent, or open. If an obstruction exists, it can be discovered. On occasion, the HSG can be therapeutic as well as diagnostic, by overcoming an existing obstruction.[94]

The HSG is performed after menstrual bleeding has ceased, but before ovulation has occurred (so as not to inadvertently interrupt a pregnancy). A speculum is inserted in order to expose the cervix. Depending on the type of instillation system used, a tenaculum may be used to grasp the cervix. Dye is instilled into the uterine cavity by passing a catheter or cannula past the internal os. The catheters are very thin—on the order of 3mm, or equal to the diameter of the cervical canal's natural opening.[95]

After an HSG, bleeding generally occurs. Usually, it represents leakage of the radiographic dye from the uterus and vagina. This fluid is blood-tinged, either from contact with the endometrium or from mixing with blood that oozes from the cervix after the tenaculum is withdrawn.[96] The bleeding that occurs from the cervix does not create a state of *niddah* based on anatomical considerations. The bleeding that is uterine in origin may create a state of *niddah*. While it should be considered traumatic in nature, we have already detailed that this may not necessarily mitigate a state

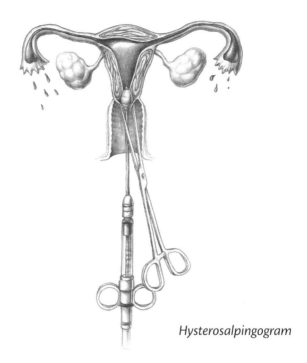

Hysterosalpingogram

of *niddah*. This issue, again, remains inconclusive. If any dilation of the cervix occurs, it is always well below the 19mm defined by Rabbi Feinstein.[97]

V. LAPAROSCOPY AND HYSTEROSCOPY

Laparoscopy is a surgical procedure that involves making a small incision in or just below the navel. A thin telescope is inserted through this incision into the abdominal cavity. This allows the surgeon to directly visualize the ovaries, fallopian tubes, and uterus and to detect any abnormalities therein. Laparoscopy can identify physical or mechanical obstructions around the tubes such as adhesions and endometriosis (sites of uterine tissue growth outside the uterus). During laparoscopy, dye may be instilled into the uterus and through the tubes as in an HSG. Using special instruments such as a laser, many pelvic reconstructive procedures, including the removal of endometriosis or repair of the fallopian tubes, can now be performed during laparoscopy.[98]

Laparoscopy is almost always performed under general anesthesia. First, a pelvic exam is performed. A tenaculum is then used to grasp the cervix and a cannula is inserted into the uterus. This enhances positioning of the uterus for proper visualization through the laparoscope. It also allows dye to be injected through the fallopian tubes during the procedure. Often, hysteroscopy is performed in conjunction with laparoscopy. This involves the insertion of a thin telescope (hysteroscope) of 6–10mm in diameter past the internal cervical os. The uterus is distended with liquid or carbon dioxide gas and its internal surfaces are visualized directly. Occasionally biopsy or other operative procedures are performed through the hysteroscope.[99]

Bleeding from the cervix caused by the tenaculum is anatomically not *niddah* bleeding. The dilation of the cervix that occurs with the cannula is well under the limits established. The only concern would be regarding uterine bleeding caused by its insertion. The issue, again, is whether such bleeding would be considered that of a *makkah*. This point remains, once again, in need of further analysis. Likewise, in hysteroscopy the telescope is of relatively small diameter.

VI. ULTRASOUND

A vaginal ultrasound is helpful in visualizing the uterus and ovaries. A probe is inserted into the vagina up to the cervix, but not beyond. It does not create a state of *niddah*, as anatomically it does not enter the uterus or even the cervical canal. Bleeding generally does not occur.

VII. ADDITIONAL DIAGNOSTIC MODALITIES

Two relatively new and advanced techniques to evaluate the patency and structure of the fallopian tubes are salpingography and falloposcopy.[100] Using small guidewires and contrast dye in a manner similar to coronary angioplasty, salpingography allows for radiologic visualization of the fallopian tubes under fluoroscopy.

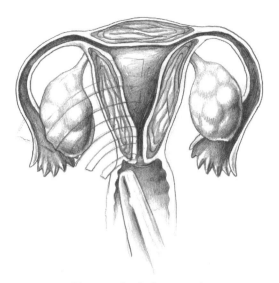

Transvaginal ultrasound

Using a flexible fiber optic endoscope, falloposcopy provides direct visualization of the interior of the fallopian tubes. The instruments used are of very narrow diameters (less than or equal to 3 mm), such that any possible dilation of the cervix would be significantly less than the minimum diameter necessary to create a state of *niddah*.[101] Bleeding can be a direct complication of either procedure, though most likely occurring within the fallopian tubes. If uterine bleeding cannot be ruled out, then the status of the woman is dependent on the previous discussions regarding *makkah* and physiologic bleeding.

Sonohysterography for evaluating uterine pathology in infertile patients is gaining popularity among some physicians.[102] It is less invasive and superior to HSG in diagnosing certain abnormalities. Using vaginal ultrasound, a thin catheter is inserted into the uterus from which saline (salt water) is infused into the uterine cavity. This causes distention of the uterine cavity allowing for a detailed evaluation by ultrasound. It is very similar to HSG except that HSG uses radiographic dyes and fluoroscopy instead of saline and ultrasound. The catheters used (less than or equal to 3 millimeters) are not wide enough in diameter to pose a problem of *niddah*.

Bleeding can occur from irritation of the uterine wall by saline or dye, but is much less likely with saline. The same principles used to determine a woman's *niddah* status with regard to HSG would be applicable here as well.

SOME QUALIFICATIONS

It is important to note that the timing of the test in regard to the women's menstrual cycle can cause halakhic complications, regardless of the procedure. For example, if a procedure is performed prior to the onset of the seven clean days, when all bleeding must have ceased, a woman cannot begin this sequence if any bleeding does occur. *Any* cause of bleeding occurring internally through the vagina simply negates the opportunity to perform an accurate internal examination. If all the bleeding that occurs, however, is observed by a physician to be entirely from outside the uterus, then the seven clean days may commence normally. Bleeding that occurs sometime after the physician has completed the procedure or examination cannot be assumed to be originating from outside the uterus, even if this is the physician's claim. These qualifications apply to the first of the seven days as well. If it is performed during the last six of the seven clean days, there is no need for concern and the days are unaffected. Rabbi Feinstein makes these points quite clear.[103]

Likewise, some authorities, including Rabbi Auerbach as quoted by Dr. Abraham, express concern regarding bleeding that occurs during or following any procedure performed around the expected time of menstruation. Their concern is that the bleeding resulting from such a procedure may actually represent menstrual bleeding when penetration of the uterine cavity with an instrument occurred. Therefore, a state of *niddah* may have been induced by the procedure. Again, this would only be of concern if the procedure were performed at the time of the expected menstrual flow, and only if bleeding was noticed by either the physician or the patient.[104] As always, a competent rabbinic authority must be consulted for practical halakhic decisions.

It should also be noted that if, during any of the procedures, the physician notices blood unrelated to the procedures, the woman is assumed to be a *niddah*.[105] It is no different than if she had examined herself and found blood on a cloth. This is true regardless of the timing within the cycle.

Sabbath Considerations

Lastly, we turn to the issue of performing certain tests or procedures on the Sabbath. The ideas developed here apply equally to the Jewish holidays, such as Passover. The Jewish Sabbath—beginning at sunset Friday evening and ending approximately ¾ of an hour after sunset Saturday evening—is one of the fundamental pillars of halakhic Judaism. Various biblical and rabbinic restrictions apply during the Sabbath. The Sabbath cannot be suspended for non-life-threatening conditions. This is certainly true regarding biblical prohibitions. Non-life-threatening conditions can mitigate the observance of rabbinic ordinances, but this is not absolute. The nature of the ordinance, the exact nature of the condition, and whether reasonable alternatives are available are factors that need to be considered. Although infertility is a serious condition, related diagnostic and therapeutic procedures do not automatically justify overriding rabbinic restrictions.[106] Therefore, both the physician and patient should be aware of how certain diagnostic procedures might be affected by the Sabbath.

It is more than likely that almost all the procedures previously described need not be scheduled for Saturdays. Also, the patient can easily schedule the procedures during non-holiday times, as these are not emergency procedures and their performance would invariably pose halakhic problems. The diagnostic procedures that are bound by tight scheduling are the postcoital test (PCT) and endometrial biopsy. During certain types of therapy, the performance of diagnostic ultrasound and blood testing may also require scheduling on the Sabbath. However, scheduling even these procedures for a Saturday or holiday is halakhically unacceptable. Even if it were permissible in certain cases to override rabbinic restrictions,

the procedures in question may very likely require biblical viola-
tions, such as the driving of a car. The use of electrical equipment
may also pose such a problem. Performing the actual PCT on the
Sabbath is probably a rabbinic violation, while the biopsy may be
a biblical one. These procedures can usually be rescheduled for a
month when no conflict will exist with the Sabbath.

Two diagnostic procedures not previously mentioned that
might have to be performed on Saturdays and holidays are: BBT
(basal body temperature) and LH (luteinizing hormone) testing.[107]
BBT is a person's temperature while at rest. Due to the hormonal
effects of ovulation, a woman's BBT rises approximately 1° F at
midcycle and remains elevated during the luteal, or second half of
the cycle (though not all women are equally sensitive to this effect).
An infertile woman who uses this technique to detect ovulation
generally measures her temperature orally every morning before
engaging in any activity, and then records it on a chart for the duration of one complete cycle. Besides yielding information regarding
the occurrence of ovulation, it is occasionally used for purposes of
scheduling a PCT and/or endometrial biopsy.

The problem with BBT testing is one of measuring, for taking
measurements and weights on the Sabbath is a rabbinic prohibition. (One reason given relates to the close association between
commerce and measurements. Engaging in acts of commerce is
prohibited on the Sabbath and holidays.) Rabbi Waldenberg, however, categorically permits an infertility patient to measure her temperature on the Sabbath with a standard mercury thermometer.[108]
His rationale includes the fact that measurements that relate to a
mitzvah (religious observance and ritual) are sometimes permitted on the Sabbath. To facilitate a couple's efforts to have children
would certainly constitute a mitzvah. Moreover, if an infertile
woman or couple is anxious to the point that the enjoyment of the
Sabbath is compromised, then measuring the temperature would
be considered in the realm of mitzvah if peace of mind would
be achieved. Secondly, Rabbi Waldenberg argues that measuring
a temperature is not at all equivalent to the typically prohibited
measuring of an object or physical space. Temperature is not a

concrete substance but a physiologic parameter. Additionally, Rabbi Feinstein and Rabbi Auerbach argue that measuring temperature is not at all associated with commerce and, therefore, is not in the same category as that restricted by the Rabbis.[109]

Although BBT measurements are permitted on the Sabbath, one must be careful not to perform associated tasks—such as smearing and squeezing—which involve their own biblical prohibitions. If the temperature is measured rectally, one must avoid applying Vaseline to the thermometer. If necessary, the thermometer may be dipped into Vaseline, but it should not be spread or smeared across the thermometer. Only if the thermometer is to be used subsequently on the Sabbath is it permissible to immerse it into alcohol. One can wipe off the alcohol with a cotton ball but should not soak or moisten a cotton ball with alcohol to clean the thermometer. It is permissible to shake down the mercury column for use on the Sabbath.[110] Recording the temperature in writing is absolutely prohibited, even with a pencil. One must wait until after the Sabbath, or use prepared number pieces. Finally, using an electronic or digital display thermometer is prohibited.[111]

In recent years, BBT charting has largely been replaced by a more precise procedure, which involves the measurement of LH levels in the urine. (LH is the hormone that triggers ovulation. If it is absent or low, ovulation is not occurring.) In a normal cycling woman, the development of a ripe egg within the ovary signals the pituitary gland to secrete large amounts of LH. This hormonal "surge" precedes ovulation by 12–36 hours and occurs around mid-cycle, or 14 days before the onset of menstruation. The urinary LH kit allows a woman to anticipate her ovulation by indicating when the LH surge is occurring, since LH circulated in the blood is rapidly excreted into the urine. The test involves dipping a small, color-coded stick in a sample of urine. The color changes that result correspond to different levels of LH in the urine. Knowing when ovulation is occurring is useful in order to time intercourse accurately. It is also useful in timing such procedures as postcoital testing, endometrial biopsy, and artificial insemination.

The problem regarding LH testing is one of dying or coloring.

(The process of dying leather, for example, constitutes a biblical violation of the Sabbath. Some forms of dying and coloring are rabbinic in nature, and still others are permissible.) Rabbi Yehoshua Yeshaya Neuwirth quotes opinions which allow the use of dipsticks on the Sabbath.[112] One mitigating factor is that the color changes are transient in that they are only noticeable for a brief period of time, after which they fade. Another reason for leniency is that, unlike the dying of leather and other materials, the patient isn't really interested in the colored paper per se, but only in the information it provides. Furthermore, the method used is somewhat indirect, in that the patient isn't applying a dye or color but only immersing the stick in the urine, which then results in color changes.[113]

However, Rabbi Neuwirth also quotes Rabbi Auerbach's view which challenges the leniency regarding dipsticks. Rabbi Auerbach argues that since the patient is interested in seeing the actual color changes in the dipstick, albeit for another ultimate purpose, this might be sufficient to constitute a Sabbath violation of dying and coloring. Rabbi Auerbach concludes, therefore, that it is preferable to effect a color change in a somewhat indirect fashion by having the urine spread through the stick on its own without being dipped in.[114] This can be accomplished by dipping the edge of the stick in the urine sample, and allowing the urine to then naturally diffuse through the stick. It should be noted that the cup of urine itself is considered *muktzeh*, or sequestered on the Sabbath from being handled and moved, once it has been used for testing. One is permitted to dispose of it after testing as long as one has not yet set the container down. Once the container has been put down, it should not be manipulated further unless its location is such that people are annoyed by its presence and odor.[115] The insertion of the dipstick into the urine does not pose a *muktzeh* problem.[116]

Conclusion

We return to our opening comment concerning the relevance of religious laws (halakhot) to the overall fertility therapy. Health professionals who are not personally familiar with halakhic observance can find it incredible that such religious restrictions could be allowed to frustrate the therapy if the couple had a real desire to conceive. Such value judgments have no place in the patient-doctor relationship.

Therapy must address the patient as a whole, and the religious commitments of a patient may be at the core of his or her personal identity. Understanding the restrictions imposed by these commitments can help the physician construct a therapeutic protocol best suited for the patient or couple at hand.

Acknowledgments

The author would like to express his appreciation to Rabbi Hershel Schachter, Rosh Yeshiva and Nathan and Vivian Fink Distinguished Professor of Talmud at Yeshiva University's Rabbi Isaac Elchanan Theological Seminary. Rabbi Schachter reviewed the halakhic material of the text, though not all the opinions expressed within are necessarily consistent with his. The author additionally thanks Rabbi Dovid Cohen, Rav of Congregation Gevul Ya'avetz, for sharing his time, opinions, and suggestions.

The author would also like to express his appreciation to Rabbi Tzvi Harari, faculty member—Shoel U'meishiv / S'gan Mashgiach—at the Rabbi Isaac Elchanan Theological Seminary of Yeshiva University, for his research assistance.

Endnotes

1. Leviticus 15:19, 25, 28.
2. *Mishneh Torah*, Hilkhot Issurei Bi'ah 6:1–4.
3. Niddah 68a. Cf. *Mishneh Torah*, Hilkhot Issurei Bi'ah 6:20.
4. Niddah 72b–73a and Rashi's commentary there. *Mishneh Torah*, Hilkhot Issurei Bi'ah 6:5–11. Cf. *Shulhan Arukh*, Yoreh De'ah 196:1. The examination is referred to as *hefsek taharah*, or conclusion in purity. Cf. Rabbi Dr. Kalman Kahana, *Daughter of Israel: Laws of Family Purity*, (English trans. by Leonard Oschry), chap. 3.

5. *Mishneh Torah*, Hilkhot Issurei Bi'ah, 6:11,13 and 7:13. Cf. Niddah 67b. Biblically, a *niddah* must wait till the end of the seventh day before entering the *mikvah* while a *zavah* need only wait till the morning of the seventh day. For both, the restrictions of intimacy are lifted only at the conclusion of the seventh day.

6. Ibid., 4:2. Cf. Leviticus 18:19 and *Shulhan Arukh*, Yoreh De'ah 195.

7. *Mishneh Torah*, Hilkhot Issurei Bi'ah 7:13 and *Shulhan Arukh*, Yoreh De'ah 197:1. See note 5.

8. Niddah 57b, *Mishneh Torah*, Hilkhot Issurei Bi'ah 9:1 and *Shulhan Arukh*, Yoreh De'ah 190:1. Cf. Resp. *Tzofnat Pane'ach*, no. 7.

9. Pithei Teshuvah on *Shulhan Arukh*, Yoreh De'ah 183:1 subscript 1; Rabbi Aharon Pfoifer, *Kitzur Shulhan Arukh Hilkhot Niddah*, chap. 5; Rabbi Feivel Cohen, *Badei Hashulhan* 183:1 subscript 5, and Rabbi Moshe David Tendler, *Pardes Rimonim*, (1988), pp. 14–15. Some authorities suggest that the second type of sensation is one of pain or discomfort associated with the bleeding. Cf. Darkei Teshuvah on *Shulhan Arukh*, Yoreh De'ah 183:1, subscripts 5, 6. See also Rabbi Avrohom Blumenkrantz, *Gefen Porioh*, 1984, chap. 1, endnote 1, where he, as does Rabbi Tendler, describes this sensation as mild uterine contractions. Rabbi Hershel Schachter has suggested to this author that the sensation described is one of something detaching from the uterine wall. Cf. Rabbi Binyomin Forst, *The Laws of Niddah*, (1997), pp. 49–51 and pp. 70–92 for a detailed discussion regarding the concept of sensation.

10. Niddah 66a and *Mishneh Torah*, Hilkhot Issurei Bi'ah 11:1–4.

11. *Shulhan Arukh*, Yoreh De'ah 183:1 and Shakh's commentary ad loc., subscript 3. Cf. *Torat Ha'Shelamim* ad loc., subscript 3.

12. *Mishneh Torah*, Hilkhot Issurei Bi'ah 11:4 *and Shulhan Arukh*, Yoreh De'ah 196:1. This period is referred to as the *shivah nekiyim*, or the seven "clean" days.

13. Ibid. in *Mishneh Torah* and *Shulhan Arukh*, Yoreh De'ah, 197:1,3,4.

14. *Shulhan Arukh*, Yoreh De'ah 190:1,5 and *Mishneh Torah*, Hilkhot Issurei Bi'ah 9:1,2. Cf. *Daughter of Israel: Laws of Family Purity*, chap. 1, par. 4 and 5. The occurrence of spotting in which there was no associated sensation (as described in the text) often requires a minimum size for the spot(s) to create a rabbinic state of *niddah*. Cf. Rabbi Binyomin Forst, *The Laws of Niddah*, chap. 7–11 for detailed discussions.

15. Ibid. 196:10.

16. Rema, gloss on *Shulhan Arukh*, Yoreh De'ah 196:11.

17. Ibid.

18. Niddah 33a,b.

19. Rema, Yoreh De'ah 196:11.

20. *Shulhan Arukh*, Yoreh De'ah 196:4,5,6. The details of the method of examination, the nature of the cloth used, and frequency of exams, are beyond the scope of this introduction. Rabbi Shimon Eider's *Halachos of Niddah* and Rabbi Dr. Kalman Kahana's *Daughter of Israel: Laws of Family Purity* provide

excellent reviews of these and other details. It is important to stress, however, that in any practical situation a competent rabbi should be consulted.

21. F.G. Cunningham, et al., *Williams Obstetrics*, 21st edition, (2001), pp. 31–48, 68–76, and A.H. DeCherney and L. Nathan, eds., *Current Obstetric and Gynecologic Diagnosis and Treatment*, 9th edition, (2003), pp. 17–20, 41–50.

22. Niddah 17b and *Shulhan Arukh*, Yoreh De'ah 183:1.

23. Niddah 40a.

24. *Mishneh Torah*, Hilkhot Issurei Bi'ah 5:2.

25. Resp. *Hatam Sofer*, Yoreh De'ah, no. 167; *Kitzur Shulhan Arukh Hilkhot Niddah*, chap. 1, sec. 1 pp. 83–84, and Rabbi Shmuel Wosner, *Shiurei Sheivet HaLevi*, Hilkhot Niddah 183:2.

26. Rabbi Avrohom Blumenkrantz, *Gefen Porioh*, 1:14, 1984, p. 9 and endnote 48, p. 190.

27. Rabbi Shimon D. Eider, *Halachos of Niddah*, vol. 1, (1981) or one vol. ed., (1999), pp. 4–5.

28. *Kitzur Shulhan Arukh Hilkhot Niddah*, chap. 1, sec. 1, pp. 83–84. Maimonides seems to define the organ of bleeding as the one in which fetal development occurs. This implies that only the uterus itself—not the cervix—would be of halakhic significance, for the cervix is non-contributory in fetal development. Cf. *Mishneh Torah*, Hilkhot Issurei Bi'ah 5:3; Tosafot, Niddah 17b, s.v. *vedam ha'aliyah*, and Beit Yosef on *Tur Shulhan Arukh*, Yoreh De'ah 183.

    The vascular (blood vessel) characteristics of the cervix are not identical to that of the uterus, as discussed in detail in the references cited in note 21. Thus, the mechanism of menstruation only occurs within the uterus itself—not the cervix. Cf. *Current Obstetric and Gynecologic Diagnosis and Treatment*, 9th ed., (2003), pp. 135–136, which describes cyclic changes of the cervix during the menstrual period, but clearly states that the process of desquamation, or shedding of the lining, that results in bleeding is exclusive to the uterus and does not occur in the cervix. See also Rabbi Yoel and Dr. Hannah Katan in *Techumin*, vol. 15, pp. 316–331 for a detailed discussion regarding medical and halakhic perspectives in relationship to cervical pathology and trauma.

29. Rashi, Niddah 41b.

30. *Noam*, vol. 7, pp. 162–165. Cf. vol. 8, p. 275.

31. Ibid. pp. 167–172. Cf. *Sidrei Taharah* on *Shulhan Arukh*, Yoreh De'ah 194:26, who makes reference to such an opinion and disproves it convincingly.

32. Cf. Rabbi Kenneth Brander, "Gynecological procedures and their interface with halacha," *Journal of Halacha and Contemporary Society* XLII, (Fall, 2001), p. 40, where he records as a matter of practice that cervical bleeding does create a state of *niddah*. However, this author feels that the sources Rabbi Brander cites to substantiate this view are equivocal.

33. *Kitzur Shulhan Arukh Hilkhot Niddah*, chap. 4, sec. 5, and n. 7. See also section 1. Cf. *Daughter of Israel: Laws of Family* pp. 40–41.

34. Niddah 21b, 57b.

35. Ibid. 21b.
36. Rashi, Niddah 21b. Cf. *Noam*, vol. 7, pp. 138–145 for a discussion by Rabbi Shlomo Zalman Auerbach.
37. *Noam*, vol. 7, pp. 143–144.
38. Ibid. p. 144.
39. Rabbenu Asher's commentary to Niddah, chap. 3, sec. 2. Cf. *Noam*, vol. 7, pp. 146–154.
40. *Noam*, vol. 7, pp. 145–146.
41. Resp. *Tzitz Eli'ezer*, xvii, 37. Cf. index to no. 37. This view is further reinforced by Rabbi Ya'akov Ettlinger (1798–1871) in *Sefer Arukh L'Ner*, Niddah 21b. He also seems to require that the entire flow occur in a normal fashion and not just be initiated by a natural cause. He argues that the lack of contact between the blood and reproductive tract is not normal.
42. *Shulhan Arukh*, Yoreh De'ah 188:3.
43. *Hidushei Haran*, Niddah 57b.
44. *Sidrei Taharah* on *Shulhan Arukh*, Yoreh De'ah 190:1 and *Noam*, vol. 7, pp. 142–143.
45. Niddah 21a,b.
46. Rashi, Niddah 21b.
47. Niddah 21a,b.
48. Maimonides, *Commentary on the Mishnah*, Niddah chap. 3, 21a. An alternative understanding is that the amount of blood may be microscopic and therefore not visible. However, Rabbi Hershel Schachter mentioned to this author that this is unlikely since any item which is microscopic is generally considered insignificant in terms of halakha. Cf. *Iggerot Moshe*, Yoreh De'ah 2:146 and *Halikhot Shlomo*, Rabbi Shlomo Zalman Auerbach, chap. 4, par. 25, n. 78 for detailed discussions regarding this concept.
49. *Sefer Hazon Ish*, Yoreh De'ah 215 and Niddah 17b. Cf. *Hidushei HaRitvah*, Niddah 18b, 21a.
50. *Hidushei HaRashba*, Niddah 21a. Cf. *Hidushei HaMeiri*, Niddah 21a.
51. *Shulhan Arukh*, Yoreh De'ah 188:3 and 194:2.
52. Resp. *Nodah Bi'Yehudah*, vol. 2, Yoreh De'ah, no. 120.
53. *Binat Adam*, sec. 23.
54. Resp. *Avnei Nezer*, Yoreh De'ah 224. Cf. Resp. *Iggerot Moshe*, Yoreh De'ah, 1:83 where Rabbi Feinstein maintains that Rabbi Danzig fundamentally agrees with Rabbi Landau's basic principle.
55. *Sefer Hazon Ish*, Yoreh De'ah, sec. 83.
56. Maimonides' explanation cited before (note 49) also emphasized that the discharge of the contents of the uterus is always associated with bleeding. Similarly, Rashi seems to imply that only the opening of the cervix during the birthing process involves bleeding. Cf. Rashi on Niddah 21a.
57. *Shulhan Arukh*, Yoreh De'ah 183:1 and Taz's commentary, subscript 1.
58. Resp. *Iggerot Moshe*, Yoreh De'ah 1:83. Cf. 1:89 and *Arukh HaShulhan*, Yoreh De'ah, 188:51. A disagreement exists as to whether Rabbi Yosef Karo, author of

the *Shulhan Arukh*, subscribed to the principle explicitly developed by Rabbi Landau. He implicitly acknowledges it, for he questions the exemption of the previously discussed tube because of the fear that the opening of the cervix by the tube will result in bleeding—albeit it is an external process of opening. See Beit Yosef on *Tur*, Yoreh De'ah 188. The suggestion has been made that the withdrawal of an instrument inserted into the uterus is equivalent to something being discharged from the uterus. See Resp. *Beit Yitzhak*, Yoreh De'ah 2:14. However, this is still not the equivalent of a specific process that involves bleeding—namely, labor and delivery in some form. Based on this presentation, the dilation or opening of the cervix by a physician constitut-ing a valid cause of a woman becoming a *niddah* is dependent on a major disagreement among the authorities.

59. *Shiurei Sheivet HaLevi*, Hilkhot Niddah 188:3 subscript 4; Resp. *Beit Yitzhak*, Yoreh De'ah 2:14.

60. *Kitzur Shulhan Arukh Hilkhot Niddah*, chap. 1, sec. 3, pp. 85–86. Rabbi Pfoifer points out that Rabbi Feinstein also seems to accept this view. However, he feels that in practice one should be stringent since it is a valid dispute.

61. *Noam*, vol. 7, pp. 168–174.

62. Beit Yosef on *Tur Shulhan Arukh*, Yoreh De'ah 188. Cf. *Hidushei HaMeiri*, Niddah 21a.

63. Resp. *Avnei Nezer*, Yoreh De'ah, 224.

64. Resp. *Iggerot Moshe*, Orach Haim, 3:100. Cf. *Nishmat Avraham*, Yoreh De'ah 194:4, and n. 55. Rabbi Feinstein's reason for leniency in terms of the diameter is partly based on the fact that Rabbi Landau's principle is a disputed one. In addition, the basic premise of bleeding being associated with any kind of opening of the cervix as presented in the Talmud is a debate among authorities. Cf. *Iggerot Moshe*, Yoreh De'ah, vol. 1, no. 89.

65. *Badei HaShulhan*, 194:2, subscript 31 and *Gefen Porioh*, chap. 1, n. 68, p. 194. Rabbi Blumenkrantz quotes Rabbi Feinstein's measurement as one half of an inch, which is 13 mm approximately. This author has not found this measure-ment in Rabbi Feinstein's responsa. Cf. *Kitzur Shulhan Arukh Hilkhot Niddah*, chap. 1, sec. 3, pp. 87–88 where Rabbi Pfoifer concludes that the leniency of these measurements is only appropriate vis-a-vis the dilation of the external os and not the internal os. Since the basic notion of dilation of the external causing bleeding is a questionable one, one can be lenient. Any dilation of the internal os, however, raises concern about bleeding from the uterus, since some opinions maintain that the minimum diameter is very small (the diameter of a match). Cf. *Shiurei Sheivet HaLevi*, Hilkhot Niddah 188:3 sub-script 4 and 188:6 subscript 5. According to Rabbi Feinstein himself, however, it is the dilation of the internal os that stimulates bleeding. Thus, it would seem that one need not be concerned even with regard to the dilation of the internal os, provided that the dilation was less than 19 mm and no bleeding was noticed by the physician or patient. Rabbi Kenneth Brander in "Gyne-cological procedures and their interface with halacha," *Journal of Halacha*

and Contemporary Society, xlii, (Fall, 2001), p. 38, states that the majority of rabbinic decisors, particularly within the Sephardic community, rule that any cervical dilation of the internal os of greater than 3 mm is halakhically problematic and may create a state of *niddah*. This author has reviewed the basic sources and has found that the majority of rulings in the *Shulhan Arukh* proper require a significantly greater degree of dilation than 3 mm. Cf. *Badei HaShulhan* 188:3,6 subscripts 37 and 93 and 194:2 subscript 31.

66. Niddah 16a, *Shulhan Arukh*, Yoreh De'ah 187:5 and Shakh's commentary ad loc., subscript 17. Cf. *Pithei Teshuvah* ad loc., subscript 22.

67. Rema, Yoreh De'ah, 187:5. Cf. *Shulhan Arukh*, Yoreh De'ah 196:10.

68. Ibid. in Rema and Shakh's commentary ad loc., subscript 26.

69. *Badei HaShulhan* 187:5 and subscripts 78 and 81.

70. Cf. Rabbi Avrohom Blumenkrantz, *Gefen Porioh*, (1984), 1:14, p. 9 and Rabbi Shimon Eider, *Halachos of Niddah*, p. 5.

71. Niddah 64b, 65b; *Shulhan Arukh*, Yoreh De'ah 193:1.

72. Resp. *Iggerot Moshe*, Yoreh De'ah 1:87.

73. Cf. *Nishmat Avraham*, Yoreh De'ah 193:2.

74. In some cases, the tearing of the hymen results in a laceration that involves a healing process such that a *makkah* was created that remains after the initial trauma. Therefore, a superficial laceration may not be exempt. Cf. F.G. Cunningham, et al. *Williams Obstetrics*, 21st ed., (2001), p. 35. The fact that this type of wound is transient is not a reason to mitigate its status as a *makkah*, though this has been suggested as the explanation as to why hymenal bleeding is exempt. Cf. *Sidrei Taharah* on *Shulhan Arukh*, Yoreh De'ah, 193:1.

75. Resp. *Iggerot Moshe*, Yoreh De'ah 2:69. Others also discuss the insertion of an instrument into the uterine cavity. Concern is expressed regarding bleeding due to the instrument itself coming into contact with blood vessels in the uterine lining. Cf. *Darkhei Teshuvah*, Yoreh De'ah 194:14; *Beit Yitzhak*, Yoreh De'ah 2:14.

76. *Iggerot Moshe*, Orach Haim, 3:100. Cf. *Nishmat Avraham*, Yoreh De'ah 194:4.

77. *Nishmat Avraham*, Yoreh De'ah 187:2.

78. Quoted in *Nishmat Avraham*, Yoreh De'ah 187:2.

79. *Hapardes*, March, 1961, 35:6, p. 33 as quoted in part by Rabbi Eider, *Halachos of Niddah*, p. 5, vol. 1, footnote 25. See note 80.

80. *Kitzur Shulhan Arukh Hilkhot Niddah*, chap. 4 sec. 11–14 and footnote 13.

81. Hymeneal bleeding caused by instrumentation, therefore, would be exempt simply because it is not uterine in origin. Only under normal circumstances of intercourse did the Rabbis institute the restrictions of *niddah* as a result of hymeneal bleeding, though it is not actually uterine in origin. Otherwise, this fact is the operative one. It should be noted that the state of *niddah* that might be imposed due to traumatic bleeding would probably be a rabbinic one. This is due to the lack of the necessary sensation required to impose a biblical state of *niddah* (see note 90). Regardless, the issue of traumatic vs.

physiologic bleeding is the most fundamental one of significance for this chapter. See note 95.

82. Resp. *Iggerot Moshe*, Orach Haim 3:100 and Yoreh De'ah 1:83. Cf. *Havot Da'at* on *Shulhan Arukh*, Yoreh De'ah 187:17 (in the Hiddushim); 187:5 and 196:3 (in the Be'urim). See also *Pit'hei Teshuvah* on Yoreh De'ah, 187:5 subscript 24 and 190:34 subscript 39.

83. Personal communication, Rabbi Hershel Schachter. Cf. *Nishmat Avraham*, Yoreh De'ah 187:8, subscript 5 for a lengthy discussion regarding the credibility of physicians and Resp. of Rabbi Moshe Feinstein as quoted by Rabbi Eider at the end of *Halachos of Niddah*, vol. 1, sec. 17. Cf. Rabbi Kenneth Brander, "Gynecological procedures and their interface with halacha," *Journal of Halacha and Contemporary Society* XLII, (Fall, 2001), p. 35, where, in an attempt to obviate this problem, he recommends that a woman should arrange for her physician or a nurse to perform the internal examination (*hefsek taharah*) prior to sunset before beginning the seven clean days. Then, after waiting a short while till nightfall, the same health care professional performs a second internal examination to satisfy the examination requirement of day one. Two issues arise from this approach. First, it is questionable as to whether anyone other than the woman herself (or someone who is similarly committed to the practice of the laws of *niddah*) is halakhically able to perform the necessary examinations. Cf. *Shulhan Arukh*, Yoreh De'ah 196:7, 8. Secondly, it is generally assumed that the examinations should be performed during the daytime. Cf. *Shulhan Arukh*, Yoreh De'ah 196:4 and *Badei Hashulhan* 196:4, subscript 79 and pp. 298–299 in the *Be'urim*. Special circumstances may, at times, allow for nighttime examinations. A competent rabbi should, of course, be consulted.

84. J.R. Scott, R.S. Gibbs, B.Y. Karlan, A.F. Haney, eds., *Danforth's Obstetrics and Gynecology*, 9th ed., (2003), pp. 487–491, and *Current Obstetric and Gynecologic Diagnosis and Treatment*, 9th ed., (2003), Alan H. DeCherney, and Lauren Nathan, eds., pp. 577–587.

85. *Darkhei Teshuvah* on *Shulhan Arukh*, Yoreh De'ah 194:19; *Kitzur Shulhan Arukh Hilkhot Niddah*, chap. 1, sec. 4. Cf. *Nishmat Avraham*, Yoreh De'ah 194:4.

86. Cf. *Nishmat Avraham*, Yoreh De'ah in preface to Hilkhot Niddah pp. 76–79.

87. Cf. *Kitzur Shulhan Arukh Hilkhot Niddah*, chap. 1, sec. 4, pp. 89–90.

88. *Nishmat Avraham*, Yoreh De'ah 194:4.

89. Rabbi Pfoifer adopts this rationale as the reason that Pap smears do not initiate *niddah* status. C.F. *Kitzur Shulhan Arukh Hilkhot Niddah*, chap. 1, sec. 4. It should be noted that any state of *niddah* that could have been created by a pelvic exam and Pap smear would likely have been rabbinic. This is due to the lack of the necessary sensation to impose a biblical state of *niddah*. This point, however, is also open to dispute. Cf. *Har Zvi*, Yoreh De'ah, no. 152.

90. Alan H. DeCherney and Lauren Nathan eds., *Current Obstetric and Gynecologic*

Diagnosis and Treatment, 9ᵗʰ ed., (2003), pp. 584–585, and James R. Scott, et al. eds., *Danforth's Obstetrics and Gynecology*, 9ᵗʰ ed., (2003), p. 492.

91. Ibid., *Danforth's Obstetrics and Gynecology.*

92. This author has discussed this central issue with two prominent rabbinic authorities. Rabbi Hershel Schachter, a Rosh Yeshiva and Rosh Kollel at Yeshiva University, has questioned the premise that bleeding resulting from gynecologic procedures is equivalent to that of *makkah*. Rabbi Schachter's view is that bleeding originating from the uterine lining creates a state of *niddah*, regardless of the cause. The only exception to be considered would be a situation in which a preexisting lesion, such as a fibroid, was identified as the source of bleeding. Cf. Rabbi Binyomin Forst's *The Laws of Niddah*, pp. 440–441, 450–461, and 467–469, where he addresses the *niddah* status of a woman undergoing various gynecologic procedures. He too reflects skepticism regarding the use of the *makkah* principle for purposes of leniency. However, Rabbi Dovid Cohen, rabbi of Congregation Gevul Ya'avetz in Brooklyn, New York, has shared a differing view. Rabbi Cohen maintains that any uterine bleeding associated with gynecologic procedures does not create a state of *niddah*, provided that two conditions are met. First, the procedure must not involve dilation of the cervical canal to a diameter of two-thirds of an inch, or 17 mm. Second, the uterine bleeding must be, in the physician's opinion, clinically attributable to the procedure. Such bleeding would thus be considered that of *makkah*. Absolute knowledge that the bleeding is not menstrual or physiologic is not required since a very reasonable and probable traumatic cause exists. If the procedure was performed at a time during her cycle when the woman would normally expect her period, then one cannot so readily disregard normal menstruation as a contributing cause of bleeding. Cf. Rabbi Yehoshua Zev Zand, *Birkas Banim*, chap. 4, par. 13, footnote 33 and *Nishmat Avraham*, Yoreh De'ah 194:2, subscript 4. See also Rabbi M. Deutsch, "Gynecologic examination and halakhah (summary and sources)" in *Emek Halakhah-Assia*, Rabbi Mordechai Halperin, ed. (1985), pp. 221–256 and for a detailed discussion regarding gynecologic procedures and *niddah* status.

93. *Shulhan Arukh*, Yoreh De'ah 184:2.

94. DeCherney and Nathan, *Current Obstetric and Gynecologic Diagnosis and Treatment*, pp. 57 and 985, and Berek, *Novak's Gynecology*, pp. 1002–1003.

95. Cf. *Nishmat Avraham*, Yoreh De'ah 194:4.

96. Personal communication, Dr. Richard V. Grazi, director, Genesis Fertility, Affiliate of Maimonides Medical Center, Brooklyn, New York.

97. Cf. *Nishmat Avraham*, Yoreh De'ah, 194:2, subscript 4 and Rabbi Moshe David Tendler, *Pardes Rimonim*, 1988, pp. 42–46 where Rabbi Tendler reviews various gynecological procedures and their import on *niddah* status.

98. Berek, *Novak's Gynecology*, p. 293.

99. Ibid.

100. Berek, *Novak's Gynecology*, pp. 1003–1004 and *Taber's Cyclopedic Medical Dictionary*, 19ᵗʰ ed., (2001), entries: falloposcopy; salpingography.

101. Personal communication, Dr. Richard Grazi, director, Genesis Fertility, Brooklyn, New York.

102. Berek, *Novak's Gynecology*, pp. 1,009–1,010.

103. Resp. *Iggerot Moshe*, Orach Hayim, 3:100.

104. *Nishmat Avraham*, Yoreh De'ah 194:2, subscript 2.

105. *Kitzur Shulhan Arukh Hilkhot Niddah*, chap. 1, sec. 4, p. 91.

106. Infertility should be defined within the category of *holeh she'ain bo sakanah*, one who is ill but not in danger of loss of life or limb. This category includes one who cannot function normally, which is an accurate description of an infertile individual. For such a person, certain rabbinic restrictions may be suspended. Cf. Rabbi Yehoshua Zev Zand, *Birkat Banim*, (1994), chap. 10, p. 249, par. 1, footnote 1 and pp. 268–270, par. 21, footnote 32, where the author convincingly defines the status of an infertile individual to be equivalent to a *holeh she'ain bo sakanah*. He specifically discusses the use of injections and oral medications on the Sabbath in the course of infertility treatment. The use of oral medications is normally in violation of a rabbinic injunction, but is suspended for someone who is functionally ill. Injections administered by a non-Jew would similarly violate a rabbinic prohibition with the same dispensation for an illness that renders the person unable to function normally. Several authorities permit the use of injections administered by a non-Jew in the treatment of infertility, clearly reflecting the categorization of infertility within the domain of *holeh she'ain bo sakanah*. Most prominently, Rabbi Zand records that Rabbi Moshe Feinstein subscribed to this view. Cf. Rabbi Yigal Shafran in *Techumin*, vol. 17, pp. 335–339, where he raises an objection to this classification of infertility. He primarily analyzes whether IVF (in vitro fertilization) and IUI (intrauterine insemination) procedures would be permissible on the Sabbath.

107. Berek, *Novak's Gynecology*, p. 995.

108. Resp. *Tzitz Eliezer*, vol. XI, no. 38 and vol. XII, no. 44:5.

109. *Iggerot Moshe*, Orach Haim, 1:128 and *Shemirat Shabbat Kehilkhata*, vol. 1, 40:2 and footnotes 2, 3. Cf. *Nishmat Avraham*, Orach Haim, 306:7, subscript 2.

110. *Shemirat Shabbat Kehilkhata*, vol. 1, 40:2 and footnote 7.

111. Cf. Rabbi Avrohom Friedlander, *Hasdei Avraham*, (1999), vol. 2, chap. 14, par. 34 and footnotes 73, 74. See also *Nishmat Avraham*, English ed., (2002), Orach Haim, chap. 19, 306:7, pp.156–158 regarding measuring one's temperature on the Sabbath in general and the use of contact thermometers in particular.

112. *Shemirat Shabbat Kehilkhata*, vol. 1, 33:20 and footnote 81. Cf. *Nishmat Avraham*, Orach Haim 318:11, subscript 2.

113. Resp. *Tzitz Eliezer*, vol. X, nos. 25:1.4 and 25:18.1.

114. *Shemirat Shabbat Kehilkhata*, vol. 1, 33:20, footnote 83 and *Nishmat Avraham*, vol. 5, supplemental section "Ha'Rofei", par. 32.

115. *Shulhan Arukh*, Orach Haim 308: 34, 35 and *Mishnah Be'rurah* ad loc., subscripts 134 and 136. Cf. *Shemirat Shabbat Kehilkhata*, vol. 1, 22:42.

116. *Nishmat Avraham*, vols. 4 and 5, Orach Haim 321:5, subscript 1 and vol. 5, supplemental section "Ha'Holeh", par. 30. Collecting and testing the urine does not pose a problem of *muktzeh*. There are several categories of *muktzeh*, one being an item which lacks purpose or function. A person's intent on using the urine for testing renders the urine non-*muktzeh* by definition until the testing is completed.

Yoel Jakobovits

A General Overview
of Male Infertility

The perception of the degree of male involvement in infertility has undergone a number of revisions in the past fifty years. Initially, and still in the minds of many, infertility was considered primarily a female problem. As we shall see however, the halakhic problems that arise in treatment are far more serious for the male than for the female.

Even now, the extent of male "liability" is hard to quantify with precision. For example, it is estimated that 40% of infertility is wholly or partly due to male factors.[1] On the other hand, there have been attempts to redefine, in a downward direction, the lower limit of "normal" sperm counts. Thus, many men who previously would have been considered as subfertile are now considered normal, and the focus has turned back again to the females.[2] Some conditions adversely affecting seminal function include changes in hormone levels, genetic or congenital anatomic abnormalities including retrograde ejaculation, drug use, toxins, infections, and surgical sequalae; some are discussed below in more detail.

Blood Tests

Subsumed under male infertility are a diagnostically heteroge-
neous group of disorders. One key basis of discrimination within
this group rests upon widely available blood tests. Chief among
these are assays of gonadotropins.[3] A defect in the production of
gonadotropins can be measured in the blood; low levels of these
hormones indicate a production problem. Approximately 9% of
infertile males belong in this category. Causes include brain tumors
and several rare congenital syndromes. Treatment by injections of
gonadotropin may be effective in selected cases.

On the other hand, patients with testicular failure will have
high levels of circulating gonadotropin hormones.[4] Such patients
comprise about 14% of the total number of infertile males. Causes
include, in particular, radiotherapy, chemotherapy, and post-infec-
tion such as after mumps orchitis. Treatment is currently not
possible.

By far the largest group of infertile males—77%—have normal
gonadotropin levels. These patients are said to have "post-testicular
dysfunction," that is impairment of the outflow or production of
sperm, in spite of normal pituitary and testicular structures. This
category encompasses men with mechanically obstructed ejaculatory ducts (6%), infections such as prostatitis and epididymitis
which are often transient, varicoceles (37%), and idiopathic (25%).

Varicocele

Varicoceles and their effects were noted as early as the first century. Celsus, a first century doctor, described superficial and deep
varicoceles and noted the presence of testicular atrophy on the
affected side. A varicocele is an abnormal dilation of veins within
the spermatic cord. This cord consists of nerves, blood vessels, and
spermatic ducts through which the testes are attached to and communicate with the body. These vein deformities probably exert their

deleterious effects on sperm production by raising the temperature around the testes.[5] As the spermatic vein is directly inserted into the renal vein on the left side, 90% of cases occur on that side. By contrast the right testicular drainage is through the vena cava, a venous system with lower resistance pressure. This asymmetric vascular arrangement may also be the basis of the halakhic ruling that injuries to the left testicle (the "weaker one") are less problematic than injuries to the right one, which can lead to restrictions in conjugal union within the Jewish community.[6]

The exact significance of a varicocele—and hence of the indications for surgical obliteration—in the management of infertility is controversial. Approximately 10–15% of males in the general population have a varicocele. There is no evidence that males with normal semen characteristics need corrective treatment even if a varicocele is present.

In men with varicoceles and documented impairment of fertility, surgical correction results in a 30–50% pregnancy rate, although this response rate is very controversial.[7] In spite of lingering questions,[8] current practice is to offer correction of varicocele in such men. Surgical interruption of the internal spermatic vein is the usual treatment for clinically apparent varicoceles; there is also a nonsurgical approach that utilizes embolization to occlude the vein.

Halakhically speaking, varicocele repair presents little difficulty. Provided that the medical risks are low and the possibilities of fertility improvement are real, one would give every encouragement to correction of this potentially significant impairment.

Sperm Evaluation

A virtual axiom in all of medicine, however, is that most infertility problems are multifactorial in origin. When the male contribution is suspected of being problematic, evaluation for varicocele is not sufficient. Men with varicoceles significant enough to factor in infertility often have specific sperm abnormalities as well.[9] The evaluation of sperm characteristics therefore lies at the center of male infertility testing—and at the crux of the halakhic concerns.

Van Leewenhoek, the inventor of the microscope, first observed sperm with his new instrument in 1677. However, it was not until 1929 that the modern era of sperm analysis really began.[10] In addition to the initial exclusive emphasis on the sperm itself, attention is now paid to the noncellular biochemical components of the seminal fluid as well.

Semen Procurement

The proper collection of sperm is described in detail in many texts. The following extract from a book on infertility testing is instructive in that it directs us immediately to some of the special problems with which Jewish law is concerned.

> The specimen may be obtained at home or in the physician's office, but it should be kept warm during transit. It is very unusual for a patient to object to masturbation as a form of inducing ejaculation. When there is an objection, coitus interruptus is an alternative method of obtaining the specimen. If the patient has religious objections to both masturbation and withdrawal, he can use a perforated plastic condom manufactured by the Milex Corporation of Chicago, and if he is of the Catholic faith, he may have the condom perforated by a priest. In the rare situation in which none of these methods is satisfactory to the patient, the physician will have to rely on postcoital examination of the ejaculate in the vagina. The patient should understand that an incomplete collection is not only worthless but also misleading.[11]

Halakhic misgivings are prompted by every option summarized in this excerpt. The collection of sperm, masturbation, coitus interruptus, and the use of condoms—they are all of concern to the halakha. Notwithstanding the strongly pro-procreative attitudes outlined earlier, (see Section II, "Introduction") there are several halakhic principles which pull in the antithetical direction, curtailing any routine or automatic authorization to investigate male infertility.

By omitting explicit prohibition of masturbation, the Torah has promoted much discussion as to its precise categorization.[12] The "improper emission of genital seed"[13] is regarded as fitting within the general heading of prohibited sexual relations by some,[14] as a "free-standing" prohibition by others,[15] or as merely of rabbinic origin by yet others.[16] In addition to these negative aspects, improper emission of seed may be forbidden as a breach of the obligation to have children.[17] However, another authority holds that the ban on conscious wastage of seed is entirely unrelated to the mitzvah of procreation.[18] Other candidates for the classification into which masturbation properly fits are the interdictions forbidding wastage in general,[19] and censuring eroticism even when only by contemplation,[20] let alone by performance.

The Torah records its condemnation of the wastefulness of seed in two historical settings. Many commentaries cite it as the sin which constituted the principal reason for the Flood in Noah's days.[21] Secondly, it was the transgression of Er and Onan, an occurrence which gave rise to the term "onanism."[22] Chief among the several sinful ingredients in Onan's act is its association with coitus interruptus, a topic which prompts apparently contradictory views in Talmudic literature.

Despite the Onan story, with its unequivocal censuring tones, there is a Talmudic record of Rabbi Eliezer's opinion actually recommending the practice of coitus interruptus![23] Of course, Rabbi Eliezer limits this recommendation to very specific circumstances, such as the protection of a lactating mother from a second pregnancy which could endanger the existing infant by diminishing the mother's milk supply. Rabbi Moshe Feinstein, the recently deceased, universally acknowledged premier halakhic adjudicator comments:

> Since this is the same Rabbi Eliezer in whose name the Talmud quotes a dictum warning against even unintentional improper emission of

seed, his endorsement of coitus interruptus for reasons of the health of the child is all the more instructive. It means that, to him at least, seed is not said to be "uselessly" destroyed if a proper purpose is served thereby, and if this is the only manner in which that purpose can now be served. Marital relations is that purpose; since normal intercourse would cause a hazard to health, the emission of seed for such relations, where there is no alternative, is not wasteful; where there is an alternative, it is, even according to him.[24]

The normative ruling, however, is in accordance with the Sages' dissenting opinion. Ergo Maimonides prohibits the practice without equivocation: "It is forbidden to destroy seed. Therefore, a man may not practice coitus interruptus, etc."[25]

The strict attitudes regarding coitus interruptus[26] should be considered alongside, and in contrast with, the somewhat more lenient attitudes toward "unnatural intercourse" (*beiah shello k'darkah*). The prevailing Talmudic view is that "a man may do with his wife as he wishes."[27] Tosafot records two notable formulae proposed by Rabbi Yitzhak to resolve the law's permissiveness in Nedarim as compared with the restrictive attitude held in Yevamot.[28] Firstly, the tolerant view sanctioning unnatural intercourse may have assumed that no semination occurs. Alternatively, semination is in fact tolerated provided unnatural intercourse is resorted to only on occasion and that the contraceptive intention of the husband is not constant.

This second answer of Rabbi Yitzhak—highlighting both "intent" and "irregularity"—may constitute broad foundation for authorization to practice unnatural intercourse within marriage when it fulfills a "purpose." Even the assuagement of the husband's or wife's sexual desire may be included within the parameters of acceptable standards of sexual relations, this being reaffirmed by many authorities.[29] All authorities emphasize, however, that this general license is controversial and certainly applies only to occasional sexual expression.[30]

There are several instances where prominent early sources sanctioned even masturbation—and the inevitable spillage of seed to which it leads—to achieve an overriding "purpose." A man may resort to masturbation in order to relieve an otherwise uncontrollable sexual desire, thereby avoiding an even graver transgression of a prohibited sexual relationship.[31] The Talmud itself recommended masturbation for the investigation of sexual impotence (erectile dysfunction), a disability which can impose severe restrictions on marriage within the Jewish community.[32] Some authorities also sanctioned masturbation in order to ascertain whether postcoital vaginal bleeding derives from the male or from the female, as postcoital bleeding in the female may pose restrictions on the resumption of sexual relations.[33]

Other specific "purposes" may also be acceptable reasons to sanction a lenient attitude. Medical considerations—though not specified—would be generally pardoned and can provide halakhic grounds for sanctioning this method for temporary birth control.[34] This is clearly articulated by Rabbi Isaiah da Trani[35] who writes: "...how [in the light of the sin of Er and Onan] did the Sages permit unnatural intercourse [as when using a diaphragm][36] when it involves [wasteful] emission of seed? The answer is: Wherever the husband's intent is to avoid pregnancy so as not to mar his wife's beauty and he does not want to fulfill the mitzvah of procreation, it is forbidden. But if his intent is to spare her physical hazard, then it is permitted. So also if he does so for his own pleasure [unnatural intercourse is permitted]...for 'a man may do with his wife what he wishes.'" Strikingly, as David Feldman points out, though this passage was written in the thirteenth century but remained unpublished until 1931, it nevertheless reflects an oft-repeated mainstream opinion.[37] It has been used to provide significant support for lenient rulings by several twentieth century halakhic masters such as the late Chief Rabbi of Israel, Rabbi Isaac Herzog,[38] and Rabbi Moshe Feinstein.[39]

It should be noted, however, that there is a notable body of extra-halakhic Kabbalistic literature which inveighs heavily against any spillage of seed under any circumstance.[40] Reflecting this view is the comment of Rabbi Yosef Karo: "Had Rabbi Yitzhak seen what the Zohar says about the gravity of *hash'hatat zera*, namely that it is the most severe of sins, he never would have written what he did."[41] Both the permissive and restrictive opinions are recorded by Rabbi Moshe Isserles.[42]

These considerations form the foundation upon which the halakhic position regarding masturbation is based. Of paramount importance is purpose. When the intention is procreation, either directly through artificial insemination and in vitro fertilization or indirectly when evaluating male infertility, there is significant room for leniency within the halakhic guidelines.

It is important to recognize that no *carte blanche* regarding the method of semen procurement, even under conditions of need and sanction, is granted. Justification for a tolerant approach exists only in special circumstances, as in the investigation of male infertility, and even there, restrictions apply in regard to method. For example, by recommending either warm perianal applications or visually evocative stimuli to arouse ejaculation, the Talmud itself appears to be deliberately avoiding any suggestion of direct penile stimulation to avoid conflict with the Talmud's express admonition against such contact in Niddah 13a.[43] A similar reluctance may have prompted the "teach us our Rabbi" phrase used to establish an acceptable method of penile evaluation. The expression assumes that there is difficulty with the seemingly obvious technique, masturbation.[44]

Specifically germane to our discussion here are the expressed rabbinic positions regarding procurement of sperm by masturbation in the medical investigation of male infertility.[45] Mindful of the pro-procreative intent of the procedure, where no other technique is appropriate, some authorities sanction such artificial collection of sperm.[46] Others, however, disagree, arguing that because of the many technical uncertainties[47] coupled with the strongly condemnatory Talmudic and, in particular, Kabbalistic, pronouncements, masturbation can never be sanctioned—even in the interest of siring offspring.[48] Similarly some have even argued that considering the severity of the sin of masturbation, one would rather recommend that a childless couple divorce and remarry someone else![49] Mindful of the limited likelihood of helpful medical intervention, several authorities are similarly disinclined to sanction masturbation even with the intention of aiding procreation.[50]

On the other hand, as mentioned, contrary, more lenient views exist as well. Chief among these opinions are the views of Rabbis Ya'akov Emden and Haim O. Grodzinski. The latter suggests that, if possible, it is better to collect seminal fluid from a condom[51] worn during intercourse, thereby avoiding masturbation. More contemporaneous decisors[52] have also suggested this method as most acceptable. In addition, Beth Shmuel,[53] citing the same Talmudic passages, also deduces a liberal attitude with respect to semen procurement in pressing circumstances. Accordingly, where postcoital bleeding is detected, he permits the non-coital ejaculation of sperm to establish whether hematospermia is responsible. This license may only be appropriate when the evaluation of the female companion is not conclusive.[54]

A leading contemporary halakhist, Rabbi Shlomo Zalman Auerbach, has ruled that "even when he has a male and a female child [the halakhic minimum] a man is permitted to obtain sperm [notwithstanding the severe restrictions which would normally apply] in order to fulfill the imperative of *lashevet* [see Part 1 "A Brief History of Fertility Therapy"] or where his wife is in significant [psychological] distress in not having more children."[55] However, the precise method of procuring sperm is not indicated.

Yet another approach might be applied in situations where investigations the infertile couple have already undertaken fail to identify any female disorder. Here it may be fair to assume that the male either has no viable sperm or has defective sperm. In either case, wastage of his seed would not constitute *zera l'vatalah*, it being likely that there is viable seed to speak of. This line of reasoning is developed by Rabbi Simcha Bunim Sofer,[56] who concludes by advising that "where it is possible, a postcoital diaphragm may be used; even during coitus one may be lenient for this purpose…. But if it is impossible [to use the semen collected] by a diaphragm, then my opinion is to be lenient [about manual masturbation]…. However, since I failed to find absolute proof, and due to the gravity of the issue, I would solicit additional [concurring] opinions…."

Summary of Semen Collection Methods

The reader may be excused if he is left quite bewildered by the foregoing account of widely differing views. A workable algorithm of graduated choices along the lines of Rabbi Eliezer Waldenberg's[57] is suggested:

> The preferred method of semen collection is from the vagina following normal coitus.[58]
>
> Where that is not possible because of technical or emotional reasons, sperm may be procured after coitus interruptus.[59]
>
> Where that is unsuitable, the collection should be made using a condom—preferably one with a perforation—worn during intercourse.[60]
>
> If that is impossible, a collecting receptacle should be placed intravaginally.
>
> Finally, if that too is impractical, sperm may be obtained by masturbation. Penile stimulation should preferably be achieved by a mechanical stimulator, though self-stimulation is also permitted.[61]

Testicular Biopsy

Occasionally biopsy of the testicle is indispensable to accurate diagnosis. It is usually recommended in azospermic men with normal-sized testes to discriminate between ductal obstruction and spermatogenic failure. In men with poor quality sperm or very low counts, histological evaluation results will rarely, if ever, alter therapy. The biopsy will assist, however, in making a definitive diagnosis that can aid the physician in delivering a reliable prognosis, thereby avoiding needless treatment in unsalvageable circumstances.

Evidently the futility of testicular biopsy was assumed by one early halakhic writer who reports that "none of the physicians of my town are familiar with such a test."[62] Nevertheless he proceeds to discuss the halakhic concerns in some detail. The obstacles relate in particular to the biblical injunction proscribing marital bonds with a genetically Jewish woman by any man who has "wounded testes or severed membrum."[63] The Talmud elaborates this injunction to include any wounding or crushing injury to the penis, testes, or cords of the testes.[64] The author concludes that as the perforation in the testes performed in a testicular biopsy heals completely, the injunction against "wounded or crushed" would not present a problem. However, he regards this method of semen procurement as "unnatural" emission of seed and therefore rules against it. He does not speak of actual biopsy of the testicle.

Some, however, allow the procedure, arguing that testicular sperm are undeveloped prior to their maturation in the collecting ducts and therefore are not subject to any restrictions on sperm emission.[65] Furthermore, the prohibition on surgical damage to the genitalia might be applicable only where the patient has reproductive capacity, a precondition clearly not extant in the investigation of an infertile male.[66] Similarly, Rabbi Feinstein also permits testicular biopsy, arguing that the Talmudic constraints are applicable only when the perforation of the testis results in infertility; nowadays the procedure has the reverse likelihood, being designed to help alleviate infertility.[67]

Endnotes

1. R.F. Blackwell, M.P. Steinkampf, "Infertility: Diagnosis and therapy," *Controversies in Reproductive Endocrinology and Infertility*, M.R. Soules, ed., (New York: Elsevier, 1989), p. 15.
2. C.M.K., Nelson, R.G. Bunge, "Semen analysis: Evidence for changing parameters of male fertility potential," *Fertility and Sterility*, 25:503, (1974).
3. Gonadotrophins are a set of hormones secreted by the pituitary gland in the base of the brain which stimulate (= trophic) the testicular apparatus (= gonads) to produce seminal fluid (= sperm and the fluids in which it is suspended).
4. The pituitary gland, trying to drive the unresponsive testes, produces hormones. It is unrestricted by the negative biofeedback which successful spermatogenesis would provide, causing the levels of circulating gonadotropins to rise.

5. Alternative suggestions—none of which have been adequately substanti-
   ated—include different concentrations of adrenal hormone exposure to the
   testes and decreased testicular blood flow. (E. Steinberg, "Male infertility,"
   Gynecologic Endocrinology, J.J. Gold, J.B. Josimovich, eds., 4th ed., [1987], pp.
   572–3.)
6. See fuller discussion in sec. 6 regarding testicular biopsies.
7. A.T.K Crockett, H. Takihara, M.J. Cosentino, "The varicocele," *Fertility and
   Sterility*, 41:5, 1984.
8. A. Vermeulen, M. Vandeweghe, "Improved fertility after varicocele correction:
   Fact or fiction," *Fertility and Sterility*, 42:249, (1984).
9. B.J. Rogers, G.G Mygatt., D.W. Soderdahl, R.W. Hale, "Monitoring of suspected infertile men with varicocele by the sperm penetration assay," *Fertility
   and Sterility*, 44:800, (1985).
10 D. Macomber, M.B. Sanders, "The spermatozoa count," *New England Journal of Medicine*, 200:981, 1929. An up-to-date discussion is provided by B.C.
   Dunphy, L.M. Neal, I.D. Cooke, "The clinical value of conventional semen
   analysis," *Fertility and Sterility*, 51:324, (1989).
11. R.J. Sherins, S.S. Howards, "Male infertility," in *Campbell's Urology*, 5th ed.,
    P.C. Walsh, ed., *et al.*, (Philadelphia: W.B. Saunders, 1986), p. 645.
12. The primary Talmudic source is in Niddah 13a (see Magid Mishnah on
    Mishneh Torah, Issurie Bi'ah 21:18).
13. Known in Hebrew as either *hotza'at zera l'vatalah* or more commonly as
    hash'hatat zera, generally regarded as interchangeable phrases. Feldman, *loc.
    cit.*, p. 109, cites Resp. *Hinnukh Beit Yitzhak*, Even HaEzer, no. 7, who proposes
    a plausible distinction between the two.
14. Rambam, *Mishneh Torah*, Issurie Bi'ah 21:18 and *Tur Shulhan Arukh*, Even
    Ha'Ezer 23:1 based upon Exodus 20:13. Cf. Rambam's *Commentary on the
    Mishna*, Sanhedrin 54a.
15. S'mak, no. 292 and Ma'adanei Yom Tov on Rosh, Niddah chap. 2, no. 40.
    Contemporary discussions: Rabbi M. Feinstein, Resp. *Iggrot Moshe*, Even
    HaEzer III, 14 staunchly reiterates the biblical nature of this transgression;
    Rabbi E. Waldenberg, Resp. *Tzitz Eliezer* IX, 51:1.1, cites various opinions but
    comes to no firm conclusion.
16. Resp. *P'nei Yehoshua*, Even Ha'Ezer II, no. 44.2 argues that the severe stric-
    tures applied by the Sages are exaggerated and were meant to underscore the
    repulsiveness with which they regarded onanism.
    An unusual analysis is suggested by *Haggaot Ezer Mikodesh* cited by
    Rabbi A.M. Babad, Resp. *Imrei Tova*, no. 33: "The [biblical] prohibition of
    wasteful spillage of seed pertains only prior to the ban on polygamy promul-
    gated by Rabbeinu Gershom ben Yehuda (c. 1000) when [by having several
    wives] it may have been possible for *each* ejaculation to achieve fruition.
    Today—especially in our countries where secular laws make [even] divorce
    difficult—the matter has changed and the halakha has changed and there
    is no more than a rabbinic prohibition here." Rabbi Babad also quotes his

uncle, the author of Resp. *Havatzelet HaSharon* (addenda to Even HaEzer. vol. 1), who concluded similarly that today spillage of seed is only a rabbinic prohibition. I am grateful to my brother-in-law, Rabbi C.Z. Pearlman of London, for directing me to these citations.

17. Tosafot Sanhedrin 59b. Those excluded from the mitzvah of procreation would therefore be free from this restriction (Rabbeinu Tam in Tosafot Yevamot 12b, s.v. *shalosh*).

18. Ramban, Niddah 13a.

19. "*Bal tash'hit*" (Deuteronomy 20:19), undoubtedly civilizations earliest conservation legislation! Rabbi Ya'akov Ettlinger in his Resp. *Binyan Tzion*, no:137 and novalle *Arukh L'Ner*, on Niddah 13b makes this tentative suggestion. He also suggests that this interdiction may be based upon a *halakha le'Moshe m'Sinai*.

20 See *Ahiezer* III, no: 24:5 based on Deuteronomy 23:10 and Avodah Zara 20b.

21. Genesis 6:12 and alluded to by Rashi on 6:11. See also *Avot D'Rab Nosson* 32:1; Zohar I, 66:2 on Genesis 7:4; Ramban and Ritvah on Niddah 13a; M. Kasher in *Torah Sh'lemah*, on Genesis 6:12, no. 150 comparing similar suggestions in Shabbat 41a.

22. Genesis 38:7–10 and the Talmud's discussion thereof in Yevamot 34b. The passage in Yevamot equates the sin of Er and Onan with unnatural intercourse (*shello k'darkah*) rather than with Rashi's assumption (on Genesis, loc. cit.) that the failing was coitus interruptus. See Ritva and Maharsha on Yevamot 34, and Ibn Ezra on Genesis 38:7, who offer a variety of approaches to reconcile these differing interpretations. See the trenchant passage in *Levush*, Genesis 38:10.

23. Rabbi Eliezer on Yevamot 34b, a position with which the majority of Sages disagree.

24. Resp. *Iggrot Moshe*, Even HaEzer no. 63, p. 154 as translated by D.M. Feldman, *Marital Relations*, p. 152.

25. *Mishneh Torah*, Hil. Issurie Bi'ah, 21:18 and so Smag, Neg. 126 and *Shulhan Arukh*, Even HaEzer, 23:1

26. Not all authorities are always strict; some advocate coitus interruptus as the desirable method to obtain sperm for analysis: Resp. *Z'kan Aharon*, vol. 1, nos. 66, 67, and vol. 2, no. 96, p. 18 n. 67.

27. Nedarim 20b. See Bet Yosef on *Tur*, Even HaEzer 25 and *Kol Bo*, Hil. Ishut, par. 76 p. 66a who counsel caution to the pious.

28. Yevamot 34b, s.v. *v'lo*.

29. *Tur*, Even HaEzer 25 and Orach Haim 240; *Yam Shel Shlomo*, Yevamot, chap. 3, par. 18, and *Haggahot HaBach* on Rosh to Yevamot 34b and others refer to a permissive ruling by Rosh on Yevamot, chap. 3, par. 6—a text deleted (censored?) in extant versions of this commentary. Similarly Drisha on *Tur*, Even HaEzer 23:1; Resp. *Maishiv Davar*, Yoreh De'ah no. 88; and Resp. *Iggrot Moshe*, Even HaEzer, no. 63, p. 156, who also records his pleasure to hear that Resp. *Tzemach Tzedek*, Even Haezer no. 89 supported this position.

30 For example, Rema, Even HaEzer, 25:2: "A man may act with his wife as he wishes, having intercourse when he wants...[and how he wants] provided he does not ejaculate. Others are lenient and rule that he may have unnatural intercourse even if he emits sperm so long as this is not habitual. However even though all this is [strictly speaking] permitted, 'He who sanctifies himself [by denying even] that which is permitted, is called holy.'"

31. Rabbi Yehuda HaHasid, *Sefer Hassidim*, no. 176; but Hiddah (*Petach Einayim*, Niddah 13) dismisses this as a case of unavoidable spillage and not of intentional masturbation.

32. Yevamot 76a.

33. *Beit Shmuel*, Even HaEzer, 25:2.

34. *Levush* on Even HaEzer, 23:5, though dyspareunia—painful intercourse—may not be an acceptable reason to suspend the restrictions (Resp. *Melamed Lehoil*, III, no. 18)

35. Tosfot RiD on Yevamot 12b.

36. Although the expression "unnatural" intercourse customarily denotes non-vaginal (e.g. anal or oral) sex, any form of frustrated or aberrant vaginal (e.g. by a diaphragm or other intravaginal device) penetration may be subsumed under this label.

37. *Marital Relations*, p. 162.

38. Resp. *Heikhal Yitzhak*, Even HaEzer, vol. 2, no. 16.

39. Resp. *Iggrot Moshe*, Even HaEzer nos. 63 and 64.

40 In particular, the Zohar on Exodus, 259a and 263b. Similarly strongly worded restrictive views are recorded by *Sefer Haredim*, III, chap. 2 by Rabbi Eliezer Azikri (1601) and in Rabbi Isaiah Hurvitz's *Sh'nie Luhot HaBrit* (Shlah), I, *Sha'ar HaOtiot* 100, a, b. The latter, on p. 102b (Amsterdam ed.) writes: "Study to observe all the laws of marital relations as enumerated in the *Tur*, Orach Haim 240 and Even HaEzer 25, omit nothing.... A man should know every word by heart—except in the matter of unnatural intercourse. In that connection I have cited (the restrictive) words of *Sefer Haredim*—to him you should listen [rather than to the *Tur*]."

41. Rabbi Yosef Karo, *Bedek Habayit* on Bet Yosef, Even HaEzer 25.

42. On *Shulhan Arukh*, Even HaEzer 25:2.

43. Normally, men with rabbinically identified anatomical disfigurement of the penis are barred from wedding a genetically Jewish spouse; undamaged anatomy and function of sexual organs are prerequisites for such relationships. Elaborating, the Talmud in Yevamot 76a states: "If a hole which had been made in the [penile] corona itself is closed, the man is disqualified if it reopens when semen is emitted; but if it does not [reopen the man is deemed] fit. Rava the son of Rabbah sent to Rav Yosef: Will our Master instruct us how to proceed [with a test when it is desired to ascertain whether the semen will reopen an occluded perforation]. The other replied: Warm barley bread is procured, and placed upon the man's anus. This stimulates the flow of semen and the effect can be observed. Said Abaye: Is everybody like our father

Jacob…because [of whose saintliness] he never before [marriage] experienced the emission of semen? [An alternative technique was offered by] Abaye who said 'no, colored [female] garments are dangled before him.' Said Rava: Is everybody then like Barzillai the Gileadite [known for his indulgences]? In fact it is obvious that the original answer is to be maintained."

44. *Yam Shel Shlomo*, Yevamot, 8:16.

45. Quite another application of the restriction of masturbation is found in the laws of circumcision. A tense penis is recommended prior to the procedure to assure safe amputation of the foreskin and thus reduce the risk of injury to the underlying glands. This is especially true in the adult. It is permissible for erection to be achieved by physical stimulation of the penis but since this can lead to *hotza'at zera l'vatalah* it ought to have been banned because of the Talmud's opposition to manual masturbation as recorded in Niddah 13a. Rabbi Shlomo Kluger (introduction to *Sefer Kin'as Sofrim*) eliminates this apparent difficulty: in accordance with the general rule that positive commandments taking precedence over negative ones, especially when the former are biblical and the latter rabbinic in origin, circumcision takes precedence over the ordinance banning masturbation. Based upon these considerations it is arguable that in spite of whatever rabbinic restrictions may exist, masturbation would still be permitted when it is performed to facilitate reproductive capability. However, a counterargument might be that in the case of circumcision, seminal spillage is not inevitable; in the case of infertility it is.

46. Rabbi C.O. Grodzinski, *Ahiezer* III, no. 24:4 partly based upon Rabbi Ya'akov Emden, Resp. *She'elat Ya'avetz* I, no. 43; Rabbi Uziel, Resp. *Mishpetei Uziel*, Even HaEzer no. 42. Resp. *Z'kan Aharon* I, no. 67 insists upon coitus interruptus rather than masturbation.

   Semen analysis and procurement are discussed in detail by many authorities, including: Rabbi E. Waldenberg, Resp. *Tzitz Eliezer*, vol. 7, 48:1.7 and vol. 9, 51:1; by Rabbi Ovadiah Yosef, Resp. *Yabia Omer* vol. 2, Even HaEzer 1:7, and Rabbi M. Feinstein, Resp. *Iggrot Moshe*, vol. 3, Even HaEzer I:70, and II:16; vol. 5, Even HaEzer III:14; vol. 7, Even HaEzer IV:27.

   A valuable review of semen destruction and contraception in general appears in the *Reb Ya'akov Rosenheim Jubilee Volume*, (New York, 1932), p. 87, by Rabbi J.Z. Horowitz of Frankfurt. He gathers the major opinions and concludes that seminal procurement for analysis intended to facilitate procreation is permissible.

47. Uncertainties include: The impediment may be in the female partner; there may in any case be no effective therapy; it may be possible for him to father children were he married to someone else; a problem with the technique of intercourse may exist.

48. *Otzar HaPoskim*, Even HaEzer, vol. IX, p. 86a (quoting in particular Resp. *Divrie Malkiel*) vol. 5, no. 157; *Vaya'an Avraham* no. 7; R. S. Engle (quoted below); etc.

49. In his Responsa, vol. 6. no. 75, Rabbi S. Engel recommends this radical answer after ten years of barren marriage have transpired. See S. Shilo, "Impotence as a ground for divorce (to the end of the period of the *Rishonim*)," *The Jewish Law Annual*, 4:127–43, (1981), for an interesting historical review.

50. Sedei Hemed "Pe'as Sadeh" in *Ma'arechet Ishut* no. 13; Resp. *Ezrat Kohen*, Hil. Ishut no. 32 by Rabbi A.Y. Kook; Resp. *Avnei Nezer*, Even HaEzer 83. They advocate empiric therapeutic trials without regard to specific diagnoses. On the other hand, Resp. *Tzitz Eliezer*, vol. IX, 51:1.2 acknowledges that modern differential diagnoses may indeed have a significant impact on treatment choices. Rabbi Eliezer of Munkacz, author of Resp. *Minhat Eliezer*, in *Darkhei Teshuva*, Hil. Niddah, agrees with the restrictive views, but would sanction the postcoital vaginal collection of sperm for analysis.

51. Rabbis Y. Newirth and S.Z. Auerbach are quoted by A. Abraham in *Nishmat Avraham*, Even HaEzer, 23:2, p. 112, as recommending that when a condom is worn a small perforation should be made, thus enabling sperm to enter the female's reproductive tracts. This would obviate concerns about wastefulness of seed in that it is possible that the coital act will result in pregnancy.

52. Rabbi Y.Y. Weiss in Resp. *Minhat Yitzhak* vol. 3, no. 108:6.

53. *Shulhan Arukh*, Even HaEzer 25:2

54. Rabbi Waldenberg, Resp. *Tzitz Eliezer*, *loc. cit.*, takes issue with *Mahatzit Hashekel*, *loc. cit.*, who maintains that the dispensation of *hatza'at shikhvat zera l'vatala* implied by Yevamot 76a is limited to when the investigation is needed to establish marriageability within the *kahal;* Rabbi Waldenberg argues that avoiding divorce is no less a reason for permissiveness. Evidence of spermatogenesis may be required to overcome restrictions which pertain to certain categories of infertile men. Such investigations, of course, must be made on the male in question. Rabbi Waldenberg cites *Taharat Yisrael*, Orach Haim 240:39, who rules that ejaculation is permitted when physicians are undertaking investigations designed to promote fertility and eventual procreation.

55. Quoted by A. Abraham in *Nishmat Avraham*, Even HaEzer 23:2, p. 111. By contrast, Rabbi Eliyahu Bakshi-Doron of Haifa (*Binyan Av*, 11 and cited in a personal communication to Dr. Joel Wolowelsky, Dec. 15, 1991) submits that the grave ban on *hatza'at zera* could not be lifted for purposes other than the mitzvah of *peru u'revu*. The rabbinically invoked mitzvah of *lashevet* would not in itself authorize annulment of this *issur*.

56. Resp. *Shevet Sofer*, Even HaEzer 1. Similar arguments are found in Resp. *Imrei Esh*, Yoreh De'ah 69 and Resp. *Levushei Mordekhai*, 111, *Orach Haim* 51. A contrasting view is that of Resp. *Rav Pe'alim* 111, Even HaEzer 2.

57. Resp. *Tzitz Eliezer*, *loc. cit.*, end of gate 1.

58. A. Abraham in *Nishmat Avraham*, Even HaEzer 23:2, p. 112 reports that Rabbi Shlomo Zalman Auerbach recommends that if possible, this be performed by a female doctor or nurse.

59. As recommended by Resp. *Z'kan Aharon* vol. 1, no. 66; but see next note.

60. Other authorities would reverse this step with the previous one.
61. In accordance with Resp. *Ahiezer*, but in contrast with Resp. *Iggrot Moshe*, which would never allow self-stimulation .
62. Resp. *Z'kan Aharon*, vol. 1, no. 66. He assumed the purpose of this test to be the analysis of the semen.
63. Deuteronomy 23:2.
64. Yevamot 75b.
65. Rabbi Y. Newirt quoted by A. Abraham in *Nishmat Avraham*, Even HaEzer 23:2, p. 113.
66. Rabbi Y.Y. Weiss, Resp. *Minhat Yitzhak*, vol. 3. no. 108:7. In view of Rabbeinu Tam's opinion, which permits even complete excision of the left testicle, Rabbi Weiss counsels that an elective biopsy be taken from the left side. Rabbi E. Waldenberg, Resp. *Tzitz Eliezer*, vol. 9, no. 51:1.2, agrees with him.
67. Resp. *Iggrot Moshe*, Even HaEzer vol. 2., 3:2. Note that Rabbi Feinstein does not make his authorization contingent upon using the left side only. See also J.A. Gordon, R.D. Amelar, L. Dubin, M.D. Tendler, "Infertility practice and Orthodox Jewish law," *Fertility and Sterility,* 28:480, (1975).

Part IV
Therapeutic Interventions

Introduction

Across many cultures and socioeconomic groups, it is widely assumed that a woman's barrenness lies in her own body. For a sexually competent man to grasp that he might be the source of his wife's barrenness is often difficult. For this reason, it is not uncommon for the evaluation of the female to completely precede the evaluation of the male. Nevertheless, there comes a point for nearly one half of infertile couples when the man must submit to investigation before the process can continue. An observant man, however, cannot proceed with an examination without first considering potential halakhic restrictions. Moreover, there are psychological reasons that may cause him to delay his evaluation.

In times of good health, men differ from women in the way that they approach their health-care needs. A young woman who has reached adulthood generally understands the need for annual exams with her gynecologist. There are many reasons for even an unmarried woman to undergo a gynecologic consultation and examination. By the time the issue of infertility arises, she likely will have already established a professional relationship with someone who she trusts to give proper counseling and guidance. The examination process itself provokes little anxiety. Going through a new testing phase is only an extension of medical interventions to which she has already been accustomed. The situation is far different for the average man facing infertility. Commonly, his last visit to a physician will have been to his pediatrician. He is not used to the consultative necessity of baring his private habits and issues to another. The prospect of having a genital exam is unnerving.

Observant Jewish men share these anxieties and more. The focus of the examination is the seed itself. But the seed is not just an ordinary cell in the body. It is considered, in a certain sense, holy. There is a direct biblical reference to wastage of seed as a sin. Although it is recognized halakhically that the sperm cell is not the equivalent of a human life, rabbinic lore is replete with allusions that this is so. Maimonides declared that wasting of the seed is equivalent to *shefihut damim*, or murder. The homonculous theory—"the finding, using the new microscopes of our day, that the entire human is contained inside the sperm" was used by later authorities to validate this precept.[1] As noted in the previous section, many contemporary rabbis have addressed the question of providing sperm for analysis in cases of infertility. Although most do not consider it "wasting of the seed," there are many differing opinions regarding the length of time that must pass prior to the examination, the methods of collection, and under what circumstances. Even a Torah scholar understands that when he is faced with infertility, he is going to need to consult with a rabbi. He must find a rabbi who is not only a good adviser but also expert enough in reproductive halakha that he can function as a *posek*, or halakhic decisor.

Notwithstanding all of this, the compelling desire to have children will eventually bring the man to the attention of a physician. This is most often an urologist, preferably one with a special interest in male fertility. In the following chapter, Dr. Nahum Katlowitz explains the process of evaluation and management from the physician's perspective.

The chapters that follow on therapy for female infertility and assisted reproduction are medically comprehensive and define the flashpoints where medical treatment and halakhic problems overlap.

This information should be of great value to couples undergoing treatment for infertility. But it is hoped that rabbis and *poskim* will also find the discussion interesting and useful. Unlocking for them the mysteries of treatment may help restore their trust in physicians. This is sorely needed in these matters, where rabbinic doubt about the trustworthiness of physicians has fueled patient anxieties. And not without cause. The world is not a perfect place, and there are people who deal unscrupulously in all walks of life. Couples seeking treatment for infertility should indeed check the credentials of the treating physicians, and should have a sense of their ethical qualities. They should feel comfortable with both the level of professional expertise and the level of personal concern that accompanies their treatment. They should be able to discuss their religious concerns without feeling embarrassed or threatened. As will be evident from the material presented, excepting rare cases, there are virtually no fertility treatments that cannot be adapted for use in halakhically acceptable ways. Couples who are being treated by physicians unfamiliar with their halakhic concerns should feel comfortable sharing this information with their caregivers. To the extent that unanticipated problems may develop, open communication between physicians and rabbis who are well informed of each others' guiding principles will facilitate care.

This approach should govern the physician-patient relationship regardless of the type of therapy that is required. When a couple feels that their physician is on their side, and that he or she has in mind their religious values as well as their ultimate goal of having a child, they can comfortably trust that physician to do the right thing for them. Others who may cast doubt on the motives of physicians will do little but add stress to an already stressful situation. On the other hand, the couple who enters therapy with confidence will be emotionally prepared to persist in that therapy as long as it takes to achieve their desired goal.

Endnote

1.   *Arukh HaShulkhan*, Even HaEzer 23.

Nahum Katlowitz

Evaluation and Treatment of Male Infertility

V ery few men are truly infertile. Even men with severely depressed sperm counts may father biological children without medical assistance if they are married to extremely fertile women. Other than cases of complete absence of sperm, or azospermia, most men who are diagnosed with infertility are actually subfertile. Absent halakhic restrictions, the ideal evaluation of husband and wife would be simultaneous, with good communication between the specialist physicians. Together they would evaluate the subfertile *couple*. As a practical matter, whether one begins with the evaluation of the woman or the man depends on the particular circumstances of their fertility problem. Certainly, the status of both husband and wife must be ascertained before either of them is subjected to any invasive procedures.

Anatomy and Physiology

In order to fully understand what is involved in the evaluation and treatment of the male, it is best to first understand the basic anatomy and physiology involved.

In the human male, the embryonic precursor of what will form the testicle appears during the fourth week of embryonic life as a small ridge toward the back of the developing fetus. Cells that will later give rise to spermatogonia, or sperm precursors, enter this ridge and fully reach their destination by about the sixth week of development. At this point a group of genes on the Y chromosome of the fetus begins to direct the production of testis determining factor, or TDF.[1] Under the influence of TDF, the ridge develops parallel sex cords within which will be found the precursors of Sertoli cells, Leydig cells, and spermatogonia. The Sertoli and Leydig cells will later support sperm production and hormonal secretion in the mature testicle, while the spermatogonia will provide the source for the actual sperm cells. These cords eventually form the seminiferous tubules, which empty into the rete testis and, later in development, into the epididymis and vas deferens. (The function of all of these components will be described below.) Abnormal development at any point in this embryologic progression may lead to future trouble with fertility. For example, if the gene that helps the sperm cells mature or the gene that helps the Sertoli cells develop is missing, one can end up without the ability to form mature sperm.

As fetal development progresses, the testis eventually releases itself from the dorsal ridge of the fetus and migrates downward into the developing scrotum. Abnormalities in descent, believed by some to be due to an intrinsic defect in testicular development, can leave the testicle in abnormal locations such as the perineum, the inguinal canal, or even inside the abdominal cavity. These abnormalities in testicular descent are relatively common, and are known as cryptorchidism. Cryptorchid testes must be diagnosed and surgically repaired early in life or they will function very poorly, if at all.

When proper testicular development is complete, the germ

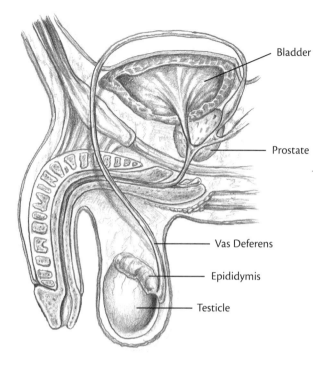

Normal male anatomy

cells in the precursor stage are located within the testicle and are surrounded by the supportive and nurturing structures of the Leydig and Sertoli cells as well as by other connective tissues such as blood vessels. In the mature testicle, the Leydig cells will produce testosterone and the Sertoli cells will support proper sperm maturation. The testicle is quiescent until puberty, at which time changes in the neuroendocrine system awaken it to undergo these final stages of development.

Pituitary-Testicular Axis

The signaling that takes place between the pituitary gland and the testicle is an example of the neuroendocrine system. That is, input from the brain (= "neuro") and central nervous system (including external environmental stimuli) can be translated and modulated via the endocrine, or hormonal, system into direct physiological events.

The pituitary gland is an extension of the base of the brain. It receives instructions from the hypothalamus, a complex array of neuronal centers near the center of the brain that respond to higher

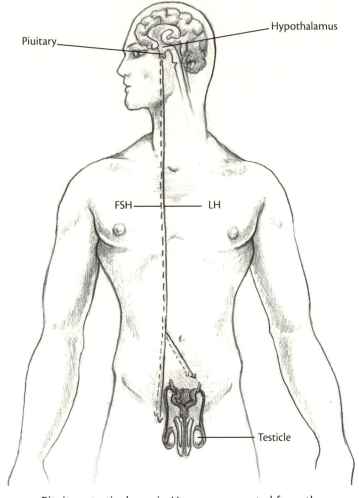

Pituitary testicular axis: Hormones secreted from the pituitary gland control sperm production in the testicles

stimuli such as emotions, environmental triggers, and the body's changing homeostatic needs. The major reproductive signal of the hypothalamus is the pulsatile release of gonadotropin releasing hormone, or GnRH. By varying the amplitude and frequency of GnRH pulses, the hypothalamus can stimulate or inhibit pituitary secretion of follicle stimulating hormone (FSH) and luteinizing hormone (LH). FSH and LH are the major determinant of testicular activity. FSH stimulates the Sertoli cell to direct the production of sperm. The Sertoli cell, in turn, produces inhibin. In what is known as a negative feedback loop, inhibin suppresses pituitary secretion of FSH.[2] LH stimulates the Leydig cells to produce testosterone, the dominant male hormone. When testosterone is converted to estrogen in other parts of the body, the estrogen then turns off pituitary secretion of LH. Leydig cells, Sertoli cells, and testosterone are all important in the progressive development of spermatogonia into mature sperm. It should be noted that the use of exogenous forms of steroids, such as testosterone or any of its analogs, for bodybuilding, or the use of other steroids such as those for medicinal needs, may alter this delicate balance and negatively impact sperm production.

In situations where the testicle cannot respond to the stimulatory signals of the pituitary gland, such as if there are no sperm precursors or if the Leydig cells are damaged, the feedback inhibition loop becomes defective and the pituitary gland will continue to produce more and more LH and FSH in an attempt to overcome the lack of response. Blood levels of LH and FSH may therefore be useful as an indicator of testicular potential. (FSH and LH are secreted in a specialized fashion that is dependent upon the sleep cycle. Proper measurement of these hormones is therefore done within several hours of waking.)

Spermatogenesis

Sperm develop inside the seminiferous tubules, long tubular structures lined by Sertoli cells, which are joined to one another with very tight connections that have the effect of isolating sperm from the blood in the surrounding network of small blood vessels. Through many different steps of differentiation, the spermatogonia within these tubules become spermatocytes, then spermatids and, finally, full-fledged sperm (spermatozoa). During this process, the DNA content of the sperm precursors is reduced from 46 to 23 chromosomes. All normal sperm carry either one Y (male) or one X (female) chromosome. The process of normal fertilization will eventually combine the sperm with a mature egg, or oocyte, which also carries 23 chromosomes, thus creating a new individual, or embryo, with the normal complement of DNA on 46 chromosomes. As all normal oocytes can only carry an X chromosome, it is the sperm that determines the gender of the new individual, i.e. the Y-containing sperm will produce a male and the X-containing sperm will produce a female.

The process of sperm maturation and differentiation takes approximately 74 days and involves many specialized cellular components. The mature sperm consists of the head, midpiece, and tail. The head contains the nuclear material—tightly wound coils of DNA that provide half of the instruction set to produce a new individual. It is surrounded by the acrosomal cap, which contains

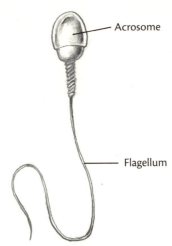

Sperm cell: Each part of the sperm is designed to deliver
DNA within the sperm head to the waiting egg

enzymes necessary to help it penetrate the mature oocyte. The tail, or flagellum, is composed of sliding microfilaments. Flagellum movement is powered by surrounding mitochondria, which are located mainly in the midpiece and provide energy for the microfilaments to slide against each other in a coordinated fashion, resulting in motility, or movement, of the sperm. The fully motile, or moving, sperm cell has the ability to move from the vas deferens to the outside world.

Sperm Maturation, Capacitation, and Transport

The rete testis is a sort of collecting station for sperm that are about to exit the testicle. From there they move to the epididymis, a long coiled tube that, if straightened, would measure 3 to 4 meters in length. The epididymis plays an important part in normal sperm development. The initial portion is the site of continued sperm maturation while the end, or distal, portion functions as a storage site. It takes approximately two weeks for sperm to traverse the entire epididymis. As they exit the epididymis, the sperm enter a thicker tube called the vas deferens. The vas is a long tube which exits the scrotum and travels into the pelvis to join with the tube draining the seminal vesicles, where the majority of seminal fluid, or semen, is produced. These two tubes join in a structure called the ejaculatory duct. The ejaculatory duct traverses the prostate and empties into the prostatic urethra. At the time of orgasm, the contents of the urethra, containing seminal fluid and sperm, are expelled out of the penis in a process called ejaculation. Depending on the frequency of ejaculation, sperm will remain viable in the epididymis for 3–10 days.

Ejaculated sperm are not immediately capable of fertilizing an egg. The process by which sperm acquire the ability to fertilize is called capacitation, and it occurs inside the female's reproductive tract. When the capacitated sperm reaches the egg, signaling from the egg causes the acrosome surrounding the sperm head to release its enzymes in a process called the acrosome reaction. The enzymes then bore a hole into the protective cover of the egg (the zona pellucida), enabling the sperm to swim through and fuse with the cell membrane of the egg. The nuclear materials of both cells then decondense and merge into one nucleus, forming a new organism—the embryo. From this newly created cell a complete and unique human being eventually will emerge.

Assessment of Male Infertility

I. HISTORY

As with any medical evaluation, the first and often the most important step is taking a careful history. For obvious reasons, the evaluation of the infertile male is a personal and sometimes very delicate matter, involving a discussion of issues not typically covered in a standard medical evaluation. Aside from the general history of past illnesses, operations, and known medical problems such as diabetes and hypertension, other issues that require addressing include:

Occurrence of puberty—Early or delayed puberty can often point to abnormal functioning of the pituitary gland or testicles. Some men may marry before puberty has been completed.

Prior surgery or other genitourinary trauma—Surgery to repair undescended testicles, hernias, or bladder problems, as well as traumatic injury to or torsion of the testicles, can all be linked to later reproductive problems.

Previous chemotherapy—Chemotherapeutic drugs used to treat a variety of cancers are toxic to developing sperm and often to testicular tissue. Although the effects of many wear off over time, some can cause irreversible sterility.

Environmental exposure—Exposure to toxic chemicals, heavy

metals, radiation, or prolonged heat, can inhibit or damage sperm production mechanisms.

Smoking—Smoking is believed to be an inhibitor of sperm production and can also adversely affect sexual ability and performance.

Recreational drug use—The use of alcohol, marijuana, depressants, stimulants and anabolic steroids for muscle building can all impair sperm production.

Prior pregnancies with the current or prior partner(s)—A positive history, even of pregnancy that did not continue to term, would indicate that the individual had functional sperm at some point in his life, suggesting that there are no major chromosomal abnormalities affecting his sperm.

Prior evaluations and or treatments—Duplication of testing is costly and wastes time. Full medical records should be available. Testing that has been performed suboptimally may have to be repeated. Examples include semen analyses done in commercial laboratories.[3]

Length of infertility—The average couple takes six months to conceive, and it is normal for conception to take up to twelve months. Some couples may be impatient in allowing nature to take its course, and be concerned about their fertility before granting a sufficient amount of time to trying to conceive. Others, on the other hand, may have allowed many years or even decades to pass without proper evaluation. Longstanding infertility is commonly due to severe sperm problems.

Sexual ability—If the man is not able to obtain and/or maintain an erection rigid enough and of sufficient duration to ejaculate inside the woman, then difficulties with conception will obviously occur.

Sexual frequency—Pregnancy can result from a single act of intercourse as many as five days prior to ovulation.[4] Coital frequency must increase, however, in order to maximize the chance for conception. In particular, frequency should increase near the time of ovulation. A minimum of once every 48 hours as ovulation approaches is optimal, although for men with normal sperm counts daily intercourse is preferable.

Lubricant use—Natural lubrication is a result of vaginal secretions produced during sexual foreplay. Hasty intercourse, fear of performance and other sources of anxiety prevent lubrication and can make intercourse difficult or even painful. When necessary, relaxation techniques should be used. If they do not work and exogenous lubrication is needed, oil-based lubricants such as Astroglide® or mineral oil should be used. Thicker lubricants such as K-Y Jelly® or Vaseline® can immobilize sperm and should not be used when conception is desired.

Marital and personal stress—Although psychological stress per se will not impair fertility, it can adversely affect coital ability, frequency, and adequacy.

Ejaculatory dysfunction—Ejaculation during intercourse may be premature, delayed, or even absent. If prior to or shortly after the commencement of intercourse the husband has orgasm, this is called premature ejaculation. Wives of men with premature ejaculation may lack sexual satisfaction and ultimately decrease the frequency of their sexual encounters, resulting in subfertility. The same can also occur if ejaculation takes too long, as a result of which intercourse becomes painful for the woman (and possibly the man as well). If ejaculation does not occur during intercourse, the couple will obviously not conceive.

General complaints—Items of general interest in the medical history would include other existing or prior urological complaints, such as voiding dysfunction and prior infections, especially urinary tract infections or those involving the testicles, such as mumps, *epididymitis* (swelling of the epididymis) or *orchitis* (swelling of the testicle).

Female factors—Although the urologist's evaluation inevitably focuses on the male, basic information regarding female factors should include the following: regularity of the menstrual cycle, any episodes of pain with menses or with intercourse, prior pelvic infections, the results of any previous evaluation, especially postcoital testing, and any previous treatments for infertility.

II. PHYSICAL EXAMINATION

After the history is completed, a complete examination should be performed. This includes general physical aspects such as demeanor, vital signs, heart and lung function. Special attention is paid to body habitus, hair pattern, and breast enlargement. The genitalia need to be carefully examined including the penis, testicles, and paratesticular tissue. The testicles are examined for their presence, size, consistency, and areas of abnormal texture that might imply prior infection. The paratesticular tissue is examined for structures that may be abnormal—such as an enlarged scrotal vein called a varicocele, or inflammation of the epididymis—or missing. An example of the latter is congenital absence of the vas deferens (CAVD), which has been described in men who carry the gene for cystic fibrosis.[5] This is a well-established cause for complete azospermia and sterility despite normal production of sperm inside the testicles, and it is correctable (see below). A rectal exam is performed to examine the prostate and feel for enlarged seminal vesicles and anal tone. A neurological and peripheral vascular exam is usually performed as well.

III. LABORATORY AND RADIOLOGICAL EVALUATION

Depending on the results of the history and physical examination, the urologist will usually request one or more of the following laboratory tests to be done. As a rule, most *poskim* have little difficulty allowing any of these.

Hormonal Testing—Measurements of FSH, LH, prolactin, and testosterone are considered standard in the hormonal assessment of a male suffering from infertility. The first three of these hormones are of pituitary origin while the third is a testicular hormone. Together, they reflect the function of the pituitary-testicular axis. These blood tests are best drawn early in the morning, within the first three to four hours of waking. Otherwise a falsely low value may be obtained. Many *poskim* request that even if there is only a remote possibility that a hormonal problem is causing the infertility, it should be ruled out before a semen analysis is done. If the testicles are smaller or softer than expected, hormonal testing becomes even more important. Blood chemistries to evaluate liver and renal function, as well as a complete blood count, may also be done.

Radiological studies—Ultrasound is a means of using sound waves to confirm or rule out the presence of abnormalities in soft tissues. *Scrotal ultrasound* can detect the presence of a varicocele. This is a common cause of male infertility. When a varicocele is present, any increase in intra-abdominal pressure—as may occur with laughing, coughing, or exercising—causes increased blood flow to the testicles through the dilated testicular vein. The excess heat and toxins that accumulate as a result of this reverse blood flow may interfere with proper sperm production. Scrotal ultrasound may also detect abnormalities of the epididymis and testicle. *Transrectal ultrasound* (TRUS) may be requested if previous testing, either by postcoital test or semen analysis, has revealed an absence of sperm. Using an ultrasound probe inserted through the rectum, the prostate and seminal vesicles can be imaged. Ejaculatory duct obstruction or absence of the seminal vesicles may be diagnosed. If the ejaculatory ducts are obstructed, a surgical procedure to relieve the blockage may allow spontaneous conception to occur. If the seminal vesicles are congenitally absent, then exploration of the scrotum with removal of sperm from the epididymis or testicle (micro-epydidimal sperm aspiration [MESA], or testicular sperm extraction [TESE], respectively) can be used in conjunction with in vitro fertilization to achieve a pregnancy.

Urine testing—Some men have a condition known as retrograde ejaculation. This means that when ejaculation occurs the sperm move backward into the bladder instead of outward from the penis. This condition is often associated with advanced diabetes and vascular disease, and may also result from certain urological procedures or medications. The only health consequence of retrograde ejaculation is infertility. In order to check for this condition, the first voided urine after ejaculation is examined for the presence of sperm. Finding a few sperm is normal; a large number of sperm in the urine is diagnostic of retrograde ejaculation.

Postcoital test—As a practical matter, it is possible to determine if a man has sperm and if they are viable from a vaginal examination of his partner after intercourse has occurred (providing that the test is done near her time of ovulation, see "General Aspects of Female Infertility"). When other clues about the origin of a couple's infertility are evident, such as when the wife has absent or irregular cycles, normal results on the postcoital test are reassuring and may allow formal semen analysis to be deferred. In such cases, most *poskim* advise that correction of the female factors should take place first and then a certain waiting period ensue prior to allowing direct examination of the semen. On the other hand, the complete absence of sperm on repeated, well-timed postcoital testing invariably points to a likely male factor. In such cases, semen analysis is necessary to ascertain the severity of the sperm abnormality. Rabbinical consultation at this point is absolutely necessary so that time is not wasted and the wife is not subjected to inappropriate interventions.

Semen analysis—The postcoital test is not a replacement for the semen analysis. It simply provides information about the presence or absence of sperm. Semen analysis, on the other hand, provides for multiple assessments of sperm that, taken together, can be used to accurately assess male fertility potential. The semen analysis provides for the measurement of the following parameters:

> *Viscosity*—an indication of how thick the semen is. In the presence

of infection or in the absence of certain enzymes, the semen can thicken. This interferes with proper movement, trapping the sperm. If increased viscosity is the only abnormality detected, then amylase suppositories for the man or sperm washing with intrauterine insemination (see "Therapeutic Solutions") may be useful.

Agglutination—a measure of clumping, or sticking together, of sperm cells. If there is a lot of agglutination, it may point to the presence of infection and/or antisperm antibodies. The coating of the sperm by these antibodies, which may be produced by the man against his own sperm or by the woman, can prevent fertilization.

pH—a measure of the acidity of the semen. Abnormal pH, especially in the basic range, is suggestive of infection.

Volume—a certain minimum (2 cc) or maximum (6 cc) volume of semen is expected. (A cc is a cubic centimeter, and is also equivalent to a milliliter, or ml.) If there is too little, it may be a result of retrograde ejaculation, obstruction, or an anatomical problem. If there is too much seminal fluid, then the sperm concentration may be relatively low, as it is diluted by the excess volume.

Motility—a measure of the percentage of sperm that are moving. Motility is decreased in men with infertility, especially in the presence of a varicocele. In most laboratories, 50% is the lower limit of normal.

Concentration—the number of sperm per cc of seminal fluid. The minimum concentration of sperm in a normal semen specimen is 20 million/cc. Most men, however, have over 50 million/cc.

Linearity—a measurement of the forward progression, or straightness, of the sperm as they swim through the semen. It is usually measured by a skilled technician on a scale of 0–4, with greater than 2 defining normal movement. Computer assisted semen analysis (CASA) is used by some laboratories to grade both linearity and velocity. The latter refers to the actual swimming speed of the sperm.

Morphology—this refers to the shapes of the sperm, which may be measured by one of two sets of criteria, or both. Criteria set by the World Health Organization (who) are commonly used in commercial laboratories, and require that 30% of the sperm be of normal shape in order for the specimen to be considered normal. In recent years, specialized andrology laboratories have used different criteria, as set forth by Kruger, to examine sperm in a more exacting fashion. The Kruger criteria require that each sperm be exactly measured against a perfect standard. Using Kruger criteria, only 4–14% of the sperm need to be morphologically normal in order for the specimen to be considered normal. The limits of normal may, of course, vary from laboratory to laboratory.

One should be aware that the semen analysis is not always an exact indicator of fertility potential. Of course, in the absence of sperm in the semen, fertility through natural intercourse is impossible. But barring that specific finding, the semen analysis is merely

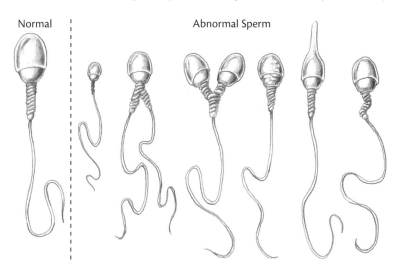

Normal   Abnormal Sperm

Sperm morphology: Sperm are found in many different shapes, but only the one at left is considered normal

a quantitative assessment of sperm. Some men who are assessed as subfertile by a standard semen analysis may initiate conception without difficulty. Likewise, some men may have apparently normal test results yet have poorly functional sperm and infertility. Results of the semen analysis therefore require interpretation by a physician thoroughly familiar with the complete clinical picture.

Note on the Procurement of Sperm for Analysis
The halakhic basis for different methods of sperm evaluation is discussed elsewhere in this book (see "Male Infertility: Halakhic Considerations"). Many couples will choose to use a seminal collection device (SCD), which is simply a medical-grade condom that, unlike commercially available condoms, is not coated with spermicide. The device is worn during intercourse and collects the ejaculated semen, which may then be submitted to the laboratory for evaluation. Some *poskim* require a small pinhole to be placed somewhere along the SCD. From the laboratory perspective, the smaller the hole and the farther back on the device it is made, the more accurate the test will be. If, how, and where to make this hole in the SCD requires discussion with a *posek*.

Depending on the clinical circumstances, some rabbinical authorities may request that semen be evaluated only during an insemination procedure. In this way there is less concern about wasting the seed, or *hash'hatat zera*.

Special Studies
When semen analysis reveals no or very limited sperm in the ejaculate, and there is no obvious cause on physical or laboratory exams, a genetic test called a Y-deletion study may be requested. This study will examine the man's Y chromosome for defects that may have led to the sperm abnormality. Chromosomes are the blueprints by which our bodies develop. All normal individuals have 46 chromosomes, consisting of 22 pairs of autosomes and one pair of sex chromosomes. Sex chromosomes can pair as either XX in females or XY in males. The Y chromosome contains the information required

for normal testicular development and function. As we now understand, some men have an extra piece or are missing a piece of their Y chromosome. These additions or deletions may not be significant enough to prevent normal male physical development but may be sufficient to impair or preclude fertility. Although some men with Y chromosome abnormalities can father children using the ICSI technique with in vitro fertilization (see "Assisted Reproduction"), they must be aware that any male children will likely be born with the same abnormality and also suffer from infertility. Sometimes the results of the Y-deletion study indicate that assisted reproduction will be necessary to produce a pregnancy. Occasionally, the results indicate that the man is not capable of fathering his own genetic child under any circumstances.

Treatment

Because treatment of infertility often involves both male and female systems, treatment by both a reproductive endocrinologist (for the woman) and an urologist (for the man) is often required. In the case of the Jewish infertile couple, this team often expands to include the rabbinical adviser.

Treatment options include situational/behavioral/functional, medical, surgical, and supportive.

SITUATIONAL/BEHAVIORAL/FUNCTIONAL

Behavioral changes are the least complicated medically but often the most difficult emotionally. On occasion, couples do not understand the timing and frequency of marital relations that would lead to an acceptable chance for conception. If, for example, as a misguided demonstration of piety the couple has sexual relations only on Friday nights during the permitted portion of the month while the wife consistently ovulates during the middle of the week, then they may both be normally fertile and never conceive. Likewise, some couples, especially those who marry very young, might not fully understand the anatomy or mechanics involved in conception and require some technical instruction. Ovulation prior to *mikvah* is a separate problem and is discussed elsewhere (See "Halakhic Considerations in the Treatment of Female Infertility").

There may also be problems with sexual performance. Couples are not always cognizant of how different the male and female sexual responses are. Ignorance of what should be expected from a partner may create stress and anxiety in both the husband and wife. For example, a normally functioning man may find that he is unable to perform sexually on the night prior to a postcoital test or in anticipation of a semen analysis. In these instances, any additional pressure from the wife is unhelpful. On the other hand, a woman may feel aroused and ready to have intercourse, but stop before completion because she experiences pain. Pain during intercourse, or dyspareunia, can sometimes be symptomatic of an underlying physical problem and sometimes be due to vaginismus, an involuntary contracting of the vaginal muscles. In either case, continued attempts to have intercourse will only result in frustration and helplessness.

Proper urological attention to any complaints of sexual dysfunction in the male is absolutely necessary. In certain instances, the same hormonal problem that is causing the sexual dysfunction can also be interfering with normal sperm production. Such cases may be receptive to medical therapy.

There are some men who are neurologically incapable of reaching orgasm during intercourse. Some may be successful in achieving ejaculation with vibratory assistance. If this and other medical therapies have failed, electro-ejaculation under anesthesia can be used to procure semen for use with insemination. Alternatively, testicular sperm extraction (TESE) may be used in conjunction with ICSI.

MEDICAL THERAPY

When hormonal problems are found as the basis of male infertility, correction should follow. Examples would include the lowering of prolactin levels in a man with hyperprolactinemia and also the replenishment of LH in an LH-deficient man. Assuming that normal sperm production follows immediately after the hormonal corrections are made, it would take approximately three months for normal sperm to appear in the ejaculate. Therefore, medical therapy should be followed by a three-to-six month waiting period to determine if the system has normalized. If it has, a further interval of waiting for pregnancy to occur should follow.

SURGICAL PROCEDURES

A variety of surgical procedures may be done in the process of evaluating or treating male factor infertility. Among the most common are:

Testicular biopsy—In the azospermic man, testicular biopsy with or without simultaneous TESE may be performed using either percutaneous (i.e. through the skin) or open techniques. The latter may be macrosurgical or microsurgical. The purpose of the biopsy is to remove a small piece of tissue from the testicle. This tissue is

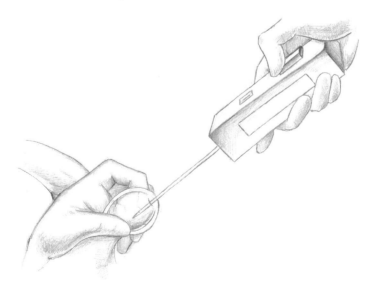

Testicular biopsy: Testicular tissue is obtained using a special tissue extractor

then examined for the presence or absence of sperm. If sperm are present, then their amount and degree of maturation are evaluated. Tissue containing mature sperm may be frozen for later use with IVF/ICSI. If there are sperm but they are not fully developed, this finding may help guide further therapy. If there are no sperm present, further microsurgical exploration or sperm mapping (see below) can be performed. If no sperm are found on all examinations, Sertoli Cell Only Syndrome (SCOS) may be diagnosed. Men with this syndrome are unable to produce genetic children through currently known methods.

Testicular mapping—In this procedure, fine needle aspirations of one or both testicles are performed. The results indicate if sperm are present and where in the testicles they are most likely to be found. Under local anesthesia, a needle is advanced through the scrotal skin into the testicle at multiple sites, using a standardized pattern. Suction is gently applied with an attached syringe in order to aspirate fluid from within the testicle. After withdrawal, the needle is

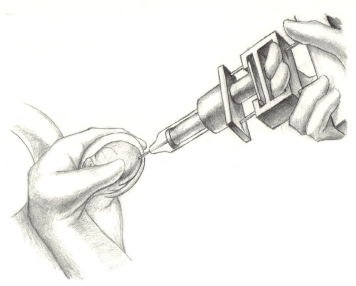

Testicular aspiration: A needle is used to asirate sperm from the testicle

rinsed with culture media and the aspirated fluid is examined for the presence or absence of sperm. If sperm are present, then the precise site from which they have been taken is noted. Eventually, a three dimensional map emerges indicating precisely where in the testicle sperm may be found.

Varicocele ligation—As described above, a varicocele may be found in as many as half of infertile men. For 40 to 60% of those, the semen analyses will normalize after ligation, or surgical tying, of the varicocele. This normalization usually takes three to six months, following which a waiting period of up to one year must follow to see if pregnancy can be achieved naturally. (Because the waiting time after varicocele ligation is long, the procedure is not recommended in older couples, where the age of the wife may preclude such a long wait.) Techniques to accomplish varicocele ligation include macrosurgical, microsurgical, and laparoscopic. A nonsurgical approach has also been described. Using x-ray guidance, a catheter can be threaded through the venous channels and used to embolize, or occlude, the varicocele. Which technique is used and when it

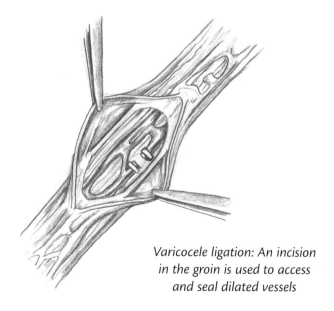

Varicocele ligation: An incision in the groin is used to access and seal dilated vessels

is performed depends on the particular clinical circumstances as well as the preference and skill of the surgeon.

Varicocele ligation is not useful in all cases of male infertility, especially when there are other significant female factors. However, it may be used even in those cases in order to prevent further deterioration of testicular function. Young men with large varicoceles and/or testicular atrophy should undergo ligation even if other methods of assisted reproduction are being considered. Likewise, painful varicoceles should be ligated no matter what the clinical circumstances.

Microsurgical epidydimal sperm aspiration (MESA)—If the man has an obstructed epididymis and either cannot, or does not, want to undergo surgical reconstruction, sperm may be removed directly

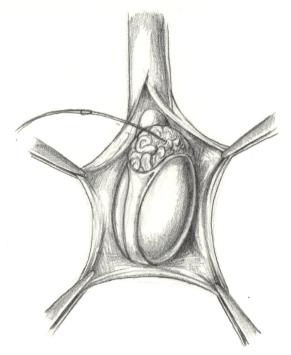

Microsurgical epidydimal sperm aspiration: The scrotum is open and the epididymal tubules are aspiarated under magnification

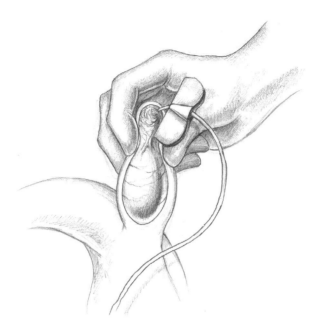

Percutaneous epidydimal sperm aspiration: A needle is placed through the scrotal skin into the epdidymis

from the epidydmis. In these men, the epididymis harbors functionally normal sperm, and therefore plenty of sperm can be obtained not only for use in a current cycle of IVF/ICSI but also for cryopreservation and later use.

Electroejaculation (EEJ)—This procedure is most often used with patients who have had spinal cord trauma, but is sometimes indicated for men who have psychogenic impotence and/or cannot ejaculate. Under general anesthesia, an electrical probe is placed through the rectum to a point near the prostate and seminal vesicles. The probe is activated with a low electrical current that causes the ejaculatory mechanism to activate.

Transurethral resection of the ejaculatory duct (TURED)—In rare cases where the ejaculatory ducts are obstructed, the obstruction can be surgically removed or resected. The operation is not very

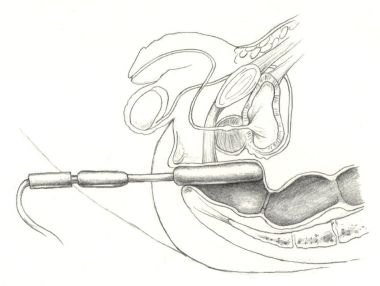

*Electroejaculation: Stimulation of the spinal
nerves cause erection and ejaculation*

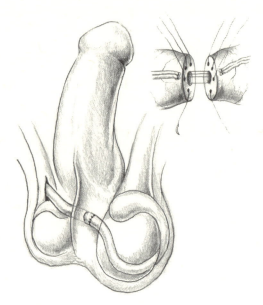

*Vasovasostomy, with inset: The obstructed segment is
removed and the open ends sutured together*

common and not without risk, but in select patients can result in a return of the sperm count to normal.

Vasovasostomy/Vasoepididymostomy—These procedures refer to the joining of the vas deferens to the epididymis or to another portion of the vas deferens. In most cases it is performed in patients who have had prior vasectomies. In some men, however, trauma or infection can result in closure of the vas deferens. Depending on the location, a microsurgical bypass of the obstructed area can be performed. If the procedure fails, MESA or TESE can be used in conjunction with IVF/ICSI.

Choosing Caregivers

Just as women commonly see a general gynecologist when they first suspect that they have a fertility problem, men will commonly see a general urologist to evaluate suspected male infertility. This is a good starting point, as most gynecologists and urologists have a basic working knowledge of how to deal with infertility. However, problems that occur in older couples, that are complex in nature, that are longstanding, or that involve the coordination of several highly technical services belong in the purview of the specialist. In such cases, and in all others that are not solved in a reasonable period of time, consultation with a reproductive specialist—either a reproductive endocrinologist or an urologist with special training in male infertility—should be sought. Today, most such specialists collaborate at centers that provide full service fertility care. In such facilities, the urologist is able to work side by side with the reproductive endocrinologist in order to expedite and optimize the outcome of treatment.

Assisted reproductive techniques such as insemination and in vitro fertilization are often used when primary treatment of the infertile male is not possible or has failed to achieve its goal. On occasion, these techniques may be suggested as alternatives to direct focus on the specific urological problem in order to overcome male infertility. Such decisions require expert evaluation by the involved specialists and communication on all matters. For Orthodox couples, these specialists include a rabbinical authority who is similarly "specialized" in matters of reproductive halakha. It is useful, in almost every circumstance, for the physicians and the rabbi to work together as a team on behalf of the best interests of the couple. Doing so assists the couple by giving them the psychological and spiritual support they require to weather the strains and stresses of treatment and to emerge successfully from their condition of infertility.

Endnotes

1. The natural, or default mode, of embryonic development is female. In the absence of a Y chromosome, or if the Y chromosome is present but is missing TDF, development will proceed as female.

2. This system of feedback control has an exact parallel in the female. In women, FSH secretion from the pituitary gland stimulates egg maturation. Granulosa cells in the maturing egg follicle produce inhibin, which then suppresses FSH secretion.

3. Commercial laboratories that process large volumes of automated tests are not always accurate in performing semen analysis, which is time-sensitive and which requires the attendance of an experienced technician. Most fertility specialists therefore have preferences for which laboratories they will accept, and many have their own laboratory facilities.

4. A.J. Wilcox, C.R. Weinberg, D.D. Baird, "Timing of sexual intercourse in relation to ovulation—effects on the probability of conception, survival of the pregnancy, and sex of the baby," *New England Journal of Medicine*, 333:1517–21, (1995).

5. Men who carry only one gene for cystic fibrosis are completely normal in every other way, and usually do not find out that they are carriers for this disease until they present with infertility.

Richard V. Grazi

Halakhic Considerations in the Treatment of Female Infertility

Although physicians commonly accept that female factors and male factors share almost equally in causing infertility, there is little question that the major focus in curing infertility is on the female. Several reasons may account for this. First, scientific understanding of reproductive physiology in women is more sophisticated than its parallel in men. As a set of biological phenomena, the mysteries and intricacies of cyclicity, conception, pregnancy, and childbirth seem to have captivated scientific attention more deeply than the static and, to a certain extent, more simple system in the male. The result is that our understanding of the two is unequal. This is also interesting from a historical perspective, as it may stem in part from the time-honored focus on the woman as the exclusive cause of infertility. As previously noted, it was not until the early twentieth century that physicians even entertained the thought that a sexually potent man may be infertile. In more recent times, the development of a medical specialty dealing specifically with male infertility lagged far behind its counterpart in gynecology.

Another reason for focusing on the treatment of women may be due to their innate biology: The cyclic system which characterizes normal female reproduction is exquisitely sensitive to stress. Not uncommonly, therefore, the experience of infertility and its accompanying stresses, regardless of the primary cause, will lead to physiological disturbances in the woman. Finally, and most obviously, it is the woman who must conceive. This means that many male disorders for which there are no direct cures require procedures to be performed on the female. Together, these factors emphasize the centrality of the woman in most fertility therapies and the crucial role which her treating physician must play.

In dealing with a problem so emotionally charged and physically challenging as infertility, strong bonds are often formed between the affected woman and her physician that go beyond the typical doctor-patient relationship. Because of the unpredictable nature of certain treatments, the physician is continuously "on call" for the patient. Office visits may be required several times a week. Addressing the anxieties that accompany treatment, phone calls may come daily and at odd hours. In return for this level of involvement, the physician may expect that instructions will be followed unerringly. As the complexity of treatment grows, the commitment of each to its success is expected to grow accordingly. It is within that framework that the demands of halakha may be perceived as obstacles to success.

Sensitivity to the halakhically committed woman may require of the physician that he or she alter modes of practice. While attention to modesty in the office is always important, it suddenly becomes even more so. Although repeated consultations with the husband may be routine, a fourth party—the rabbi—must now also be consulted. These changes in the style of practice that are made in order to accommodate halakhically committed couples may be perceived as intrusions that indirectly question the physician's competence or integrity. More importantly, the physician is given a new set of restrictions under which treatment must be designed. At times, those restrictions may actually prevent rather than promote pregnancy. It is exceedingly important, therefore, for the physician to understand and anticipate the needs of the Orthodox patient. Likewise, the patient must understand the limitations within which the physician must function. This chapter is written with these goals in mind. Building on the concepts developed in previous sections, it translates halakhic principles into practice.

Artificial Insemination

Although artificial insemination is used in most instances to treat male infertility, a discussion of this procedure rightfully belongs in this chapter on treating infertility in the female. This is mainly because the procedure is performed on the woman, no matter where the problem lies. Also, on occasion, artificial insemination is specifically used as therapy for female factors. Most important of all, however, is the frequency with which artificial insemination may be used to overcome halakhic obstacles to fertility therapy. As we shall see in subsequent sections, this procedure often arises as an option during therapy. But first, some definitions:

Artificial insemination refers essentially to the placement of sperm in the female reproductive tract, usually the cervix, by means other than intercourse. The procedure is simple, requires few instruments, little training and, in fact, can even be done by the husband himself. It is meant to simulate what would otherwise happen during natural intercourse.

In the past, artificial insemination with the husband's sperm (AIH) was used to enhance fertility under a variety of circumstances, in particular male subfertility. Studies eventually determined, however, that in the case of male infertility, AIH does not have more of an effect than intercourse alone. Today, AIH is rarely done. It is reserved for those rare cases when an anatomical or psychological obstruction to intercourse cannot be corrected.

The type of insemination most commonly performed today

is called intrauterine insemination, or IUI. IUI refers to the placement of the husband's sperm directly into the uterine cavity. It requires, first, that sperm be separated from the rest of the semen after ejaculation. This is because semen contains substances called prostaglandins which, when in contact with the uterine wall, may cause violent cramping. Also, seminal fluid is a potential source of infection. The procedure for separation of sperm cells from semen is called "sperm washing" and is usually performed in a laboratory under strictly sterile conditions. (Responsible laboratories maintain a variety of safeguards to make sure that semen samples cannot be switched.) After the sperm are isolated and concentrated in a small volume of a nutrient liquid, the suspension is injected into the uterus through a long, soft catheter that traverses the cervical canal. The procedure is rarely painful and takes only minutes to perform. The utility of the procedure lies in the placement of large numbers of sperm high in the uterus, just near the opening of the fallopian tubes—a place few sperm would reach after normal intercourse.

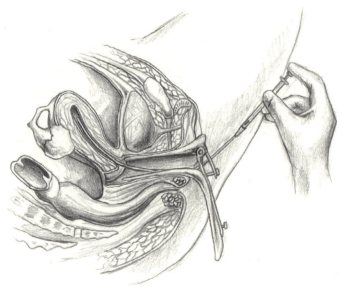

Intrauterine insemination: Sperm is injected through a soft catheter into the upper reaches of the uterine cavity

It is believed that by increasing the numbers of sperm that reach the upper reproductive tract, fertility is enhanced. Although IUI is primarily used to treat male factor infertility, it is also often used to treat infertility that is unexplained by either male or female factors. IUI is most successful in the absence of a male factor, when normal sperm are used to overcome a cervical barrier to infertility.

In vitro fertilization (IVF) involves the joining together of sperm and egg in a laboratory dish. This is a type of insemination, albeit one that occurs completely outside the body. The specifics of IVF and other forms of assisted reproduction are discussed in the next chapter (see "Assisted Reproduction").

Not all halakhic authorities allow artificial insemination, even though the husband's sperm is being used. In addition to the problems concerning sperm procurement (See "Male Infertility: Halakhic Considerations"), some authorities simply do not trust the physician not to substitute the semen of another man in order to guarantee a "success." Needless to say, a good relationship between the doctor and rabbi goes a long way in allaying these concerns. In general, though, most halakhic authorities are willing to allow artificial insemination if it is clear that no alternatives exist for overcoming the couple's infertility. Despite the fact that sperm loss must be recognized as an inevitable consequence of all forms of insemination, whether natural or artificial, many authorities regard sperm procurement for artificial insemination as purposeful, and therefore not considered *hotza'at zera le'vatala*.

Several finer points warrant consideration. For example, Jewish law proscribes conjugal relations during the *niddah* interval. Several authorities insist that insemination with the husband's sperm be confined to the non-*niddah* days, i.e. during the *tahara* interval, of the wife's menstrual cycle. On the other hand, Rabbi Moshe Feinstein permits insemination even while the wife is *niddah*. However, if insemination is done during the *niddah* interval, procurement of the sperm is an obvious problem, as most rabbis prefer that sperm be obtained through intercourse (with the aid of a condom for collection purposes, or using coitus interruptus). In this case, sperm must be collected in the cycle prior to insemination and frozen for later use. Medically, better results can usually be expected from fresh sperm; halakhically, there can be some objection to further manipulating the natural process. This dilemma highlights the importance of close and deliberate consultation between the rabbinic authority, the physician, and the couple in treatment.

Some authorities maintain that the child conceived through IVF has no halakhic relationship to the genetic father, as the conception takes place "unnaturally" outside of the mother's body. If this is so, the husband cannot fulfill the mitzvah of procreation through this procedure and there are therefore no halakhic grounds for allowing the semen to be procured. Most authorities, however, have concluded that the child conceived through IVF has the same relationship to its genetic father as it would had the conception occurred naturally (See "Assisted Reproduction"). Physicians should encourage their patients to consult with their halakhic authority on these matters.

Menstrual Cycle Disorders

ANOVULATION

The basic mechanisms involved in producing cyclic ovulation have already been described in Part III, "General Aspects of Female Infertility." Not uncommonly, these mechanisms break down. The result is that ovulation ceases (anovulation), or becomes irregular and unpredictable (oligo-ovulation). Disorders of ovulation are among the most common causes of infertility in the female. Fortunately, they are also among the most successfully corrected causes.

Depending on the cause of anovulation or oligo-ovulation, the physician may choose to use a variety of different ovulatory agents. These are all designed to manipulate the levels of follicle stimulating hormone (FSH) and luteinizing hormone (LH) which, in turn, control egg development in the ovaries. The use of these agents for ovulation induction is discussed below, along with the halakhic considerations that must accompany treatment with each particular medication.

(a) *Clomiphene*

Clomiphene citrate is the most commonly used medication for induction of ovulation. It was approved for use in 1962. It is currently available as Clomid® or Serophene®. Millions of babies have been born after ovulation induction with clomiphene, and numerous clinical studies have attested to its safety. Clomiphene is an anti-estrogen whose main effect is in the hypothalamus and pituitary gland. There, it stimulates FSH and LH secretion. During the time that clomiphene is administered, levels of these hormones rise dramatically, stimulating egg maturation within the ovary. If this process is successfully completed, ovulation occurs and pregnancy may result.

Most women who are treated with clomiphene, however, are anovulatory and therefore menstruate irregularly or not at all. This chronic absence of normal menstruation can lead to undesirable changes in the uterine lining, including ones that render it unsuitable for implantation. To begin a treatment cycle, therefore, menstruation is usually induced with either natural progesterone (available as progesterone vaginal suppositories, progesterone cream [Crinone®] or injectable progesterone in oil) or with a synthetic progesterone such as Provera®. Typically, a 50 mg tablet of clomiphene citrate is taken orally beginning on the fifth day of the menstrual period and continued through cycle day 9. Ovulation can be monitored in a variety of ways, including basal temperature charting, urine testing for the "LH surge" or ultrasound tracking of egg development in the ovaries.

When a halakhically committed woman requires clomiphene to ovulate, she should begin taking it later in the cycle than day 5. This will ensure that her ovulation takes place after she has gone to *mikvah* and normal marital relations are permitted. This is especially important in normal-weight or thin women, who may be very sensitive to the effects of clomiphene and in whom ovulation may occur rapidly. Because there is no natural ovarian cycle to contend with, delaying the start of clomiphene is ordinarily an easy thing to do. In fact, clomiphene can even be started after the *niddah* interval is completed, provided that the physician is assured that the woman's hormonal status has not changed by this time.

Two potential halakhic problems may arise during clomiphene treatment. The first relates to midcycle uterine bleeding, which can result from the anti-estrogen effects of clomiphene. When this occurs, it does not inherently interfere with the fertility-inducing effects of the medication. However, if as a result of such bleeding the woman becomes a *niddah* and intercourse is prohibited, the end result is the same. There are two ways to manage this problem. The first is artificial insemination with the husband's sperm (AIH or IUI). If rabbinic approval is forthcoming, this can be accomplished during the same cycle in which the problem was discovered. If such approval is not forthcoming, then that cycle will be wasted. This does not mean, however, that clomiphene treatment must be stopped. Often, the addition of small amounts of estrogen (e.g. oral Premarin® or Estraderm®, a transdermal patch) just after clomiphene has been completed will prevent midcycle bleeding. If it does not, adjusting the dose of clomiphene may do the trick. If all of these maneuvers are unsuccessful, clomiphene should be discontinued and a different agent used.

The second problem with clomiphene also involves its anti-estrogen effects. Not uncommonly, women treated with clomiphene will have a seemingly perfect response but will not conceive because the medication has interfered with their normal production of cervical mucus. This secretion, which is easily detected in cycling women and is a sign of impending ovulation, acts as a reservoir for sperm and as a conduit for their movement through the female reproductive tract. When absent or reduced, fertility is impaired. It has been estimated that 15% of women treated with clomiphene will suffer from poor or absent cervical mucus production.[1] While estrogen treatment of the type described to overcome midcycle bleeding may sometimes overcome this problem as well, this is usually not the case. More commonly, insemination of sperm past the cervical canal (IUI) is necessary to overcome this clomiphene complication. Here, too, if rabbinic approval is given, IUI can be used effectively during the same cycle in which the mucus problem is detected.

(B) *Gonadotropins*

The term "gonadotropins" refers to a general class of hormonal medications that are identical in composition to natural LH and FSH. Unlike clomiphene, which is a synthetic, estrogen-like compound, gonadotropins are natural hormones. Generically called human menopausal gonadotropins, they have been available for treatment of infertility since 1968. Unlike clomiphene, which can be taken orally, all gonadotropins preparations currently in use must be injected into the body. Like natural LH and FSH, the gonadotropins used for ovulation induction are cleared rapidly from the body and have no effect on the developing fetus. They are highly potent and highly effective. Two general classes of gonadotropins are used today. The first is a combination of LH and FSH (human menopausal gonadotropins); the second is composed of FSH only (human follitropin).

Human Menopausal Gonadotropins (*h*MG)—The first *h*MG preparation that became widely available for clinical use was Pergonal®. Many laypersons familiar with fertility treatments are familiar with the name. This drug stands alone in the history of infertility treatment not only because it was the first such medication, but also because it was the only one available for 25 years after its first introduction to the medical community in 1968. Facing competition from other, more convenient hormone preparations, such as Repronex®, production of Pergonal ceased in 2004.

*h*MG is derived from the urine of postmenopausal women. It contains a combination of the pituitary hormones LH and FSH. These hormones are naturally found in both men and women, but postmenopausal women have an abundant amount. When concentrated as an injectable preparation, hMG is a direct and potent stimulator of egg development in the ovaries (and, in some cases, of sperm production in the testis).

During the purification process used to produce Pergonal, certain proteins remain in the resulting material that are irritating to the surrounding tissues under the skin. Because of this, Pergonal was given as an intramuscular injection. Repronex, like Pergonal, is a combination of urinary LH and FSH. However, because of further elimination of the irritant proteins during its production process, it can be taken as a subcutaneous injection. Most women find subcutaneous injections significantly more comfortable. As a result, Repronex has replaced Pergonal when treatment with hMG is indicated.

Urinary FSH—Another historical milestone in the development of gonadotropin therapy was reached with the elimination of LH from hMG. The presumed benefit of such a drug was that many women who need ovulation induction, particularly those with polycystic ovary syndrome (PCOS), already have high levels of LH, and therefore need only FSH to induce ovulation. Some studies also suggest that too much LH might decrease pregnancy rates or increase the chances of miscarriage. The makers of Pergonal, Serono, were the first to introduce Metrodin®, which they marketed as "pure" FSH. Of course, this preparation was hardly pure. It was simply the same Pergonal from which the LH had been removed, and it retained the same urinary proteins that required it to be given by intramuscular injection. Further purification of Metrodin eventually led to the development of Fertinex®, which was the first gonadotropins preparation—this time, containing FSH only—that could be given by subcutaneous injection. Urinary FSH is presently available in the United States only as Bravelle®.

Recombinant FSH—One of the disadvantages of using gonadotropins extracted from menopausal urine is that there is a limited supply of urine available from which to extract these hormones.[2] With the advent of the assisted reproductive technologies, which require gonadotropins treatment of normally ovulating women, pharmaceutical companies foresaw a need to develop a new source of gonadotropins. Recombinant DNA technology provided the answer to this problem. By inserting the exact gene that codes for human FSH synthesis into living mammalian cells, scientists at these companies created a "biological machine" that could produce an exact replica of the human hormone with nearly perfect purity and in large quantities. Gonal F® and Follistim® are the result of such technology. Because of their high purity, they can be injected subcutaneously.

Human Chorionic Gonadotropin—The use of hMG or FSH is highly effective in stimulating follicle development within the ovary. However, because of certain alterations in the dynamic interplay of hormones between the ovary and the pituitary gland, treatment with either of these gonadotropins is not sufficient to stimulate actual ovulation. In order to affect the final maturation process within the egg itself and its extrusion from the ovary, human chorionic gonadotropin (hCG) is required. This hormone mimics the LH surge that commonly precedes natural ovulation, and it is sometimes used with clomiphene therapy as well. Virtually all women will ovulate within 36–38 hours after hCG is administered. As is the case with other gonadotropins, some hCG preparations are given by intramuscular injection and some by the subcutaneous route.

Other Gonadotropins—For practical purposes, gonadotropins can be used interchangeably for most clinical situations. Most women with ovulatory disorders will respond to hMG or to FSH, no matter how those medications are prepared.[3] It is expected that other gonadotropin preparations will eventually enter the market, and that some in current use will eventually disappear. This is common fare in the medical world. As experience with these medications grows, and as new technologies are developed, more precise combinations of hormones will be used to achieve the desired result. One gonadotropin preparation that will likely be introduced soon is recombinant LH. When this is accomplished, reproductive endocrinologists will be able to use precise quantities of LH and FSH to produce the desired effect in the ovary. It is hoped that this will increase the effectiveness of gonadotropin therapy while minimizing side effects.

Unlike clomiphene, gonadotropins do not have anti-estrogenic side effects. Therefore, some halakhic problems associated with the side effects of clomiphene (e.g. midcycle spotting and decreased cervical mucus production) are not relevant to gonadotropin therapy. Certain other problems may arise, however, and when they do, they can be particularly distressing. This is because treatment with gonadotropins is more expensive, more physically demanding and more psychologically stressful, by several orders of magnitude, than treatment with clomiphene. Aborting a cycle of treatment because of an unexpected halakhic problem may be devastating for the couple.

Traditionally, gonadotropins have been used to induce ovulation in women who do not ovulate and who have failed to become pregnant with clomiphene. When used for this purpose, the concerns regarding early ovulation are similar to those discussed for clomiphene. If, as is standard practice, gonadotropins injections are begun on the third day of an induced menstrual period, the rapid egg development that occurs may lead to ovulation before the *niddah* interval is completed. Therefore, it is best to begin therapy later in the cycle, around day 7. This virtually assures that the woman being treated will have been to *mikvah* in time for her most fertile phase.

It may also be helpful for some women to completely delay gonadotropin treatment until after going to *mikvah*. This is because physical contact between the couple is restricted when the wife is a *niddah* and some rabbis will not permit husbands to administer the injections. This strategy is only helpful, however, for women who do not ovulate on their own. If they do, and the goal of gonadotropin treatment is to stimulate multiple egg production, therapy must begin as soon as possible after menstruation begins. It is helpful at these times to use subcutaneously injected medications, as these can be self-administered more comfortably than those given by intramuscular injection.

(c) *Gonadotropin Releasing Hormone* (GnRH)
In certain cases of anovulation, where the cause resides in failure of the hypothalamus to secrete its hormone GnRH, this hormone may be replaced by either intravenous injection or injection just below the skin. Natural GnRH needs to be administered through a special computerized pump which delivers a small dose every 60–90 minutes. The advantage of this type of hormonal therapy is that because it very specifically replaces the missing hormone, it requires minimal monitoring, and there are virtually no side effects. Because the therapy induces a normal menstrual cycle or one in which ovulation is slightly delayed, there are few specific halakhic problems relative to this therapy. The only common problem has to do with the delivery system itself. That is, the pump needs to be attached to an indwelling plastic catheter, inserted either sub-cutaneously or intravenously. The hookup must be dismantled to allow immersion in the *mikvah*. For this reason, it is preferable to begin therapy only after *tahara* has begun.

(d) *Oophorotomy*
In certain circumstances, a physician and patient may together decide that medications need to be avoided altogether. This is most likely to occur when anovulation is the result of PCOS. In this syn-drome, egg development within the ovary never gets past its initial stages. As a result, multiple small follicles, or cysts, develop within the ovary. These cysts create a local hormonal environment within the ovary that is unfavorable for ovulation, and thereby exacerbate the condition. Several reports have indicated that elimination of the cysts at laparoscopy, either by vaporization with a laser or by electrocautery, may result in normal ovulation for up to one year *without the use of medications*. This strategy needs to be remem-bered and used when the halakhic problems surrounding the medi-

cal induction of ovulation render such therapy overly cumbersome or frankly unfeasible.

(E) *Insulin-sensitizing Agents*

It has been demonstrated that most women with PCOS have an underlying metabolic defect that involves resistance to insulin. This insulin resistance is not, however, sufficient to render them diabetic. Instead, they compensate metabolically by producing large amounts of insulin, which keeps their blood sugars in the normal range. But having chronically high insulin levels is not without cost. The insulin is able to bind to cells in the ovary, stimulate male hormone production and suppress ovulation. The net effect is the typical clinical characteristics of PCOS, including hirsutism, acne, irregular menstrual cycles, and infertility.

The management of anovulation resulting in PCOS has changed considerably since the introduction of insulin sensitizing agents as a viable treatment option. Many medications of this type are available and are being developed, but metformin has been studied most widely. Although its precise mechanism of action is unclear, it appears to lower insulin resistance and improve glucose utilization, and is most widely prescribed for the treatment of Type II ("Adult Onset") Diabetes. Its usefulness in the treatment of PCOS has been well established.

Many protocols are available for the use of metformin, alone or in combination with clomiphene or gonadotropins. Aside from some gastrointestinal side-effects, which are usually well tolerated if proper protocols are maintained, the only significant disadvantage of metformin therapy is that it can take some time to work. The first ovulatory cycles will usually manifest in three to four months, and pregnancy typically will occur in about six months. The advantage of metformin is that, when it works, it induces a physiologically normal ovulation, which does not confer the additional risk of multifetal pregnancy. There is no anti-estrogen effect to contend with, and ovulation is almost never accelerated. As a result, there are rarely any halakhic issues to contend with. Occasionally, a woman who is starting metformin therapy may report irregular bleeding, but this usually resolves once the full effect of the metformin is established.

One of the interesting features of infertility resulting from anovulation is that, in most cases, it is a condition that can be anticipated by a woman. Very often, young women who are in the planning phase of their marriage anticipate that they will have difficulty conceiving because of their history of irregular cycling.[4] Sometimes, they will present for treatment very soon after their marriage, even within the first year. When PCOS is identified in such young women, who have short histories of infertility or who only anticipate infertility, there is no question that an insulin sensitizing agent is the initial treatment of choice.

CONTROLLED OVARIAN HYPERSTIMULATION

In recent years, indications for giving clomiphene and gonadotropins have expanded widely. There are now numerous situations in which women who cycle naturally are advised to take these medications. The goal of therapy may be simply to repair a suspected dysfunction in the ovulatory cycle or, in other situations, to stimulate the ovaries to produce as many eggs as possible—an effect called controlled ovarian hyperstimulation (COH). Examples include the following:

(1) Luteal phase defect, a condition where ovulation occurs but the hormonal output from the ovary is too weak to sustain a pregnancy. Generally, this condition is first treated with progesterone supplementation or clomiphene. However, certain women who do not respond successfully must then resort to gonadotropins.

(2) Male factors, which can include a variety of conditions in which sperm production is inadequate to achieve a pregnancy in the natural way. Usually, ovulatory agents are given and intrauterine insemination is performed in the same cycle in order to increase the numbers of both sperm and eggs interacting within the fallopian tubes.

(3) Ovarian adhesions or scarring around the ovaries, which can prevent entry of the egg into the tube after its release from the ovary. If the tubes are normal and at least some portion of the

ovaries is in contact with the tubes, COH may be tried in order to increase the likelihood that an egg will be released in the direction of the tubes.

(4) Unexplained infertility, a diagnosis that is given to at least 10% of infertile couples. In this situation, where all diagnostic tests have failed to reveal the cause of infertility, clomiphene or gonadotropins are often used empirically (that is, without the intention of treating a specific problem) in order to induce pregnancy. Medical treatment using COH is usually coupled with intrauterine insemination as well.

(5) Assisted reproduction, a global term for a variety of high technology procedures, the most well known of which is in vitro fertilization. Most women undergoing assisted reproduction have ovulatory cycles naturally but are given gonadotropins in order to increase the number of eggs available for fertilization in the laboratory. The success of in vitro fertilization is, to a certain degree, dependent on the number of eggs harvested from the ovaries during a particular cycle.

One of the problems with clomiphene is that it may hasten an otherwise well-timed and normal ovulation. A woman undergoing treatment may, for example, change from ovulating on day 14 to ovulating on day 10 or 11, while she is still a *niddah*. One must be careful to anticipate this situation and to plan accordingly. Of course, if artificial insemination prior to *mikvah* is permitted, and if a *heter* is given to procure sperm by masturbation, this alleviates the major concern. Even so, it is helpful to determine this before starting the cycle so that last minute, emergency rabbinical consultations—and the stresses they involve—are avoided.

Many women will not receive rabbinic approval for early insemination. This does not necessarily rule out treatment with clomiphene, since some women will not experience any change in the timing of their ovulation, and will not require insemination. If ovulation is advanced into the *niddah* interval and clomiphene therapy must for some reason be continued, it is best to delay the initiation of therapy until day 7 of the cycle, to allow the time of *mikvah* to approach as closely as possible. If this is done, however, it should be understood that delaying the start of clomiphene therapy most often results in the ovulation of only one egg, which may be contrary to the desired effect. Ultrasound monitoring of egg development provides useful information in such cases.

Gonadotropins are almost always the drugs of choice when COH is performed in preparation for assisted reproduction. The halakhic problems accompanying the assisted reproductive technologies will be discussed separately. With regard to the use of gonadotropins for *in vivo* fertilization in the otherwise cycling woman, the halakhic issues are similar to those regarding clomiphene and mainly relate to the frequent occurrence of ovulation prior to the completion of the *niddah* interval. Again, it must be stressed that the medical concept underlying this type of therapy is to increase egg production. In order to accomplish this, gonadotropin injections must be initiated as early in the cycle as possible; beyond about the third or fourth day, one egg will already have been selected to ovulate and no amount of gonadotropins will induce others to mature. As the average length of gonadotropin treatment is about seven days, it is not unusual for the gonadotropin-stimulated ovary to be poised for ovulation on day 10. For the Orthodox woman so treated, the problem is obvious.

This problem is also an important one for the physician, and not only because the treatment may fail. In many gonadotropin-treated women, estrogen levels rise dramatically higher than in the natural cycle or with clomiphene. If, at a certain point, ovulation does not occur, the estrogen level will continue to rise and may pose a serious health hazard. This condition, known as ovarian hyperstimulation syndrome, may become severe and has been fatal in some women. It can be quite discomfiting for the physician to watch as his patient heads toward hyperstimulation, unable to let her ovulate because halakhic restrictions forbid intercourse for another day or two. This is a situation that no one wants to be in but which occurs frequently. Again, anticipation of this problem and discussion of various solutions prior to commencing treatment are invaluable.

The ways in which the problem of early ovulation can be

solved depend on each couple's specific halakhic position. As with the clomiphene-induced early ovulation, acceptance of early artificial insemination with a semen specimen produced by masturbation allows for the most straightforward approach. Some authorities do not object to insemination prior to *mikvah*, but do not allow masturbation. If this is the case, a true catch-22 situation results: insemination is allowed, but only if semen can be obtained through intercourse, and intercourse is not allowed. One possible solution is to have semen from the husband frozen in advance and available for use during a subsequent cycle. This may be obtained by intercourse during any previous, non-treatment cycle (with the use of a special collection condom or coitus interruptus). If ovulation must be induced prior to *mikvah*, the sample can then be thawed and used for insemination.

Not all authorities permit the freezing of semen for this purpose. For couples who have no *heter* for insemination prior to *mikvah*, or for couples who find themselves in the catch-22 described above, therapy with gonadotropins need not be completely avoided. One may embark on a treatment cycle, understanding that ovulation may occur at an inopportune time. Often this will not occur. If it does, having been prepared beforehand limits, to a certain degree, the emotional impact of the failed cycle.

GnRH ANALOGS

Repeated early ovulation in the gonadotropin-treated woman who cannot be inseminated presents a most frustrating dilemma to that woman and to her physician as well. By the time that the problem becomes obvious, both have expended considerable energy in managing her treatment. As the fertile period has been missed consistently, neither know if the therapy had a chance of working. Still at square one, both feel more stress than ever. Fortunately, the use of a second medication that allows additional control of the ovulatory process may offer a solution. These are called "gonadotropin releasing hormone analogs," or "GnRH analogs."

Produced in a central area of the brain called the hypothalamus, GnRH is, reproductively speaking, the master hormone. It controls pituitary production and release of LH and FSH which, in turn, control egg maturation in the ovary. GnRH analogs are hormones that are nearly identical to the natural GnRH hormone, but with minor modifications that allow them to selectively bind to the pituitary gland and exert the exact opposite effect, i.e. they *turn off* the secretion of LH and FSH. Without these two hormones, egg production in the ovary essentially shuts down. Estrogen levels, which are a reflection of egg production in the ovary, fall to basal levels and all menstrual cycling ceases.

Two classes of GnRH analogs are currently available for use. GNRH agonists (e.g. Lupron®) initially activate and then suppress pituitary function. It takes approximately one week for the suppressive effect to begin. GnRH antagonists (Anatagon®, Cetrotide®) cause suppression of pituitary function immediately upon administration. It is the GnRH agonist that may be very useful in solving the problem of early ovulation.

Earlier, it was intimated that the Orthodox woman who takes gonadotropins is sometimes better off if she is anovulatory than if she cycles normally. Normal cycles mean that the complex interplay of internal hormones is fully functional, and that egg production in the ovary is proceeding at the appropriate innate pace. Women who cycle may respond less than optimally to gonadotropins because the drug needs to override that operational setting. Gonadotropins meet no such environment in a woman who does not ovulate. When she uses them, the gonadotropins are doing all the work, and are in total control. If ovulation needs to be delayed, it can be done reliably, simply by delaying the start of therapy.

Pretreatment with a GnRH analog such as Lupron is a means by which the cycling woman can be made to stop cycling, thus becoming more responsive to gonadotropins. When the ovulatory system is interrupted, she becomes like any other woman who does not ordinarily ovulate; that is, the default operational mode of her cycle is canceled, leaving her more sensitive to the gonadotropins. As a result, ovulation timing during therapy with gonadotropins can be controlled. Using this strategy, even a woman who cycles normally can be given gonadotropins and reliably be made to ovulate after *mikvah*.

The following example illustrates how this strategy works. In a woman who menstruates every 28 days, ovulation presumably occurs on day 14. One week later, on day 21, progesterone production from the ovary that released the egg reaches its peak. On that day, Lupron therapy should begin. The initial outpouring of hormones (FSH and LH) will not be perceived in the presence of progesterone. By the time the progesterone levels fall, toward the end of the cycle, Lupron's effect will already be established. When menstruation occurs, hormonal functioning in the ovaries will have been eliminated. In this scenario, gonadotropin therapy can be started any day afterwards. Day 3, Day 7, Day 17—each is the same as the next. (It is not recommended to start gonadotropins too far beyond immersion in the *mikvah,* however, because the effects of too little estrogen begin to be felt about then.) When Lupron is used in combination with gonadotropins, there is virtually no gonadotropin-timing problem that cannot be solved.

Though a potent tool in solving the problems with gonadotropin therapy for Orthodox women, the addition of Lupron is not a perfect solution. As previously mentioned, during Lupron therapy, the ovaries are functionally asleep by the time menstruation occurs. Because estrogen production is minimal, the lining of the uterus may not heal properly, and bleeding may be prolonged. If left untreated, this continuous bleeding would negate the entire purpose of the Lupron. In this situation, therefore, one could add estrogens (either orally or by transdermal patch). With estrogen treatment, bleeding ceases promptly. The estrogen should be continued during the first several days of gonadotropin administration, until blood testing reveals estrogen levels are adequate to sustain the uterine lining (>100 pg/ml). This is a process that can take up to a week to occur, but eventually estrogen levels will be sufficient to regrow the uterine lining in every cycling, Lupron-treated woman. With estrogens handy as a solution to Lupron-induced bleeding, the Lupron-gonadotropin combination seems perfect.

PREMENSTRUAL STAINING

Staining that repeatedly occurs a few days prior to menstruation may result from a condition called luteal phase insufficiency. In this condition, the hormone progesterone is inadequately produced during the luteal, or second phase of the cycle. This relative deficiency of progesterone results in poor development of the uterine lining and premature shedding. While not a particularly serious problem in most women, luteal phase insufficiency may be a cause of infertility. Infertile women who experience premenstrual staining should therefore be investigated for this condition.

The diagnosis of luteal phase insufficiency is generally made by endometrial biopsy just prior to menstruation. (Some doctors simply check progesterone levels at various intervals after ovulation, but this method of diagnosis is controversial.) If a luteal phase deficiency is suggested, a confirmatory biopsy during a subsequent cycle is usually recommended.

Not uncommonly, the biopsy results are normal and suggest that the premenstrual staining is not pathological. It may simply reflect the sensitivity of the uterine lining to falling levels of progesterone. In such women, the bleeding is a minor nuisance and does not need to be treated. For the Orthodox woman, however, even this minor amount of bleeding may pose a problem because it renders her a *niddah*. For her, progesterone supplementation by vaginal suppository should be given just prior to the expected time of bleeding. It is then continued until the time that true menstruation begins.

When the diagnosis of luteal phase insufficiency is suggested, two forms of treatment are generally available. Progesterone supplementation may be given by vaginal suppositories or cream (and sometimes by injection) just after ovulation occurs, and there are no halakhic consequences. Alternatively, ovulation induction with clomiphene may be performed. If the latter is chosen, attention should be paid to the concerns raised in the previous section on ovulation induction.

MIDCYCLE BLEEDING

In a normal menstrual cycle, estrogen and progesterone are produced within the ovary by the corpus luteum after ovulation has occurred. These hormones sustain the uterine lining and prepare it for pregnancy. When pregnancy occurs, hormonal signals sent by the developing embryo cause the ovary to maintain its production and release of estrogen and progesterone, a process which continues until the placenta is completely formed and able to take over. In the absence of pregnancy, on the other hand, these hormones are no longer produced. In response to the decline in estrogen and progesterone levels, the uterine lining loses its hormonal support and begins to break down. That breakdown is experienced as menstrual bleeding.

Even as menstrual bleeding is occurring, the ovary is preparing itself for its next ovulation. Within its substance, one egg is emerging once again as dominant over the rest. As it grows, it produces increasing amounts of estrogen, which serve to repair the uterine lining and begin anew its preparation for pregnancy. It is estrogen from the developing egg, therefore, that is the major reparative hormone. When it is produced and released in normal amounts, menstrual bleeding is normal and self-limited. When deficient, menstrual bleeding may be heavy and prolonged.

Deficient estrogen release and sustained menstrual bleeding are the hallmarks of the non-ovulatory cycle. Varying ways to induce ovulation in women who do not ovulate have already been discussed. But estrogen deficiency may also accompany ovulatory cycles. In particular, two types of such estrogen deficiency are common, and both produce midcycle bleeding or staining.

Normally, at ovulation, release of the egg and disruption of the surrounding cells cause estrogen levels to fall transiently. (Shortly afterward, those cells become the corpus luteum and begin to produce estrogen and progesterone efficiently.) In most women, there are no consequences to that brief withdrawal of estrogen. Some, however, are very sensitive to this and experience midcycle bleeding. Although this does not impair fertility in any way, for an

Orthodox woman, this type of bleeding is an obstruction to conception because it prevents her from having sexual relations during her most fertile time of the cycle. It causes "halakhic infertility."

Midcycle bleeding may also represent a truly pathologic process. The developing egg may be truly deficient in estrogen production and, at midcycle, the normal decline in estrogen levels is therefore exaggerated. Under these conditions, progesterone production after ovulation will likely also be deficient. This type of luteal phase insufficiency is a known cause of infertility. It is especially important, therefore, for women who consistently bleed at midcycle to determine whether or not they have this disorder. (For a discussion on diagnosing and treating luteal phase insufficiency, see section on luteal phase insufficiency) Errors in diagnosis may lead to incorrect treatment and possibly to numerous religious obstructions to conception.

When no abnormalities are detected, it may be assumed that the midcycle bleeding is a result of the normal midcycle estrogen drop, and that fertility is otherwise normal. In such cases, attention need only be given to removing the halakhic barriers to conception. To do this, estrogens should be administered just prior to the time when bleeding usually commences and continued until after ovulation (usually days 9–16). It is important to use a low dose of estrogen so that pituitary functioning is not altered. The dose may be adjusted upward, however, if midcycle bleeding persists. Transdermal estrogens (e.g. Estraderm® 50 µg) should be used because it delivers the natural estrogen (estradiol) at a continuous and steady rate. Cessation of midcycle bleeding is usually prompt, and fertility easily restored.

CONTINUOUS BLEEDING

On occasion, a woman may experience bleeding every day, continuously and without interruption. It may change in intensity from day to day—she may even notice when actual menstruation is occurring—but it never completely subsides. As a result, she remains a perpetual n*iddah*. Even when fertility is not desired, the resulting disruption in normal sexual functioning may cause profound marital stress. For the Orthodox woman with this problem, aggressive attempts at correction are therefore urgent.

Under these circumstances, the most important factor to be ascertained is whether or not ovulation is occurring. Many high-tech methods for detecting ovulation are available, but the simplest and best for this problem is the basal body temperature chart. With this method, a woman records her temperature (taken orally, to within 0.1° F) every morning upon awakening. Over time a pattern emerges that is easily recognizable and will suggest that ovulation either is or is not occurring. If it is not, or if there is some other evidence to suggest a disorder of ovulation, induction of ovulation will usually reverse the bleeding and restore fertility. For those not wishing to conceive, estrogen/progesterone cycling—either with birth control pills or with cyclic estrogen and progesterone as given to menopausal women—will also safely reverse the bleeding but without restoring fertility.

A woman who bleeds continuously but who ovulates cyclically presents a different set of problems. Because the pattern cannot be explained by variations in estrogen and progesterone, other sources must be looked for. Certainly, a complete blood count should be checked and any anemia resulting from sustained bleeding should be corrected by dietary iron supplementation. At the same time, disorders of blood clotting, thyroid function, and prolactin production should also be looked for. If normal, or if the physician is suspicious, endometrial biopsy should also be done. In this case it is done not in order to test for a luteal phase insufficiency but in order to rule out uterine cancer or its precursors. (Although uterine cancer is generally a disease of older women, it is sometimes seen in younger women, especially those who are significantly overweight.) If the biopsy is normal, uterine x-ray (hysterosalpingogram), sonohysterogram, or hysteroscopy should be done to elucidate the internal uterine anatomy. Often, a polyp or fibroid will be found; removing these will stop the bleeding.

If no source for the bleeding is found, it must still be corrected so that the couple may resume marital relations. Again, the method here depends on the goal of the couple. If fertility is desired, daily administration of a GnRH analog such as Lupron should first be given. This will cause all hormonal output from the ovaries to cease. The uterine lining will shrink almost totally, and bleeding will stop. After an interval sufficient to allow normal resumption of intercourse, gonadotropins may then be added to induce a controlled ovulation. If used properly, bleeding will not recur unless there is no conception, in which case it will be normal menstrual bleeding. The Lupron-gonadotropins regimen should be repeated until pregnancy occurs. If pregnancy is not desired, birth control pills should be tried first. As a backup, Lupron may be given continuously daily or once monthly in its depot form. After bleeding stops, it may be continued for up to six months. When the drug is finally withdrawn, normal cycling may resume and the bleeding problem may not recur. If it does, Lupron may again be used but, because of concern for its effect on bone content, estrogens and progesterone should be added cyclically. This so-called "add back" regimen may be continued indefinitely.

EARLY OVULATION

Not uncommonly, a woman may find that she consistently ovulates before going to the *mikvah*. While a nonobservant woman with a similar cycle would not suffer any impaired fertility, for an Orthodox woman, this is another form of "halakhic infertility." Of course, a most straightforward solution is to perform intracervical insemination (using her husband's sperm) at the time that ovulation is detected, without regard to her *niddah* status. When there are no other obstructions to fertility, conception is virtually certain to occur. (This is an instance where a seldom-used procedure takes on great importance for the Orthodox couple.) Rabbinic consultation is necessary before commencing with this type of therapy.

Even if approval is obtained, timing the insemination may present a technical problem. Generally speaking, inseminations are timed to the woman's ovulation. In order to detect ovulation most precisely, urine testing is done daily in order to detect the LH surge. Typically, inseminations are performed on the day following the surge and/or on the subsequent day. This means that if the surge occurs on a Friday, a Saturday insemination would have to be scheduled. However, observant women will not be able to travel to the office on the Sabbath. In order to avoid this, LH testing on Friday should always be done as early as possible. If the surge is detected, and the physician's schedule permits, insemination should be done on that day in order to have sperm available in the cervical mucus during the most fertile time. Insemination may then be repeated on Sunday, as would normally be done. Similar precautions should be taken in anticipation of any holiday where religious restrictions prohibit traveling to visit the doctor.

If there are rabbinical objections to insemination during the *niddah* interval, or regarding sperm procurement, manipulation of the menstrual cycle in order to delay ovulation becomes necessary. Unfortunately, delaying ovulation in an otherwise normally cycling woman, while conceptually straightforward, is not always an easy thing to do. The pituitary gland, which ultimately controls egg development and ovulation, must be harnessed and manipulated in order to slow down the process. Clomiphene is commonly used for this purpose. The experience with clomiphene, however, has been mixed. While successful in some women, it can actually *hasten* ovulation in others. Also, clomiphene has side effects, not all of which are easily detected. Among these are disruptions in the uterine lining and alterations in the secretion of cervical mucus, both of which may themselves cause infertility. If clomiphene is chosen as first line therapy for early ovulation, therefore, two things must be checked. First, ovulation testing (BBT charting or LH testing) must be done to confirm that the medication is having the desired effect of delaying ovulation. Second, postcoital testing should be done to ensure that the medication is not disrupting cervical mucus production. If ovulation is successfully delayed and the postcoital test is normal but pregnancy does not occur, strong consideration should be given to performing endometrial biopsy to rule out any detrimental effects of clomiphene on the uterine lining.

As clomiphene is equally likely to hasten ovulation as to delay it, other types of therapy must also be considered. Estrogens, which suppress the pituitary gland's production of FSH (the hormone that stimulates the eggs to mature), can also suppress or delay ovulation. When given continuously, as in birth control pills, ovulation stops completely. If given for a limited period of time very early in the menstrual cycle, estrogens will also halt the ovulatory process, but only enough to delay it a few days. For example, conjugated estrogens (e.g. Premarin®) taken during day 2–6 of the cycle consistently delays ovulation. There is, however, a problem with this type of treatment as well. Not infrequently, as the uterine lining is very responsive to estrogen, bleeding develops when the estrogens are withdrawn, and it can be prolonged. So while ovulation may be successfully delayed, for example, from day 10 to day 15, the secondary bleeding that occurs delays the visit to the *mikvah* until day 17. If this happens, not much has really been accomplished.

These problems can often be overcome by the use of transdermal patches that deliver natural estrogen (estradiol) instead of an estrogen pill. Unlike a daily pill, which causes undulating blood concentrations of estrogen, the patches deliver a steady dose of estrogen throughout the day and night. Also, they are packaged inside a reservoir that gradually dissipates over time. A typical patch will deliver the stated dose of estrogen for three or seven days, following which the dosage falls, necessitating removal and replacement. The estrogen patch can be used early on in the menstrual cycle, beginning on day two, in order to suppress pituitary FSH secretion. After the expiration day of, for example, the seven-day patch, the patch is left in place for an additional three days. During this last interval estrogen delivery diminishes gradually. This gradual diminishing of blood estrogen concentrations prior to removing the patch is sufficient to prevent estrogen-withdrawal bleeding of the type that can occur with an estrogen pill. This seems to be the most effective way to delay early ovulation.

A somewhat more complicated but very effective treatment combines the strengths of both clomiphene and estrogens. In this regimen, estrogens are given on days 2–6 of the cycle. On the last day, clomiphene is added and given through day 10, in order to stimulate egg development and thus prevent bleeding. When this regimen is followed, it is important that egg development be monitored by ultrasound in order to detect precisely the day of ovulation. As already mentioned, postcoital testing and endometrial biopsy should also be considered.

OVARIAN FAILURE

The spectrum of menstrual cycle disorders ranges from normal ovulatory cycling with minor bleeding disturbances on one side, to complete ovarian failure and absent bleeding on the other. While ovarian failure, or menopause, may be considered a natural state in that all ovaries are eventually depleted of their egg supply, when this occurs before the age of 35 it is considered to be a pathological event. Moreover, no matter at what age it occurs, if fertility is still desired, the only alternative is using an egg from a donor. This is discussed in "Assisted Reproduction."

Anatomical Infertility

TUBAL INFERTILITY

Closure or malfunction of the fallopian tubes may result from infection, endometriosis, or previous pelvic surgery. When the tubes are open but surrounding scar tissue prevents them from working

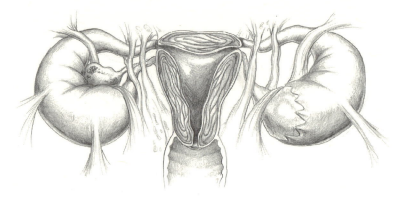

Tubal disease: The ends of the tube may be dilated or closed

properly, simple laparoscopic surgery may be all that is needed to repair the damage. In more severe cases, as when complete blockage and extensive scarring exist, a more extensive laparoscopy or microsurgery may be required. In either case, Orthodox women should encounter no specific religious problems related to their treatment. Most surgical procedures are accompanied by bleeding that is uterine in origin. Although this may induce a state of *niddah*, the bleeding is usually limited and will almost always subside by the following menstrual period. With clear instructions from the operating surgeon, the couple may then resume attempts at conception in the natural manner. The same holds true for any type of reproductive surgery, no matter which part of the internal tract is involved. Tubal disease leads to halakhic problems only when surgery to treat it has failed or when surgery is deemed to be inappropriate. In such cases, only in vitro fertilization (IVF) can offer a couple hope for a biological child.

UTERINE FACTORS

Tubal damage accounts for the overwhelming majority of cases of anatomical infertility in women. Rarely, infertility may be a result of anatomical distortion or absence of the uterus, cervix, or vagina. These cases are almost always congenital, meaning that they developed while the affected woman was still a fetus. Other than in cases of some minor defects involving the uterus (so-called "fusion defects"), surgical correction is indicated. Depending on the severity of the defect, a fully functional reproductive tract may be achieved; alternatively, as with congenital absence of the uterus and vagina, reproductive capacity cannot be achieved and surgical reconstruction is done mainly to allow normal sexual functioning. In such cases, providing that the woman has retained her ovarian function, a biological child may be produced with the use of in vitro fertilization and a gestational surrogate. Gestational surrogacy is also the only means by which a woman who has undergone hysterectomy may produce a biological child. Of course, this requires that the ovaries still be intact and functioning.[5]

A final syndrome which affects the uterus and causes

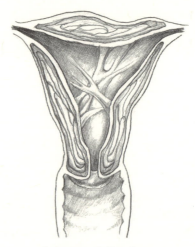

Asherman's Syndrome

infertility is one which is a complication of dilatation and curettage (D&C), one of the most common surgical procedures performed on women. Called Asherman's Syndrome, this condition develops when the curettage, or scraping, of the uterine lining during surgery has been vigorous and caused scarring. The scarred lining is incapable of responding to the ovarian hormones, which are otherwise normal. As a result, growth and shedding of the lining cannot occur and menstruation is absent. Modern surgical management includes the use of a thin fiberoptic telescope (hysteroscope) to cut away the scarred lining. Usually, this is followed by hormonal treatment designed to allow regrowth of a healthy lining. Providing that proper management of this condition is given, no particular halakhic concerns are evident. If treatment has failed, however, gestational surrogacy may again be the only option for production of a biological child.

ENDOMETRIOSIS

Endometriosis is a condition in which the lining of the uterus implants and grows outside of its normal location, usually elsewhere in the pelvis. Retaining its sensitivity to the ovarian hormones estrogen and progesterone, it grows and bleeds with each monthly cycle. This process can cause severe pain, with or without scarring of the tubes and ovaries. Doctors have believed for many years that endometriosis develops as a result of retrograde or upstream menstruation through the fallopian tubes and into the pelvis. However, this phenomenon is known to occur in most young women, and clearly most do not all develop endometriosis. Researchers now believe that the disease may reflect a breakdown in the body's immune system, but this is still only a theory. Endometriosis is also a perplexing disease, in that a woman who has only minor degrees of endometriosis may suffer from excruciating pain, while one with the most severe form may experience no pain at all. In either case, endometriosis can cause infertility. Eliminating or circumventing endometriosis is therefore a major focus of fertility specialists.

Endometriosis is usually treated with surgery, medication, or a combination of both. Most surgery for endometriosis currently involves using laparoscopy to either remove or destroy the abnormal tissue, including cysts (endometriomas) that may grow in one or both of the ovaries. Open abdominal surgery (laparotomy) is sometimes necessary, as when scarring and congealing of the pelvic organs makes laparoscopy difficult or unsafe.

As discussed in the section on tubal disease, there are no particular halakhic concerns regarding surgery in the pelvis. Although it may cause bleeding, this bleeding does not induce a state of *niddah* and, in any case, usually resolves by the next menstrual cycle. In regard to current medical treatment, there are also no special concerns. Although in the past a depot progesterone preparation was used, which caused prolonged and troublesome uterine bleeding, modern medical therapy relies instead on the prolonged administration of GnRH analogs. These are available as intranasal, subcutaneous, or long-acting depot forms. The latter is probably the easiest to take. When given properly, a "medical menopause" develops. There is no egg development in the ovary, and there is also no uterine bleeding. As with a natural menopause, hot flashes are the most common side effect, and they can be annoying. Sometimes, the uterine lining becomes so atrophied that continuous light spotting occurs. This is enough to render

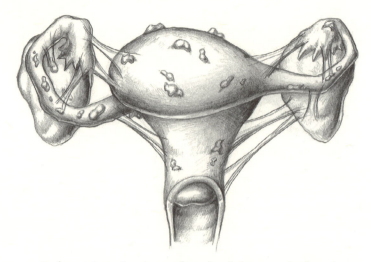

Endometriosis: Implants of uterine lining may be found anywhere in the pelvis, with or without scarring

a woman a *niddah*, and this problem may persist as long as the medication is given. If this occurs, a low dosage of estrogen, orally or by transdermal patch, should be given in order to repair the uterine lining and stop the bleeding. This amount of estrogen is not sufficient to stimulate regrowth of the endometriosis, and it may be continued for the duration of treatment with the GnRH analog. (A further benefit would be the disappearance of hot flashes.) If estrogen therapy is to be prolonged, however, one should discuss with one's physician the desirability of taking progesterone monthly or every other month, in order to allow the normal uterine lining to be shed periodically.

Medical therapy using GnRH analogs should be reserved for women with endometriosis who have been surgically treated and who are not planning to conceive or who wish to delay pregnancy. For those who wish to pursue pregnancy right away, medical suppression is not indicated and may be counterproductive. This group is best served by "expectant management," meaning no further intervention postoperatively. If the severity of endometriosis is such that pregnancy has a low chance of occurring even after surgical treatment, then treatment with ovulation induction or in vitro fertilization should be discussed with the treating physician.

Endnotes

1. F.H. Taney, R.V. Grazi, G. Weiss, C. Schmidt, "Detection of premature luteinization with serum progesterone levels at the time of the postcoital test," *Fertility and Sterility* 55:513, (1991).

2. The Serono Corporation originally obtained its urine supply through contract with convents throughout Italy, which were a reliable source of menopausal urine from presumably uninfected women. It should be noted that there is no danger of transmitting any infectious diseases using a urinary-derived product.

3. One important exception is hypothalamic amenorrhea, which is a rarer form of anovulation that responds only to hMG but not to FSH.

4. The anticipation of infertility is a halakhic problem in itself, as it brings up the question of disclosure to the intended husband. For ethical as well as halakhic reasons, many young women will disclose their irregularity, only to be besieged by questions from the intended in-laws about their capacity to bear children. In this situation, the physician plays a crucial role in educating the parties concerned and dispelling baseless concerns about permanent sterility. After permission is obtained, a well-considered letter or phone call is usually all that is needed to keep all parties calm.

5. Many women are confused by the term "total hysterectomy." Medically speaking, this refers to the removal of the uterus and cervix only. Removal of the tubes and ovaries—called "bilateral salpingo-oophorectomy"—does not always accompany total hysterectomy in younger women.

Richard V. Grazi

Assisted Reproduction

In the early 1960s, a brilliant and little known biologist by the name of Robert Edwards was studying the mammalian reproductive system, focusing on the mechanisms of fertilization and implantation. Over time, he developed a laboratory culture system in which mammalian sperm and eggs could be fertilized *in vitro*, literally "in glass" (the material from which petri dishes were then made). This work caught the attention of Dr. Patrick Steptoe, a gynecologist who had pioneered the use of the laparoscope in the evaluation and treatment of infertile women. Steptoe had a specific interest in diseases of the fallopian tube as a cause of infertility in women, and he was the first to realize that the laparoscope would be a useful tool to collect eggs from those women. If he could subject those eggs to Edwards's technique, a route for human fertilization that bypassed the damaged fallopian tubes could be established. Sperm collection, of course, posed no obstacle. In 1978, after a decade of failed attempts, Steptoe and Edwards reported the first birth of a baby born after conception outside the womb.[1] Louise Brown became the first human conceived using in vitro fertilization (IVF).[2]

In the early days of IVF, the technique was used solely in

the treatment of tubal factor infertility and, because the success rates were low, it was reserved for only the most desperate cases. Over time, however, many developments in the technique of IVF made its performance less risky, more successful, and more broadly applicable. In sequence, these developments were as follows:

(1) Ovarian stimulation prior to IVF enabled the retrieval of many eggs; this replaced the original technique of retrieving a single egg during the natural cycle.

(2) Ultrasound-guided retrieval of eggs replaced laparoscopic retrieval.

(3) Cryopreservation of excess embryos became possible.

(4) Egg donation for women with premature menopause (ovarian failure) was reported, with reliably high success rates.

(5) The use of intracytoplasmic sperm injection (ICSI) to surmount sperm abnormalities was reported, overcoming all but the most severe problems.

(6) Testicular sperm retrieval became possible for many men with azospermia, with ICSI used to initiate pregnancy.

It is important to appreciate that each of these scientific advances depended on a collaborative effort by researchers and physicians that involved years of patience and the willingness of thousands of patients to undergo treatment with an emerging, and not fully tested, medical technology. As a result of that process the 5% success rates that characterized the early days of IVF have now given way to much higher numbers. At many centers today, young couples fitting certain diagnostic criteria can expect a 50% chance of having a baby with each attempt at IVF. Nationwide, pregnancy rates from IVF continue to climb yearly. Juxtaposed to the expected *natural* fertility rate of 20% per month, the efficiency of IVF as currently performed is truly astounding.

During this same time period, other spin-off techniques similar to IVF were also developed, including GIFT, ZIFT and TET (respectively gamete intrafallopian transfer, zygote intrafallopian transfer, and tubal embryo transfer). Collectively subsumed under the category of assisted reproductive technologies, or ART, each of these techniques has its own indication and anticipated success.

All have been overshadowed, however, by the enormous success of IVF.

Indications for IVF

One need only consider the causes of infertility to appreciate the value of IVF in overcoming infertility. In women, tubal blockage, endometriosis, and severe adhesions are often surgically irreparable. In those cases, IVF is indicated. Although most ovulatory disorders can be treated medically, some will remain resistant to traditional therapy and, when treatment fails, IVF is indicated. Miscellaneous causes, such as cervical or immunological disorders, are not always easily overcome, but can be successfully treated using IVF. In men, factors leading to even severely depressed sperm counts are treatable by IVF with ICSI. Finally, for unexplained infertility, which is neither a specific male or female factor, traditional therapy with ovulation induction and insemination is successful approximately 30–40% of the time, depending on the age of the female. For the rest, IVF is indicated.

Ultimately, there are no causes of infertility other than complete azospermia (absence of sperm) or ovarian failure (absence of eggs) that are not potentially cured by IVF, with or without

Indications for IVF	
• Tubal Factor	16%
• Ovulatory dysfunstion	12%
• Endometriosis	7%
• Other	8%
• Unknown	9%
• Male Factor	18%
• Multiple Factors	30%

Indications for IVF as reported by the Centers for Disease Control, 1999

ICSI. This explains the steep rise in the demand for IVF over the last decade. It should be expected that, as success rates for IVF increase, IVF will become the treatment of first choice for many causes of infertility.

Efficacy and Efficiency

Traditionally, clinical researchers were trained to look at the efficacy of certain treatments—i.e., the likelihood of success for any given treatment. In the field of infertility, this translated into the number of couples with specific causes of infertility who conceived after a certain treatment was applied. Given the expected endpoint—a healthy pregnancy—results were measured over time. Thus, for example, women with tubal disease who had surgical repair had an expected success rate of 25% over 18 months. Couples with unexplained infertility who had ovulation induction and intrauterine insemination had a success rate of 40% over six treatment cycles. These success rates were measures of the treatments' efficacy.

Efficiency, on the other hand, is a measure of the efficacy of a certain treatment *over time and accounting for its cost*. Using the above examples, a theoretical IVF success rate of 25% would make it a far more efficient treatment for a woman with tubal disease, given that the cost of one cycle is approximately the same as the cost of surgery and the same result would be expected within a month of therapy instead of 18. For couples with unexplained infertility, the decision to use IVF is more complicated, as, using the same expected success rate, it would take two or even three cycles of IVF to reach a comparable success rate to ovulation induction and IUI, and the cost would be higher. On the other hand, for the 60% of couples who do not conceive after the latter therapy, the necessity for using IVF after six failed cycles makes the cost of achieving pregnancy that much higher.

In recent years, researchers have developed treatment pathways—called algorithms—which direct physicians toward certain clinical decisions based on the most efficient course of therapy.

These treatment algorithms take into account the age, diagnosis and expected success rates for the individual patient, based on the best current evidence. They also account for the expected cost of therapy and, as such, represent an attempt to streamline patient care. Although IVF is expensive, it is also the single most efficacious therapy per unit of time. Under certain circumstances, therefore, it is also very efficient. It is not surprising, therefore, that many pathways lead to IVF, either primarily or secondarily, if the primary treatment is not quickly successful. Common algorithms used for treating infertility are provided at the end of this chapter. For a more detailed explanation of treatment algorithms and their use, see "General Aspects of Female Infertility."

Success with IVF

The development of in vitro fertilization techniques has been the defining achievement in the field of modern reproductive medicine. Two aspects of IVF combine to achieve each pregnancy: clinical management of the couple on the one hand and the laboratory science that makes pregnancy possible on the other. Clinically, the art and science of ovulation induction has improved because of several factors: (1) the sheer numbers of couples who avail themselves of this technology, which has provided clinicians with vast experience in performing controlled ovarian hyperstimulation, (2) the reliability of ovarian reserve testing to exclude those with unfavorable prognoses from ART, (3) the bioengineering of natural hormones, (4) the development of GnRH analogs (both agonists and antagonists), and (5) improvements in the techniques of embryo transfer.

In the laboratory, the techniques that have improved have been: (1) tighter control of the environmental conditions, mainly air quality and culture media, that are used for manipulating and storing gametes, (2) greater experience in the performance of ICSI, (3) increased ability to select embryos with the best chances for implantation to transfer to the uterus and (4) embryo cryopreservation which, when feasible, greatly increases the efficiency of individual IVF cycles. In addition, the combined clinical and laboratory effort that is used in treating men with severely depressed or absent counts (using testicular sperm retrieval) has opened up this technology to more patients.

Before detailing the specific steps in the IVF process, it is worth looking at each of the above in greater detail.

Clinical Developments

I. EXPANDED INDICATIONS FOR IVF

In the early years of IVF, the main indication for IVF was tubal factor infertility. However, diseases of the fallopian tube can be caused not only by recurrent tubal pregnancies, as in the case of Louise Brown's mother, but also by infection, post-surgical adhesions (scar tissue) and/or endometriosis. These became the next indications. As the techniques and simplicity of performing IVF were refined, indications then expanded to other female factors. Once ICSI was developed, the indications spread to male factors as well, meaning that IVF would be done on women with inherently normal fertility.

To a certain extent, IVF can be used to treat all of the various causes of infertility (see table below). There are occasions, for example, when ovulatory disturbances simply do not respond to traditional medical maneuvers. Ovulation may be induced in the anovulatory woman, yet she may repeatedly fail to conceive. Endometriosis and/or pelvic adhesions may be surgically removed, but without resultant pregnancy. Not uncommonly, infertility is idiopathic or unexplained. In such cases, IVF may be used judiciously not only as treatment but also as a means to reveal the couple's reproductive physiology in a more detailed way. The ability to see the gametes directly can give the treating physician insight into a particular couple's problem that would be hard to achieve in any other way. The best example for this is when using IVF for male factor infertility. When sperm counts are very low, direct intracy-

Sources of Infertility	
• Male Factor	30%
• Female Factor	30%
– Ovulatory	
– Anatomical	
• Unexplained	20%
• Combined	20%

toplasmic sperm injection (ICSI) can result in normal fertilization and implantation. Quantity aside, success with the ICSI technique is the ultimate way to distinguish between sperm with normal and sperm with abnormal capacity to fertilize the egg.

The use of IVF with ICSI is particularly relevant in the observant Jewish community, as there exists a relative preponderance of male factor cases within this community (see Part III "General Aspects of Female Infertility"). What accounts for this is the relative paucity of some other causes of infertility among observant Jews. For example, because halakhically observant women tend to marry younger, they have less time to develop problems such as poor ovarian function and endometriosis. There is also less promiscuity and, consequently, a lower prevalence of tubal infections. Finally, the relatively sedentary lives, especially of *haredi* Jews, predisposes to weight problems in these communities. In men, obesity commonly diminishes sperm production.

These expanded indications for IVF, as well as its efficiency in producing pregnancies, have led to its increased utilization over the last decade. Whereas ten years ago IVF was used for approximately 2% of patients seeking care for infertility, in certain groups of patients utilization rates have climbed tenfold. The large number of patients who have undergone IVF has allowed reproductive specialists who perform IVF to accumulate considerable knowledge and experience in the field. Statistics from the CDC indicate that, in 2001, more than 100,000 IVF procedures were performed in some 400 clinics across the United States alone.[3] Success rates for

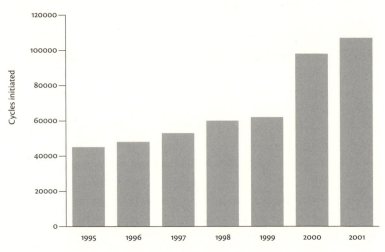

Cycles of ART initiated, US Centers for Disease Control

IVF have steadily increased since rigorous yearly reporting began in 1995. No doubt, physician experience is partially to account for this phenomenon. Today, the typical couple in need of IVF services can count on their physicians having already treated hundreds, if not thousands, of couples with this technology. It is expected that success rates will continue to rise as the practice of IVF keeps helping investigators elucidate the physiologic details of reproduction.

II. PATIENT SELECTION

In 1987, Navot et al. described the usefulness of testing follicle stimulating hormone (FSH) on day 3 of the menstrual cycle as a way of determining "ovarian reserve" in infertile women.[4] Ovarian reserve refers to the quantity and quality of the eggs existing in a woman's ovaries, and directly correlates with her ability to respond to the stimulants used to prepare her ovaries for IVF. When ovarian reserve testing reveals that the quantity of eggs is depressed, the quality is also poor and the prognosis for success with IVF is severely limited.[5]

Although often referred to as "day 3 testing," from a practical perspective the test for ovarian reserve is reliably performed on day 2, 3 or 4 of the menstrual cycle. This is important to know in the event that day 3 of the cycle falls on the Sabbath; in such cases the test may be done on Friday or Sunday.

Ovarian reserve is reflected in several hormones, including FSH and E2. FSH is the pituitary hormone that controls egg development in the ovary. (Note that it is *development* and not *production*. As every woman is endowed with her complete egg supply at birth, nothing can stimulate further egg production.) When the egg supply is healthy, there is no need for significant output from the ovary and the FSH level is therefore low. Over time, however, the egg supply diminishes continuously. This depletion of eggs is a genetically predetermined process that cannot be interrupted by any known means, including pregnancy, lactation, and the use of oral contraceptives. Paralleling this decline in the egg numbers, basal FSH levels rise, reflecting the need for the pituitary gland to increase its output of the tropic hormone in order to maintain egg development in the ovary. Beyond a certain threshold, an elevated FSH level indicates that the woman has no or very few healthy eggs remaining and that her fertility is therefore severely compromised.

Estradiol levels must always be measured along with FSH. The reason for this is that many women who are perimenopausal will begin their menstrual cycle with a very high FSH level, which in turn causes the rapid maturation of the egg. The maturing egg will cause E2 levels to rise, an event which secondarily causes a depression in the FSH level. An elevated E2 level on day 3 of the cycle, despite a normal FSH, is therefore also a sign of diminished ovarian reserve.

Women with poor ovarian reserve generally are unresponsive to the medications used to stimulate egg maturation for IVF. Pregnancy rates in these women are so low that in most fertility centers they are not considered candidates for IVF. Alternative forms of therapy are also usually unsuccessful in this population of women, and they are often advised to use donor eggs in order to conceive.

It is important to note that poor ovarian reserve is most often found in infertile women who have regular ovulation with normal menstrual cycles. This finding is also somewhat independent of age. That is, although it is most prevalent in women who are over 40 years old—and the rule beyond the age of 44—it is also commonly found in younger women, even in their twenties and thirties. The diagnosis is often accompanied by shock and disbelief, especially as there are usually no explanations for how the egg depletion has occurred. Women facing this diagnosis will commonly request that IVF be done using the one egg that they ovulate, or the few that they may develop in response to ovarian stimulation. The reason they may be denied IVF is because the diminished quantity of eggs goes hand in hand with diminished quality. Under those circumstances, IVF is almost never successful.[6]

It has become standard to test ovarian reserve in most women prior to instituting any fertility therapy. By excluding the group of patients with expected high failure rates from IVF, success rates in the population undergoing the procedure automatically rises.

III. NATURAL HORMONES

As already noted, FSH, secreted from the pituitary gland, is the major hormone controlling egg development. Together with luteinizing hormone (LH), FSH stimulates the recruitment, maturation, and ovulation of the egg.

In the late 1950s, researchers first isolated LH and FSH from the pituitary glands of cadavers and found that these substances could stimulate ovulation in women who lacked their own pituitary LH and FSH.[7] Subsequently, it was found that FSH and LH could be extracted from the urine of postmenopausal women who, because of their lack of eggs, had high circulating levels of these hormones. For the next three decades, urinary-derived FSH and LH (human menopausal gonadotropins, or hMG), were the dominant form of hormones used in fertility therapy.

Two developments, one medical and one scientific, led to a change in the source of FSH for ovulation induction. The first was the finding by clinicians that the stimulated development of multiple eggs (this is done by controlled hyperstimulation of the ovaries) prior to egg retrieval could enhance the chances for success with IVF. Essentially, the more eggs retrieved, the more embryos would potentially develop for transfer to the uterus; the more embryos transferred, the more likely it was that an embryo would implant and pregnancy would develop. (This was especially true in the 1980s, when culture techniques were not as accommodating to normal embryo development.[8] Today controlled ovarian hyperstimulation is also used, although largely to improve the efficiency of IVF.) Getting more eggs to develop meant greater use of hMG, often at high doses, prior to egg retrieval. As indications for IVF expanded, the demand for hMG around the world skyrocketed. Clearly, the supply of menopausal urine would not meet the expected future demand.

Fortunately, at the same time that IVF was developing, the science of molecular biology was also changing the pharmaceutical industry. Using recombinant DNA technology, it became possible to "bioengineer" an exact copy of a human hormone by inserting the gene that controls its production into a biological system. In this way the native, or natural, FSH molecule could be synthesized without the need for urinary extraction. Furthermore, the hormone produced is highly purified and free of the protein contaminants that usually accompany urinary-derived product. These proteins, which are potentially irritating to surrounding tissues, are the reason that urinary product must be given as a deep intramuscular (IM) injection, usually by someone other than the patient. The highly pure, synthetically produced FSH, in contrast, can be delivered by subcutaneous (SQ) injection, an easier procedure that any woman can be taught to perform on herself.

In developing the subcutaneous route for delivering hormones, the pharmaceutical companies did more than simplify the process of undergoing IVF. Unwittingly, they also solved a problem that Orthodox couples commonly faced when using gonadotropins: administration of gonadotropins typically begins early in the cycle, during the *niddah* phase, which meant that in many cases, the husband could not administer the injection, necessitating the recruitment of a third party into the treatment. As the subcutaneous route allows the woman to self-inject, it solved this *niddah* issue.

The use of bioengineered hormones does more than increase the comfort level of patients undergoing IVF. It also ensures that

Ovarian stimulants		
• hMG (human menopausal gonadotropins)		
– Pergonal	IM	urinary
– Humagon	IM	urinary
– Repronex	IM / SQ	urinary
• hFSH (human follitropin)		
– Fertinex	SQ	urinary
– Follistim	SQ	recombinant
– Gonal F	SQ	recombinant
• hCG (human chorionic gonadotropin)		
– Novarel	IM	urinary
– Profasi	IM	urinary
– Ovidrel	SQ	recombinant

a steady supply of hormones will be available to meet the growing demands of a population in need. However, one of the limiting problems with the use of these medications is their expense, often running into thousands of dollars per cycle of treatment. It is hoped that with the entry of competition into this market, the prices for these medications will fall within the reach of the average couple.

IV. GnRH ANALOGS

Although biologists of the past honored the pituitary gland as the "master gland" because of its control of many organ systems, including the reproductive system, we now understand that the pituitary is no master. It is rather the servant of a higher center in the brain called the hypothalamus. Responding to external as well as internal stimuli, it is the hypothalamus that controls the functioning of the pituitary gland and, indirectly, many other organ systems. In women, a properly functioning hypothalamus is crucial for normal ovulation and menstrual cyclicity. Without proper stimuli from the hypothalamus, the pituitary secretion of LH and FSH decline and ovulation ceases. The result is amenorrhea, or absent menses.

In 1977, Andrew Schally and Roger C.L. Guillemin shared the Nobel Prize in Medicine for their isolation and description of gonadotropin releasing hormone, or GnRH. GnRH is the signaling hormone secreted by the hypothalamus and transported to the pituitary to stimulate LH and FSH (gonadotropins) secretion. The secretion of GnRH occurs in pulsatile bursts, which allows the receptors in the pituitary to respond and reset themselves for the next stimulus. Any disruption in the synthesis or pulsatile secretion of GnRH results in failure of the pituitary to secrete LH and FSH and consequent cessation of ovarian function.

Since the mid-1980s, reproductive specialists have used GnRH agonists to turn off pituitary LH and FSH secretion in women undergoing ovulation induction for IVF. These medications work by binding to GnRH receptors on the pituitary cells that make LH and FSH and ultimately desensitizing them (by a process called downregulation) to the natural GnRH hormone. Because the agonists initially stimulate the pituitary, they are typically started one week prior to menstruation. By the time menstruation occurs, the pituitary is profoundly suppressed. The most commonly used GnRH agonist in the United States is Lupron®, but other preparations are commonly used in other countries.

There are three major reasons for the widespread use of GNRH agonists: (a) using it to suppress the ovaries prior to stimulation with gonadotropins appears to sensitize the ovary and to result in the development of more eggs, (b) inhibition of the natural LH surge from the pituitary gland prevents premature ovulation and therefore decreases the risk of needing to cancel a treatment cycle and (c) disruption of the natural cycle permits the physician to program the treatment cycle more effectively, so that the day and time of egg retrieval can be better controlled. This last point is especially important in large programs, where all parties have an interest in evenly spreading out the schedule of egg retrievals so that there are not too many on any given day.

One problem with the use of GnRH agonists has been the over-suppression of ovaries, especially in women with diminished ovarian reserve and older women. One possible solution is the use of the more recently developed GnRH antagonists (Cetrotide®, Antagon®). The virtue of these antagonists is that they shut off the pituitary secretion of LH and FSH shortly after administration,

---

Ovarian suppressants

- Birth control pills
- GnRH agonists
  - Leuprolide acetate
  - Buserilin
  - Nafarelin
- GnRH antagonists
  - Cetrotide
  - Antagon

---

bypassing the initial stimulatory effect that always accompanies agonists. Because they do not require the lead time of the GnRH agonists, the antagonists may be started later in the cycle, after ovulation induction has already begun. By then it is too late for the drug to have a suppressive effect on egg development, but there is still plenty of time to prevent premature ovulation. Although GnRH antagonists are still not routinely used in preparation for IVF, they appear to be ideal for women who respond poorly, whether because of age or other factors, to standard protocols using GnRH agonists.

V. EMBRYO TRANSFER TECHNIQUES

Embryo transfer is where the science and clinical practice of assisted reproduction come together. After all that has been done by the clinicians to obtain good numbers of quality oocytes, and after the scientists have provided the proper conditions for insemination, fertilization, and growth of the embryos in vitro, the two must collaborate to select the best embryos for transfer and place them into the proper environment for implantation. In actuality, the procedure of embryo transfer is a very simple one, so simple in fact, that in the early days of IVF little attention was given to how crucial a role it played in the establishment of pregnancy. More recently, however, it has been recognized that meticulous technique is one of the keys to success. Subsequently, many studies have characterized the variables that are associated with success or failure.

From the technical point of view, it has been found that successful embryo transfer is associated with the use of very soft catheters placed non-traumatically through the cervix to minimize uterine contractions. Great care is taken to minimize contamination, mucus plugging of the catheter and bleeding from the uterine lining. But perhaps the most helpful finding has been that ultrasound guidance of the catheter tip improves embryo placement and maximizes implantation rates.[9] This technique is also helpful in minimizing backflow of embryos into the fallopian tube, which may result in ectopic pregnancy.

It is now common practice in most ART clinics that every woman preparing for IVF undergoes a trial, or mock, transfer prior to the initiation of her treatment cycle. The purpose of this is to measure the depth of the uterine cavity in order to assure exact placement at the time of the actual embryo transfer. In addition, the trial transfer helps identify women with certain anatomical irregularities—such as a uterus which lies in an anomalous position, or an unusually curved cervical canal—which may cause difficulties in embryo transfer. Advance knowledge of the anatomical landmarks can help the physician prepare special catheters or other instruments that will maximize the chances for a non-traumatic embryo transfer. In cases where the cervix is completely closed (cervical stenosis), pretreatment dilation of the cervical canal, with or without removal of adhesions by hysteroscopy, greatly facilitates the future transfer and maximizes the chance of pregnancy.

Developments in the Laboratory

I. LABORATORY CONDITIONS

In the early days of IVF it was not uncommon for egg and embryo culture to be performed in open culture dishes placed directly into CO_2-regulated incubators. Cultures from many patients were placed into the same incubator, which was opened many times during the course of the day. Crude media preparations were adapted from animal IVF work. Maternal serum was used as a protein source

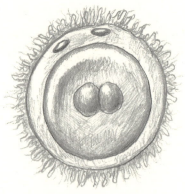

Pronuclear embryo: Normal fertilization is evident by the appearance of two pronuclei, one each from sperm and egg

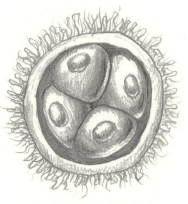

Four cell embryo: The embryo reaches four cells by the second day after fertilization

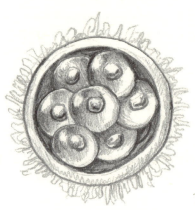

Eight cell embryo: By the third day after fertilization, the embryo may reach eight cells

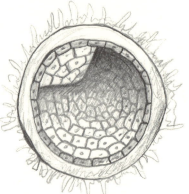

Blastocyst: By the fifth day after ferilization, the embryo has differentiated into different sections. The "inner cell mass" becomes the fetus

for media, and it varied widely in its quality and ability to support embryo growth. Although some women conceived even in those conditions, the great improvements that have occurred over time can be traced, at least in part, to the ever-increasing knowledge of the needs of human gametes and embryos. This knowledge has been the basis of many steps that have been taken to optimize laboratory conditions.

Media are now commercially prepared and tested for their ability to sustain embryonic growth. There is little batch to batch variability, which allows most laboratories to sustain constant conditions for long periods of time. As the embryo experiences changing metabolic requirements during its development, media that is competent to support fertilization may not be optimal for later, cleavage-stage development. This has led to the development of sequential media.

Atmospheric conditions within the incubators must be precisely controlled, especially with regard to their CO_2 content and pH. Most laboratories currently use multiple incubators, some as "working incubators" and others solely for the purpose of embryo culture, so that the embryos remain undisturbed under constant temperature and atmospheric conditions. Special filtration systems are used to separate out particulate matter and other toxins that may be present in room or in incubator air. Great attention has been paid to establishing maximum air purity in most IVF laboratories. This has been accomplished by the installation of positive pressure ventilation systems as well as restricting the flow of personnel traffic in and out of the lab areas.

II. INTRACYTOPLASMIC SPERM INJECTION

When physicians first began using IVF to overcome male factor infertility in the 1980s, the results were very disappointing. Although IVF could clearly be used to bring eggs into close proximity with sperm, overcoming the quantitative defect of low sperm count, this was generally not good enough to overcome the *qualitative* defects that most often accompany this condition. Too often, the eggs would fail to fertilize. In the late 1980s, embryologists began to explore ways to ease the penetration of sperm through the *zona pellucida*, the relatively hard shell that encircles the oocyte. Initial techniques involved boring a hole through the zona, so-called "zona drilling," prior to exposure of the oocyte to sperm. Subsequently, the technique of injecting a few sperm beneath the zona, in the space just outside the oocyte membrane, called subzonal insertion (SUZI), was developed. Both of these techniques were an improvement on standard IVF, but the fertilization rates were still low and very often more than one sperm penetrated the egg. This condition, polyspermy, is incompatible with normal embryonic development.

In 1992, Palermo et al. reported that direct injection of a single sperm into the oocyte could result in normal fertilization, implantation, and pregnancy.[10] This initial success was repeated in other IVF clinics, and intracytoplasmic sperm injection, or ICSI, quickly became the standard for treating recalcitrant male infertility. Although the technique is the ultimate circumvention of "natural selection," the outcomes of ICSI appear to be excellent.[11] Current data indicate that the performance of ICSI in cases of male factor infertility yields pregnancy rates comparable to standard IVF in cases where no male factor is involved. (There is no place for the use of ICSI routinely, in cases where no male factor is involved.) This appears to be so even when sperm counts are extremely low, as when testicular retrieval of sperm is required.

In contrast to standard IVF techniques, which rely on the ability of the sperm to bind to and penetrate the egg's membrane, ICSI eliminates the need for sperm binding at all, and only requires that there be as many live (but not necessarily motile) sperm present as there are mature eggs. Using a sophisticated microscope with state-of-the-art optics, each oocyte is stripped of all of its surrounding cells (the "cumulus") and held in place with a finely drawn out glass micropipette (the "holding" pipette). The embryologist then takes a second, narrower pipette (the "ICSI" pipette) and draws up one sperm from the processed semen sample. The ICSI pipette containing the sperm then pierces the outer zona pellucida and oocyte membrane and, with the aid of fine mechanical controls, the sperm is deposited near the middle of the oocyte. The ICSI pipette is then removed from the oocyte.

The great level of success with ICSI indicates that, even in cases of severe sperm deficiency or abnormality, the DNA content of sperm remains intact. In other words, these problems result in infertility only because the *apparatus* for delivering the sperm into the egg cytoplasm is dysfunctional. However, when this problem is circumvented through the ICSI technique, fertilization and embryo development may proceed normally. Because ICSI has become so routinely successful, even in cases where only rare, dysmorphic sperm are usable, it has changed the way clinicians view male infertility. With ICSI available as treatment, men either have or do not have sperm; all other considerations are irrelevant. Of course, this does not mean that the urologist has lost his role in the treatment of male infertility. Urologists, and in particular urologists who specialize in treating male fertility, are still required to help men with infertility optimize their sperm quality. They must also be available as part of the IVF team for those cases where sperm retrieval is necessary.

There is little doubt that ICSI is a marvelous tool for IVF in cases involving a male factor. However, like any other technology, it is not without its drawbacks. While thousands of babies have

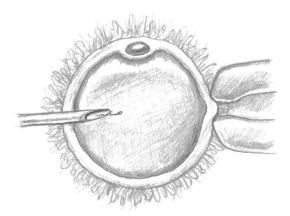

Intracytoplasmic sperm injection: A single sperm in injected directly into the cytoplasm of the egg

been born with the use of ICSI, it is still uncertain whether children (particularly male children) born from ICSI will inherit a genetic basis for infertility. Although both male and female children born through ICSI appear to have a similar percentage of minor and major birth defects as children conceived naturally, these children have not yet reached sexual maturity. Two other drawbacks to the use of ICSI are the additional cost to the couple and a small risk of damage to the oocytes. Approximately 2–5% of the eggs injected after ICSI will not survive, presumably from the physical trauma of the injection. While this is a small risk, it is a risk not associated with standard IVF insemination techniques.

III. EMBRYO SELECTION

The strict attention that is now paid to culture conditions has resulted in greater embryo viability during longer periods of time in culture. Because embryologists can now keep embryos in vitro for longer periods of time, their ability to select the better from the worse embryos has also improved. For many couples, simply moving the transfer day from day 2 to day 3 has resulted in better pregnancy rates. The later stage provides the embryologist with more information about how the individual embryos are faring. Although on day 2 most fertilized embryos are at the 3–4 cell stage, by day 3 the gap widens, with the most viable at the 6–8 cell stage and the least viable with 5 or less cells.

Physiologically speaking, the accepted practice of transferring embryos back to the uterus 3 days after oocyte retrieval is not a natural situation. Under normal circumstances, embryos that are 72 hours old are still in the fallopian tube and have not yet reached the uterus; an asynchrony may therefore exist between the age of the embryos and the developmental stage of the uterine lining.

In recent years, great attention has been given to the technique of blastocyst transfer. The embryo generally reaches the blastocyst stage on the fifth or sixth day after fertilization. At this stage, it has at least 100 cells and has begun the process of differentiation. In normal, in vivo fertilization, this is the stage when the embryo usually enters the uterine cavity and prepares for implantation.

Intuitively, it makes sense that in vitro fertilized embryos placed into the uterus during this phase would have a greater potential for implantation. Indeed, this has been borne out in an almost universal increase in the implantation rate reported by IVF clinics using this technology. Higher implantation rates mean that fewer embryos need to be transferred to maintain a good pregnancy rate.

Blastocyst transfer is not without its disadvantages, however. Only a small percentage of all fertilized eggs will develop to the blastocyst stage in culture. Moreover, despite an increased *implantation* rate, data are conflicting as to whether the overall *pregnancy* rate is significantly improved. While blastocyst transfer appears to be useful in minimizing the risk of multifetal pregnancy, it appears at this time that pregnancy rates are not different than with day 3 transfers. In addition, there are patients for whom extended culture of embryos is probably not beneficial. Couples who produce very few, or poor-looking embryos are not good candidates for this methodology because they may end up with no blastocysts formed and therefore not have a transfer at all. Older women (age 40 or above) also tend not to be good candidates, given the observations from many labs of a negative correlation between blastocyst formation and maternal age. In these situations, the uterus will provide a much better environment to sustain embryo growth than a laboratory incubator, so earlier transfer is indicated.

IV. CRYOPRESERVATION

Embryo cryopreservation is an established technology in most IVF clinics. While the stage at which embryos are frozen may differ from clinic to clinic (zygotes, cleaved embryos, blastocysts), the process of saving spare embryos from a stimulated cycle has become routine for several reasons. First, the use of frozen embryos eliminates the need for the patient to go through another cycle of ovarian stimulation should her initial cycle fail. Besides the obvious advantage in terms of patient comfort, it is also more cost-efficient to use already created banked embryos than to initiate another entire cycle of medications and oocyte retrieval. Secondly, there are instances when a woman may have her eggs retrieved but, for medical reasons, it is not safe for her to have the embryos that result transferred back to her. The most common example is when a woman produces too many eggs and has a very elevated estrogen level; pregnancy would predispose her to develop severe ovarian hyperstimulation syndrome. In such a case, freezing all the embryos is a way of salvaging what might otherwise have been a canceled treatment cycle. Women who are diagnosed with serious chronic illnesses such as cancer also sometimes anticipate that treatment might destroy their ovarian function. A woman choosing to undergo IVF under this circumstance would typically have her embryos frozen and banked, with the anticipation that they will be transferred once she has recovered from her illness.

The ability to cryopreserve embryos allows the clinician to maximize egg development in the ovary and to create many fresh embryos without worrying about needing to transfer them all. Instead, one to three may be transferred, keeping the risk of multifetal gestation low. Excess embryos or blastocysts created during the fresh cycle are then frozen, but only providing that they are of good quality. If the fresh cycle fails, the frozen embryos can be thawed at a later date in hopes of establishing a pregnancy. It is also commonplace to use frozen embryos a year or two after a successful fresh cycle, so that the patient may conceive a "twin" embryo previously created. It is important to emphasize that not all leftover embryos are frozen, only those that meet certain criteria for quality. This assures that the pregnancy rate using the frozen embryos will be high. Depending on the quality of the freezing program, the pregnancy rate using thawed embryos varies between 25–40%.

Sperm cryopreservation is often done prior to an IVF or IUI cycle to ensure that there will be sufficient sperm available on the day of the oocyte retrieval or insemination, respectively.

Understanding the Statistics

Because success rates with IVF can be reported in many different ways, it is important to understand some of the terminology used to describe pregnancy rates with IVF. Without a clear understanding of what the numerator and denominator of a percentage mean, the data from any one clinic can be misleading and confusing. The following glossary of some of the important terms that are commonly used to describe a clinic's "success rate" is helpful in deciphering the data presented by a variety of clinics.

INITIATED CYCLE: Fertility medication is begun in order to stimulate the ovaries to produce many eggs.

OOCYTE RETRIEVAL: Oocytes (eggs) are aspirated from the ovaries using a minor surgical procedure.

CANCELLATION: The cycle is cancelled after fertility medications have been initiated, but prior to the oocyte retrieval.

EMBRYO TRANSFER: Embryos are placed in the uterus using a catheter.

BIOCHEMICAL PREGNANCY: A transient and unsustained rise in the pregnancy hormone hCG (human chorionic gonadotropin). Clinics generally do not report these cases as pregnancies.

CLINICAL PREGNANCY: A gestational sac in the uterus is visualized by ultrasound. Some clinics use this term to refer to the detection of a fetal heartbeat by ultrasound.

LIVE BIRTH: Like naturally occurring pregnancies, those that occur as a result of IVF or any other ART may miscarry at any stage. Therefore, not all clinical pregnancies will result in the birth of a viable baby.

SUCCESS RATE: A percentage made up of two numbers. The most common way for clinics to report their pregnancy rates is to use the number of patients with a clinical pregnancy (at least one sac in the uterus) as the numerator (the top number) and the number of patients having embryo transfers as the denominator (the bottom number). This statistic automatically eliminates those patients who, because of poorly responsive ovaries, have been unable to undergo egg retrieval. Such cycle cancellations typically occur in 10–20% of patients, depending on the age group. Women who have undergone egg retrieval but who have had no embryos produced are also eliminated from this statistic. This is a relatively uncommon occurrence except with blastocyst transfer.

The percentage of live births per retrieval is a good measure of a clinic's success rate. Couples undergoing IVF should discuss this or other statistics prior to proceeding with treatment in order to have realistic expectations about their treatment. It is crucial to note, however, that clinic to clinic comparisons are virtually meaningless. This is because clinics differ widely in the types of patients that they see and treat. Even within defined age categories, pregnancy rates will differ on the basis of the underlying diagnosis, the general health of the patient, and her body weight. As an example, obesity appears to have a negative influence on pregnancy rate. Because obesity is more prevalent in lower socioeconomic groups, clinics that treat only couples who can afford to pay out-of-pocket for their treatment by definition deal with a group more likely to conceive. Another factor that must be taken into consideration is the multifetal pregnancy rate, especially the rate of triplets or more. Clinics that have high pregnancy rates because they transfer more embryos per patient may be doing a disservice to their patients if, as a result, too many of their patients have high risk, multifetal pregnancies. Indeed, multifetal pregnancies have become epidemic in the last decade because of the intense focus on keeping pregnancy rates high. Given the excess morbidity and poor neonatal outcome that is associated with all multifetal pregnancies, including twins, it may be better to choose a lower chance of multifetal pregnancy even if that comes at the expense of a lower chance of pregnancy altogether. Of course, there are also economic considerations that must be weighed. In countries where assisted reproductive services are provided free of charge, single embryo transfer is becoming the rule. While per cycle pregnancy rates are relatively low, the virtual elimination of twin and triplet pregnancies is of great benefit to the society as a whole. In the United States, where most couples requiring assisted reproduction have either no or limited coverage, the pressure for success with the initial cycle is intense, making single embryo transfer a rarely chosen option.

Nearly all ART providers report their statistics to the Centers for Disease Control (CDC) on an annual basis. This reporting program is overseen by the Society for Assisted Reproductive Technologies, or SART. Because of the issues described above, SART mandates that every clinic that advertises a success rate also post the following notice:

A comparison of clinic success rates may not be meaningful because patient medical characteristics and treatment approaches vary from clinic to clinic.

IVF Specifics

No matter what the indication is for using IVF, couples going through treatment typically experience a great deal of stress. Often they see their entire future dependent on the outcome of one treatment cycle. So after wading through the rigors of diagnosis and past failed treatments, patients preparing to move to IVF are almost always sent for counseling. The purpose of the counseling is to set expectations realistically, to help the couple anticipate their emotional needs during the treatment process, and to provide them with strategies to cope with the ups and downs that have come to define IVF. The couple is then ready to move through the various steps that are integral to treatment by IVF. These are:

A. *Ovarian stimulation*—Louise Brown has the distinction of being one of the few individuals conceived by IVF during a natural ovulatory cycle. In the early days of IVF, doctors monitored the woman for her own, single ovulation by measuring LH levels in her blood and retrieving the egg after the surge was detected. But, as it turned out, IVF is a very inefficient way for women to reproduce. In order to improve that efficiency (i.e. the likelihood that any one cycle will result in a successful pregnancy), more eggs were needed. Over time, doctors learned how to add ovarian stimulants to increase the "egg harvest" from each cycle. Today, natural gonadotropins are routinely used to stimulate egg development in preparation for IVF. In addition, nearly every woman is treated with either a gonadotropin releasing hormone (GnRH) agonist or antagonist, which virtually eliminates the possibility of a premature ovulation. Gonadotropin stimulation is highly effective in producing multiple egg development in most women.

B. *Egg retrieval*—When monitoring of the ovarian stimulation regimen reveals that a sufficient number of mature eggs is available, human chorionic gonadotropin (hCG) is given by intramuscular injection in order to promote the final process of egg maturation, and egg retrieval is planned 34–35 hours later. In the early days of IVF, egg retrieval was performed by laparoscopy. This technique has the disadvantage of requiring general anesthesia and all of

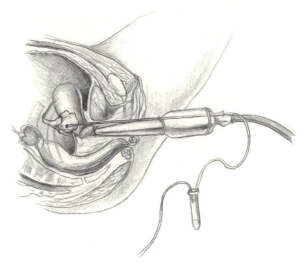

Egg retrieval: Under ultrasound guidance, a needle is placed through the vaginal wall directly into the ovarian follicles

336

the well-known risks of laparoscopic surgery. Today, egg retrieval is done by means of transvaginal ultrasound. Using ultrasound guidance, a thin needle is guided through the vaginal wall into the ovary, allowing all follicles to be drained. The fluid is rapidly examined microscopically and the ova, or eggs, are isolated and incubated in culture medium. This procedure can be done under sedation, usually in 10–15 minutes, and requires minimal recovery. Any vaginal bleeding is usually the result of bleeding from the vaginal wall, rather than from the uterus.

C. *Sperm procurement*—Following egg retrieval, a semen sample must be obtained. The sample is processed, or washed, in order to separate sperm cells from seminal fluid. This processing generally leads to the isolation of a highly concentrated, highly fertile suspension of sperm. In cases where there is a male factor, harvesting of motile sperm from the ejaculate can be more complicated. In some cases, a urologist assists by surgically extracting sperm directly from the epididymis or testis.

D. *In vitro fertilization*—Once eggs and sperm have been isolated, the actual fertilization process is performed. In standard IVF, this means incubation of each egg separately with approximately 50,000 sperm. In cases of male factor requiring ICSI, a single sperm is injected into each egg. In either case, the gametes are allowed to incubate from 2–5 days. The morning after IVF, the eggs are inspected for signs of fertilization. The detection of two pronuclei indicates that normal fertilization has occurred. During subsequent days the embryos are inspected and graded according to the number of cell divisions that have occurred and the morphology of the cells within each embryo.

E. *Embryo transfer*—Although pregnancy rates are good when embryos are transferred to the uterus two days following egg retrieval, transfer is generally delayed until the third day. As already discussed, the higher implantation rates associated with blastocyst transfer on day 5 or 6 allows for the transfer of fewer embryos and

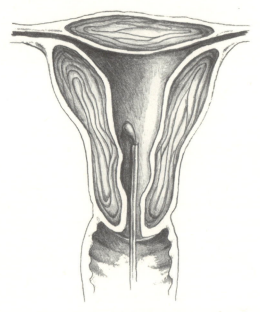

Embryo transfer: A soft plastic catheter delivers one drop of fluid containing the microscopic embryo midway to the uterine cavity.

thus a lower incidence of multifetal pregnancy. For many technical reasons, blastocyst transfer has not yet, however, become the standard. In either case, the embryos or blastocysts selected for transfer are loaded into a very soft catheter by the embryologist and then advanced transcervically and atraumatically into the uterus by the physician. The procedure is virtually painless. There is generally no uterine bleeding associated with embryo transfer.

F. *Cryopreservation*—The number of embryos transferred is generally dependent on the patient's age. Two to five is standard, with younger patients usually using the lower number. As pregnancy rates have risen, it has become more common to transfer fewer embryos in order to lower the chance of multifetal pregnancy. It is hoped that in the future, the higher rate of implantation will permit physicians to transfer only one embryo routinely. Spare embryos, if available, may be cryopreserved, or frozen, in liquid nitrogen providing that they appear morphologically normal in every respect. They may be used at a later date if the couple fails to conceive or if they successfully conceive and subsequently wish to have another child. The upper time limit for successful frozen storage of embryos is currently unknown.

Aligning IVF Treatment to Halakha

Generally, most modern halakhic authorities permit the use of IVF. However, at every stage of the process, specific halakhic issues may arise that must be addressed:

A. *Ovarian stimulation*—One of the most common questions couples face is whether or not a husband may give his wife injections while she is *niddah*. This is because gonadotropins are commonly administered during the beginning of a menstrual cycle. Until recently, gonadotropins were available only for intramuscular injection, requiring administration by the husband or, when not feasible, the recruitment of a third party into the couple's treatment routine. Fortunately, the recent development of highly purified preparations of FSH using recombinant DNA technology, allows for subcutaneous administration. This has largely solved the *niddah* problem, as a woman may self-administer by the subcutaneous route.

At present, the only preparation that is necessary to routinely administer by intramuscular injection is human chorionic gonadotropin, or hCG. However, as this is given at the very end of the stimulation regimen, the woman is most often no longer a *niddah*. What is more, hCG, like other gonadotropins, has also recently become available as a purified preparation (Ovidrel®) that can be self-administered. Even so, the question of the husband injecting his wife while she is *niddah* is still an important one, as some women are unable to inject themselves with medication. Solving this problem requires discussion with a rabbinic authority.

Other potential problems related to this phase of treatment

have to do with restrictions that take hold because of the Sabbath (Shabbat) or Jewish holidays. The couple should consult with their rabbi to ascertain if injection is permissible on Shabbat, and whether or not there is a difference between intramuscular and subcutaneous injection. More complex problems might arise if the couple is requested to undergo follicular monitoring on Shabbat in preparation for IVF. Follicular monitoring consists of transvaginal ultrasound and blood drawing for estrogen levels. Particularly during the later phase of ovarian stimulation, monitoring may be crucial in determining the success of the cycle.

Some of these problems can be avoided if the problems that might arise are clarified at the very beginning, and the treatment modified accordingly. At Genesis, our practice is to pretreat most halakhically observant patients with GnRH agonists in order to gain maximum control of the cycle and to minimize conflicts due to *niddah* and Shabbat. This strategy permits the commencement of gonadotropin therapy at a convenient time. If there is a *niddah* issue, therapy can even be delayed until after the woman has immersed in the *mikvah*. This is usually not necessary. Instead, prior to beginning gonadotropin stimulation, a sufficient number of days is allowed to elapse from the onset of menstrual bleeding so that follicular maturity will be achieved reliably only after the *niddah* interval has been completed. To avoid Shabbat issues, gonadotropins are always begun on a Friday, Saturday or Sunday. This start day almost always results in retrievals occurring on the following Sunday, Monday, or Tuesday (with embryo transfers therefore on Wednesday, Thursday, or Friday, respectively). For medical reasons, monitoring on Shabbat is almost never required. Situations where egg retrieval would be medically indicated on a Shabbat have not been encountered. During Jewish holidays, (*yamim tovim*), when two or even three consecutive days may be unavailable for monitoring purposes, IVF treatments are not be planned for observant couples. This is a convenient time to close the IVF program. Periodic lab closures are needed in any event, so that scientists can perform routine quality control.

B. *Egg retrieval*—As noted, there are ways to ensure that egg retrieval is not necessary on Shabbat. However, not all observant couples will be treated in clinics sensitive to this timing issue. On occasion, a situation may arise where the ovaries are full with ripe eggs and retrieval on Shabbat is required for the cycle to be successful. Waiting an additional day may not be a viable alternative because, with each day that passes, the estrogen levels rise and increase the risk of severe ovarian hyperstimulation syndrome. This is a potentially grave complication of gonadotropin therapy, but will almost never occur in the absence of the final hCG "trigger" injection. Therefore, the only alternative to a Shabbat retrieval is withholding the hCG injection and cancellation of the treatment cycle. A full discussion of the laws of Shabbat as they relate to ART can be found in "Fertility Treatment on the Sabbath and Festivals."

Another question relating to egg retrieval concerns the bleeding that inevitably follows. As already mentioned, this bleeding is vaginal and not uterine, and therefore should never render a woman *niddah*.

C. *Sperm procurement*—The most widely used method of sperm procurement among halakhically observant couples is the medical condom. Unlike other, commercially sold condoms, this condom is specifically manufactured without a spermicide. It allows for sperm to be collected during normal intercourse. Some rabbis tell couples to bore a small hole in the condom so that some of the sperm will escape. The exact source for this recommendation is unknown. Another, less acceptable alternative is intercourse with withdrawal (coitus interruptus). The third and least favored is self-stimulation.

One of the practical realities of IVF is that many observant couples require IVF for male factor infertility. Some husbands have sexual difficulties prior to going into IVF; even if they do not, they are at risk—as all men are—for developing such difficulties during the IVF process. Stress is usually the culprit. Not uncommonly, condoms and withdrawal simply will not work. For such men, vibratory stimuli or electroejaculation can be used. The latter is a technique that requires general anesthesia, but it is very effective in getting sperm without any operative intervention. Clinics that care for observant couples must be able to offer this technique. Rabbis should be aware that such techniques seem extreme when compared with the alternative of masturbation.

One of the accommodations that should routinely be made for the observant couple undergoing IVF is cryopreservation, or banking, of sperm prior to the actual treatment cycle. There are several reasons for this: (a) On the day of the retrieval it is not uncommon that, because of stress, the husband will be unable to produce a sperm specimen. One should understand that, because of the restrictions on self-stimulation, production of sperm translates into the need to have intercourse the morning of the egg retrieval, which is precisely timed and needs to happen at an exact hour. There is no room for saying, "We are having difficulty, so we'll come back in a couple of hours." It has to be done at a certain time. And the stress is sometimes overwhelming. By this time, the woman will have been pretreated with gonadotropins for an extended period of time, with medications that may cost $3,000–4,000. No one involved cares to be in the predicament where there are eggs but no sperm. For this reason, it is helpful to have a specimen available in the bank. (b) Because IVF is so frequently done to treat male factor infertility, it is not uncommon that the sperm specimen produced on the day of the egg retrieval is too poor for use in the laboratory. If this happens, the couple must have intercourse an additional time, a fact that often comes to light after the eggs have been retrieved and the woman is having post-operative bleeding. Even though she is not considered a *niddah*, she may be too uncomfortable to have intercourse, making the cryopreserved sperm very valuable. (c) Finally, even when the husband can reliably produce, and when his sperm are good enough for in vitro fertilization, there are occasions when, in the midst of preparing for IVF, the woman will have unexpected bleeding, rendering her a *niddah*. In such situations, sperm procurement becomes problematic. Here again, it is helpful to have that previously stored specimen.

Of course, there are also halakhic problems that may arise because of this specific accommodation. In most instances, the frozen specimen will not actually be used. Methods of properly disposing of unused sperm should be discussed with a competent halakhic authority.

D. *In vitro fertilization*—When the concept of ICSI was introduced, many believed that it simply would not work, on the grounds that overriding the natural selection process would inevitably result in abnormal embryonic development and failed implantation. But fertilization rates with ICSI have been nearly as good as with standard IVF, and the implantation rate is the same. This means, at least in theory, that pregnancy can be achieved as long as there is even a single sperm available. Pregnancies may even occur when there is azospermia, or complete absence of sperm in the ejaculate. This is possible as long as sperm are present somewhere in the testicle or in the ducts. For example, men who are carriers for cystic fibrosis also have congenital absence of the vas deferens. In these men, testicular production of sperm is completely normal. (This type of azospermia is known as *obstructive azospermia*). Using the technique of epididymal sperm aspiration, normal sperm can be retrieved and used with standard IVF. In men who have non-obstructive azospermia, sperm may be harvested by direct aspiration or biopsy from the testes and used for ICSI. Sperm retrieval is commonly done the day prior to egg retrieval, in order to allow the sperm to recover, acquire motility, and capacitate.

Sperm retrieval involves one of two techniques: one is open biopsy, the other is fine-needle aspiration directly from the testes. Both techniques cause wounding of the testes, evoking questions of *petzuah daka*. One should consult a competent *posek* for rulings in this area. Fortunately, an extensive halakhic discussion of this matter has already occurred. (See "Male Infertility: Halakhic Considerations.")

E. *Embryo transfer*—For most couples, the same pregnancy rates are achieved regardless of whether embryos are transferred on day 2 or day 3. This is another opportunity to modify standard protocol for observant couples. If day 3 happens to fall out on Shabbat, transfer should be arranged for day 2. Alternatively, blastocyst transfer on day 5 or 6 may be considered.

The number of embryos to transfer is a difficult issue. While it does seem clear that the more embryos that are transferred, the higher the chances of pregnancy, multiple embryo transfer also raises the risk of multifetal pregnancy. Infertile couples, as well as fertility specialists, may be complicit in taking such risks. Staff in the IVF unit may feel pressured to achieve success even when it comes at the expense of a multifetal pregnancy. Couples may feel that multifetal pregnancy is actually desirable, as a compensation of sorts for lost time. In their zeal to achieve parenthood, they often forget the considerable risks that carrying more than one fetus entails. This issue bears addressing by our professional society, and also by the lay public. There is certainly no room for the advice to have as many embryos transferred as are available, using fetal reduction as a fail-safe measure if too many fetuses result. The ideal number of fetuses in pregnancy in one and, ideally, only one embryo would be transferred in any given IVF cycle. Indeed, many programs in Europe operate under just such guidelines. Of course, the financial pressures on patients elsewhere are considerable, making single embryo transfer a difficult choice. If further improvements in blastocyst culture are realized, and patients could routinely get their embryos to grow to this stage, the high implantation rate of blastocysts would make single embryo transfer more realistic.

The halakhic issues pertaining to multifetal pregnancy reduction are discussed later (see "New Ethical Issues"). While it is clear that halakha permits reduction in order to minimize physical dangers to the mother and the remaining fetuses, not all rabbinic authorities are comfortable with this solution. Advances in the medical management of prematurely born infants have permitted the healthy development of many sets of triplets and even quadruplets. Although such pregnancies represent extreme hazards at many levels, the exact number of fetuses that make a reduction procedure halakhically justifiable is not clear, and in fact may change depending on certain characteristics of the mother. With no clear guidelines, some rabbinical authorities shy away from allowing the procedure. The best solution, of course, is to prevent multifetal pregnancy in the first place. To the extent that blastocyst transfer can facilitate that goal, it is a good example of using a developing technology to help Orthodox couples avoid halakhic dilemmas.

Many potential problems exist for Sabbath observant staff who work with embryos. For example, if an alarm sounds in the laboratory indicating that liquid nitrogen levels are dangerously low and either the cryopreserved embryos or sperm specimens are in danger of thawing, is this grounds for desecration of Shabbat? What happens if the incubator harboring fresh embryos breaks down on Shabbat? Is there any time that one may violate Shabbat in order to take care of these "embryological emergencies"? Some principles for dealing with these questions are presented in "Fertility Treatment on the Sabbath and Festivals."

F. *Cryopreservation*—The final step in the process, if feasible, is embryo cryopreservation. Top quality clinics use very strict criteria to identify embryos suitable for freezing. Embryos that are morphologically less than perfect should not be frozen, as that might lead to additional treatment of the couple, who most often will not be able to conceive with these imperfect embryos. Adaptation of strict freezing criteria assures high pregnancy rates from frozen/thawed embryos.

It should be noted that many frozen embryos will never be used. Halakhically committed couples who own unneeded frozen embryos need to discuss their disposition with their *posek*. Because untransplanted embryos have no specific halakhic status, and are certainly not considered human life, there are a variety of options to consider. Embryo donation would be one, although it is unclear if it is permissible to donate to a non-Jewish couple. Embryo research would be another consideration. The National Institutes of Health of the United States operates under a longstanding moratorium that disallows the funding of human embryo research. Most embryo research, like IVF in general, has been driven by private medicine and industry. The need for embryo research is pressing. Alternatively, couples may feel that their embryos should be discarded. Doing so under halakhic supervision is generally requested.

Other ART Procedures

ASSISTED HATCHING

The creation of healthy embryos in a laboratory and their atraumatic transfer into the uterus unfortunately does not always guarantee a successful cycle. The embryos must implant in the uterus if a fetus is to develop. In order for such implantation to take place, the embryos must first shed the zona pellucida. Usually when the embryo reaches blastocyst stage, around day 5 or 6, the zona thins significantly as the embryo begins to cavitate and increase in size. However, under certain circumstances, some embryos may need a little help escaping ("hatching") from the zona. Assisted hatching is a technique whereby a small hole is created in the zona pellucida by physical piercing, either with a laser, or by exposure of a tiny area of the zona to a very acidic solution.

In most laboratories, assisted hatching is not routinely

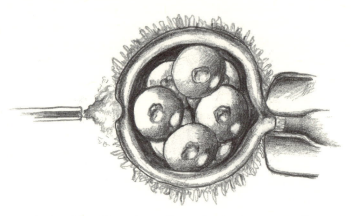

Assisted hatching: A small opening in the surrounding zona pellucida is made chemically or with a laser

practiced. There are, however, some instances when it may prove helpful in encouraging implantation. Assisted hatching may be recommended for older patients (38 years and above), for women found to have thickened zonas (often appreciated at the time of ICSI) and for patients who have had several unsuccessful cycles with no defined reason. As with ICSI, assisted hatching poses a small risk of damage to the embryo.

GAMETE INTRAFALLOPIAN TRANSFER

In 1984, Dr. Ricardo Asch introduced a therapeutic alternative to IVF which he termed "gamete intrafallopian transfer," or GIFT. It gained widespread popularity for a number of years but has largely been superceded by IVF, for reasons explained below. The GIFT procedure involves the injection of eggs and sperm directly into the fallopian tubes, and is performed by laparoscopy.[12] Pretreatment of the woman with fertility drugs in order to achieve multiple mature eggs is necessary, as in IVF, but in the GIFT procedure the eggs are not fertilized in vitro. Instead, after they are aspirated from the ovary, they are mixed with a suspension of sperm and immediately reinserted into the fallopian tube, where fertilization subsequently occurs *in vivo*. One key aspect of the GIFT procedure, as is evident from this description, is that it requires that the woman have at least one normally functioning fallopian tube.

GIFT has mainly been used for cases of unexplained infertility, or when infertility is due to mild depressions in sperm count. The preliminary experience with GIFT suggested that it was superior to IVF for these indications. The purported advantage that GIFT holds over intrauterine insemination is that it ensures that the eggs and sperm arrive simultaneously at the point in the fallopian tubes where fertilization normally occurs. In effect, GIFT substitutes incubation in the petri dish, the fundamental basis for IVF, with incubation in the reproductive tract.

One major disadvantage of GIFT is that it lacks the diagnostic capacity of IVF. That is, when the procedure fails, no further information is available on the ability of sperm and eggs to undergo fertilization, or about embryo quality. Its limitation mainly

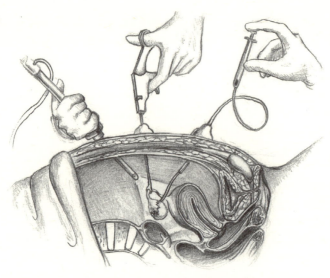

Gamete Intrafallopian Transfer (GIFT): Using laparoscopy, sperm and eggs are placed into the end of the fallopian tube

to treating cases of unexplained infertility also handicapped this procedure, especially as pregnancy rates with IVF were becoming reliably high, even with the most severe forms of tubal and male factor infertility. Although the initial successes with GIFT were born out by the yearly SART pregnancy data as reported by the CDC, it soon became evident that patients treated with IVF and with GIFT were distinctly different in many ways. In fact, for unexplained and male factor infertility, pregnancy rates similar to GIFT's can likely be achieved using a combination of ovulation induction and intrauterine insemination. Over time, therefore, the increased costs and discomfort (from laparoscopy) associated with GIFT, in addition to concerns related to the more frequent occurrence of tubal pregnancy, caused the procedure to fall from favor. Today, less than 1% of ART procedures nationwide involve GIFT.

As GIFT has become an interesting historical footnote, so have the halakhic discussions that accompanied the procedure in its heyday. At that time, many Orthodox patients were sent to Dr. Asch's clinic in California on the advice of their rabbis, specifically because the GIFT procedure appeared to circumvent some of their halakhic concerns. Rabbi Waldenberg's concerns, specifically, seemed to be addressed by GIFT: (a) the eggs were not removed from the body for a significant period of time and were fertilized in their natural location, thus avoiding the problem of establishing maternity, (b) excess sperm could be inseminated into the woman at the time of the procedure, thereby avoiding the problem of *hash'hatat zera*, and (c) the avoidance of the incubation period in the laboratory mitigates concerns about the unscrupulous switching of gametes by physicians. At the time, there was also a budding interest in the use of the GIFT procedure in the context of egg donation: the transference of the unfertilized egg to the fallopian tube conferred on the procedure the appearance of organ donation and, as in any organ donation, the halakhic "owner" was established beyond doubt. Ironically, all such interest came to a halt when Dr. Asch himself was indicted for illegally using the eggs from some patients to create embryos for others (See "A Brief History of Fertility Therapy").

ZYGOTE INTRAFALLOPIAN TRANSFER
This procedure, initially described in 1986,[13] involves the use of in vitro fertilization, followed by the placement of the developing embryo into the fallopian tube via laparoscopy. The theory behind the potential benefit of ZIFT was that the embryos were transferred to the fallopian tube as soon as possible after fertilization. This meant that they could further develop in the natural site of fertilization, rather than in the laboratory incubator. At the time, the major indication for ZIFT was to confirm fertilization in cases of male infertility, thus circumventing the obvious problem posed by GIFT. To date there is no proven benefit of ZIFT over IVF, and IVF can be done without the discomfort of laparoscopy.

TUBAL EMBRYO TRANSFER
Like ZIFT, tubal embryo transfer (TET) involves placement of the developing embryo into the fallopian tube via laparoscopy. The purpose of TET, however, is not to bypass the laboratory phase of embryo growth. TET is done on the same day that embryo transfer

would ordinarily be done transcervically. It is indicated when an anatomical variation of the cervix—absence, stenosis, or otherwise difficult to cannulate—makes it difficult or impossible to perform the transfer through the cervix. In judiciously chosen cases, TET can be done faster, with less discomfort and more successfully than a difficult transcervical embryo transfer.

PREIMPLANTATION GENETIC DIAGNOSIS

Prior to its transfer to the uterus on day 3 after fertilization, the embryo remains in a highly undifferentiated state. This means that each of its eight cells is identical to the other. Each cell—called a blastomere—carries the entire genetic information that will be used to grow the fetus and each cell separately retains the capacity to grow into that fetus. This is best demonstrated from time to time in naturally occurring pregnancies, when splitting of the embryo at this stage results in two perfectly normal, and genetically identical, human beings.

Because the early embryo is undifferentiated, removal of a single blastomere has no effect whatsoever on subsequent development of the embryo or its ability to implant and form a normal fetus. In the early days of IVF, researchers theorized that biopsy of the embryo by removing a blastomere might give insight into the genetic health of the embryo. Unfortunately, this single cell could provide only a minute amount of DNA, much less than what is needed to study the cell's genetic makeup. This dilemma was eventually solved with the invention, by Karry Mullis in 1983, of the polymerase chain reaction (PCR). A method of amplifying DNA, PCR multiplies a single, microscopic strand of the genetic material billions of times. It requires no more than a test tube, a few simple reagents and a source of heat. Beginning with a single molecule of DNA, the PCR can generate 100 billion similar molecules in an afternoon. The usefulness of this technique in studying DNA is so widespread that PCR has been hailed as one of the monumental scientific techniques of the twentieth century. (Mullis was awarded a Nobel Prize for his invention in 1993.)

In 1992, researchers described how they used PCR to analyze

the genetic material from blastomeres prior to embryonic implantation in order to avoid transmission of the cystic fibrosis gene.[14] This technique, called preimplantation genetic diagnosis (PGD), opened the door for IVF to be used in couples at risk for genetic disease. Since that time, many diseases for which the genetic basis is known, such as Tay-Sachs, have been successfully detected in embryos, allowing couples at risk to conceive with unaffected, healthy embryos and thereby avoid the dilemma of possibly needing to abort a diseased fetus.

Not all genetic problems involve single genes. Many involve rearrangements of entire chromosomes, such as Trisomy 21, or Down Syndrome. Chromosomes are tightly packaged structures containing DNA, the basic building blocks of life. All normal individuals have 46 chromosomes: 23 from each parent. Of each pair of 23 chromosomes, 22 are autosomes and 1 is the sex chromosome, X or Y. Genetic diseases may affect the autosomes or the sex chromosomes. In Down Syndrome, there is a third copy of the 21st chromosome, resulting in the typical features associated with this condition. Such abnormal numbers of chromosomes is a condition called aneuploidy. Except for rare instances such as Down Syndrome, aneuploidy nearly always results in early embryonic

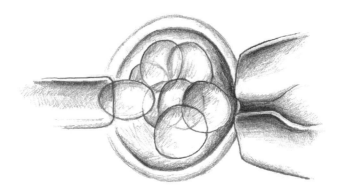

Blastomere biopsy: A single cell may be removed from the eight cell embryo to test it genetically

loss or fetal death. In fact, aneuploidy accounts for approximately 60–70% of all miscarriages.

As it happens, aneuploidy is much easier to detect than single gene disorders, because DNA analysis by PCR is not necessary. Instead, scientists have developed the technique of fluorescent in situ hybridization, or FISH. FISH utilizes different fluorescent colored probes to examine the intact blastomere. Each probe is specific for a given chromosome, and each chromosome is distinguished by a fluorescent color that can be detected using a special microscope. The various color combinations allow embryologists to distinguish normal cells from cells with aneuploidy.

Although PGD was initially used to help couples at risk for genetic disease conceive healthy pregnancies, the realization that many failed IVF attempts in genetically normal couples were due to embryonic aneuploidy has led some IVF centers to offer PGD to all couples with infertility. Although the usefulness of PGD in overcoming infertility that has been refractory to standard IVF has not been solidly established, it appears that it will be increasingly used in the future in order to select genetically normal embryos and thereby increase the implantation and ongoing pregnancy rate.[15] Women 35 years or older, in particular, are at risk for producing embryos with aneuploidy, explaining why pregnancy rates fall and miscarriage rates rise dramatically with increasing maternal age. Performing genetic analysis prior to embryo implantation could prevent the initiation of abnormal pregnancies or offer explanations for recurrent miscarriages or implantation failures. In the future, routine use of PGD in this population may increase the chance of a successful pregnancy and delivery of a healthy newborn.

It seems clear at this time that most halakhic authorities permit PGD to prevent transmission of genetic disease. The use of PGD electively carries additional concerns. Certainly, the use of PGD solely for the purposes of sex selection, while eminently feasible scientifically, would be considered a frivolous use of IVF and prohibited by most *poskim*. This is discussed further in "New Ethical Issues." The use of PGD to improve the chances of pregnancy, however, is a more recent notion and has not yet been addressed halakhically.

EGG DONATION

Oocyte (egg) donation is a variation of in vitro fertilization that enables a woman with absent or poorly functioning ovaries to conceive. Clear indications for egg donation include absence of ovaries from birth (as in the case of Turner's Syndrome) and premature ovarian failure (early menopause) which may have resulted naturally or after certain types of cancer treatment. In the past, egg donation was also indicated to circumvent genetic disorders in the female, although with the use of PGD this is less frequently required. Finally, and most commonly, egg donation is used in cases where a woman responds poorly to other treatment, including IVF with her own eggs. There are many reasons why a woman may fail to conceive with her own eggs, or to even reach the stage where egg retrieval can be performed. Surgery on the ovaries for benign conditions such as ovarian cysts and endometriosis may involve removal of the egg-containing tissues of the ovary, resulting in a depletion of the egg supply. No doubt, however, the most common indication for which egg donation is used is to establish pregnancy in women who are at or near the end of their reproductive capacaity. In such women, ovarian reserve is absent or severely compromised, resulting in their inability to achieve proper egg maturation. Alternatively, they may mature some eggs but repeatedly fail to conceive because of persistent embryonic aneuploidy, a direct result of biological aging.

In the technique of egg donation, the egg donor undergoes controlled stimulation of her ovaries similar to the regular preparation for IVF. After her eggs are retrieved, however, she drops out of the clinical picture. Her eggs are then combined with the recipient husband's sperm in the laboratory. Over the ensuing days, the eggs will fertilize and start dividing the way that they would in standard IVF. Meanwhile, the oocyte recipient is taking estrogen and progesterone so that the lining of her uterus is at the same stage as that of the donor. At the appropriate time, the embryos are placed inside her uterus, where they may implant and establish a pregnancy.

A woman's body cannot distinguish between an embryo that has developed from her own eggs or from those of a donor. The pregnancy derived from a donor oocyte will therefore develop like any other pregnancy resulting from IVF, except that the recipient will need to remain on estrogen and progesterone therapy until the end of the first trimester. From that point, the pregnancy will produce all of the hormones that it needs in order to be maintained. The results of IVF using egg donation are typically excellent, equaling those of younger women who use heir own eggs.

Most IVF programs recruit volunteers who donate their eggs anonymously. Usually, these volunteers are young women who are not yet ready to have children of their own. Many of them have seen friends or family members go through the pain of infertility and feel that it would be an act of great charity to help alleviate the suffering of an infertile couple. (Because of the natural process of egg attrition, the eggs that are donated would have otherwise

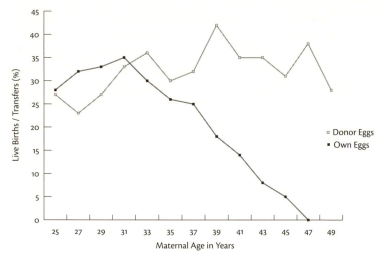

Live births with standard IVF and donated eggs

have been lost. In other words, donors are not compromising their future fertility.) Of course, all donors are screened for genetic and family history, general and reproductive health, infectious diseases and psychological stability. Potential recipients undergo a thorough medical history, physical examination and extensive laboratory testing. Every attempt is made to match each recipient with a donor of a similar physical and ethnic background. After a suitable donor is found, an individualized medication regimen for synchronizing the development of the lining of the recipient's uterus with the egg donor's cycle is developed, and the IVF cycle is initiated.

Egg donation produces remarkable results, enabling women who had no alternative years ago to become pregnant fairly easily. But for the Jewish patient, the procedure raises a serious halakhic question: who is the child's mother? Is it the woman who carries the child for nine months in her uterus and gives birth to the child? Is it the woman who provides the egg with the genetic material for the child? Or does the child have two halakhic mothers?

The halakhic status of the donor and recipient has crucial implications regarding the Jewishness of the child. If the donor has no halakhic status, then it is irrelevant whether she is a Jew or a non-Jew. If the donor has some status, then if she is not Jewish, the child may be required to undergo a modified conversion, including ritual immersion. As will be explained later, the status of the egg donor remains halakhically unresolved. Because the conversion process has become somewhat problematic in Orthodox circles, most rabbis who currently permit egg donation specifically request that the donor be Jewish. In this way the halakhic status of the child as fully Jewish is unquestioned.

However, this ruling raises another: one particularly difficult issue in making egg donation available to Jewish couples is finding Jewish donors. A common precept of those *poskim* who allow the procedure is that the donor should not be someone who, were she to conceive naturally with the recipient's husband, would create a child that would be a *mamzer* because of the prohibition of *arayot*.[16] This means that the use of a sister of the recipient as an egg donor—a common practice in the secular world—is off limits to Orthodox couples. It also means that the donor must be single.[17]

Another consideration is ascertaining that the donor herself is indeed a Jew. In general, halakha reasons that if a person states that he or she is Jewish, the statement itself is sufficient to establish their actual Jewishness. However, many rabbinic authorities today are concerned that, because of the way the Reform movement has defined Judaism (i.e. accepting patrilineal as well as matrilineal descent), it is preferable to have the donor state that her parents were both Jewish. Having the donor write this on her personal history form is sufficient. As a practical matter, Israeli women who state that their parents were married by the *rabbanut* are reliable in their Jewishness, as that government body will not marry couples if both husband and wife are not Jewish.

The issue of disclosure is controversial, for it is expected that many couples who conceive with the use of egg donation will never reveal to the child the circumstances of conception. When the egg donor is Jewish, this raises the possibility that the child may inadvertently marry a half-sibling, either a child produced through a subsequent donation by the same donor or a full biological child of the donor. For this reason, those authorities who permit egg donation usually request that the recipient be provided with *nonidentifying* medical and family history information about the donor. The expectation is that such information will be useful when the child is ready to marry, hopefully ruling out for the recipient couple the remote possibility that the intended partner might be a halakhic relative. In New York State, donor and recipient records must be kept for 25 years, although matches are closely guarded and confidentiality cannot be broken. The very fact that there exists a potential for clarifying a situation of questionable *arayot* is sufficient grounds for some authorities to discount this as a significant halakhic concern.

GESTATIONAL SURROGACY

As in the situation of egg donation, with gestational surrogacy the genetic mother and the birth mother are two different individuals.

Much of the medical treatment is also the same, albeit with the roles reversed. With surrogacy, however, the birth mother (the recipient in this case) has no intention of keeping the child. She merely lends out her womb to facilitate embryo implantation and development. Once the child is born, he or she is given back to the genetic parents (the donor in this case) for rearing. Gestational surrogacy is used mainly for women who have normal ovarian function but who have either no uterus or one incapable of carrying a pregnancy to term.

The halakhic issues surrounding gestational surrogacy are similar to those arising in egg donation, except that it is even clearer that the birth mother must be Jewish in order to prevent the need for conversion and ritual immersion. Although gestational surrogacy has been sanctioned by the rabbinate in Israel and is also legally permitted, the stipulation that the gestational surrogate be unmarried makes it difficult indeed to find suitable volunteers. In New York State, it is currently illegal to financially compensate surrogates for their services, so it is rarely practiced. Recent legal decisions indicate, however, that compensating surrogates is allowable if treatment occurs in a state where surrogacy is legal. Most IVF programs insist, with good reason, that surrogates have experienced at least one full-term pregnancy. As a practical matter, this further complicates the recruitment of potential Jewish surrogates.

The above notwithstanding, there may be room, according to some *poskim*, to permit the use of a non-Jewish woman as a surrogate.[18] Couples wishing to engage in this treatment must consult with a rabbinical authority who is fully conversant with the complex issues involved.

Summary

There are many open halakhic questions pertaining to the use of reproductive technologies. From a practical viewpoint, many modifications may be made to accommodate observant couples undergoing in vitro fertilization and other forms of ART. First and foremost, direct rabbinical consultation with the treating physician should take place in order to establish that ART is appropriate from all perspectives. Secondly, whenever possible, a sperm sample should be frozen before the couple undergoes their treatment cycle. Thirdly, the choice of medications and protocols needs to be modified in order to make sure that couples will have no difficulty administering medications and that no one will end up with egg retrieval or embryo transfer scheduled on Shabbat or Jewish holidays. Start times for ovarian stimulation have been standardized to reliably avoid such problems. Timing of embryo transfer can also be modified in order to take into consideration the couple's religious concerns without compromising pregnancy rates. Finally, rabbinical oversight may be added at the patients' request, so long as logistical problems are addressed beforehand and all staff involved understands the need for such accommodations.

Programs in which care is given to large numbers of observant couples would do best to close the IVF lab at certain times of the year, i.e. during the *yamim tovim*. During these intervals there are too many consecutive days that couples cannot be present for monitoring. Embryologists may make use of this time for important tasks such as quality control, quality assurance, standard laboratory cleaning, etc. In this way, the accommodations made for couples will also yield increased productivity and benefits for the program involved.

There is no question that the assisted reproductive technologies, especially IVF, are with us for the long run and will continue to bring great benefit to the traditional Jewish community. With the details of treatment now fully explained, it is hoped that the community will attain a higher degree of comfort with the techniques that are employed. Although opinions on the use of this technology vary from *posek* to *posek*, it is a sign of how vibrant the halakhic process is that there continues to be an active and lively discussion of all matters relevant to ART. With the passage of time, the newness of the current technology will eventually feel routine, and consensus in the Torah observant community will hopefully be reached.

Common Algorithms for the Treatment of Infertility[19]

ALGORITHM 1. INFERTILITY DUE TO TUBAL FACTOR

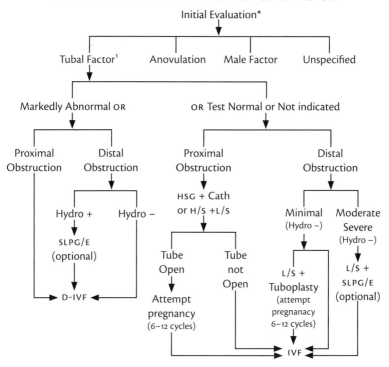

OR = ovarian reserve; Hydro + = hydrosalpinx present;
Hydro − = hydrosalpinx absent; HSG = hysterosalpingography;
Cath = cathererization; H/S = hysterography; L/S = laparoscopy;
SLPG/E = salpingectomy; D-IVF = donor oocyte *in vitro* fertilization;
IVF = *in vitro* fertilization (own eggs).

* Comprehensive history and physical examination, plus hysterosalpingogram
(HSG) to evaluate fallopian tubes, confirmation of ovulation by history BBT.
serum progesterone or detection of LH surge, pelvic ultrasound, and semen
analysis.

[1] Abnormal HSG; assumes documentation of ovulation and normal pelvic
anatomy and normal semen analysis.

ALGORITHM 2. INFERTILITY IN AN ANOVULATORY WOMAN

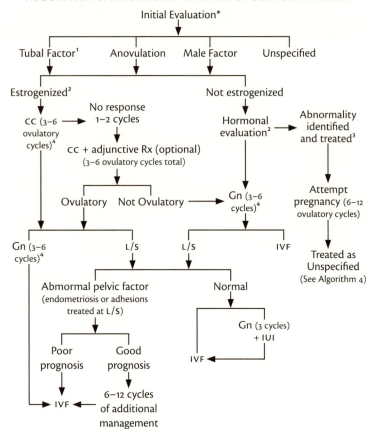

cc = clomiphene citrate; w/wo = with or without; DEX = dexamethasone; Gn = gonadotropins; L/S = laparoscopy; IVF = *in vitro* fertilization (own eggs); IUI = intrauterine insemination.

* Comprehensive history and physical examination, plus hysterosalpingogram (HSG) to evaluate fallopian tubes, confirmation of ovulation by history BBT, serum progesterone or detection of LH surge, pelvic ultrasound, and semen analysis.

[1] Ovulation not documented; assumes normal pelvic anatomy and semen analysis. HSG may also be performed.

[2] Studies could include FSH, LH, TSH, prolactin and others as clinically indicated.

[3] Specific abnormalities may include hyperprolactinemia treated with a dopamine agonist or treatment of a hormonal tumor; any condition identified should be followed independent of infertility treatment.

[4] IUI may be considered after three successful ovulatory cycles.

ALGORITHM 3. MALE FACTOR INFERTILITY

Initial Evaluation*

Tubal Factor   Anovulation   Male Factor‡   Unspecified

Urologic Consultation[1]

Hormonal[2]   Varicocele epididymal / testicular abnormality[3]   Retrograde ejac, ejaculatory duct[4]

Nonspecific Treatment

Correct Abnormality   Varicocele repair / surgical correction   Correct Abnormality

Semen parameters above IUI threshold   Semen parameters below IUI threshold

Semen still abnormal

IUI (3–6 cycles)[5]

Donor insemination   IVF + ICSI

IUI = intrauterine insemination; IVF = *in vitro* fertilization (own eggs); ICSI = intracytoplasmic sperm injection.

* Comprehensive history and physical examination, plus evaluation of female as indicated.

‡ Abnormal semen analysis on at least 2 occasions

[1] Consultation with a urologist or other clinician who is extremely well versed in male factor infertility by a virtue of training and experience.

[2] Performed if sperm concentration is less than 10 million/mL, impaired sexual function, other clinical findings suggestive of a specific endocrinopathy.

[3] Evaluation may include post-ejaculatory urinalysis or transrectal ultrasound.

[4] May include scrotal or testicular ultrasound.

[5] Ovulation indication may considered after three successful cycles.

ALGORITHM 4. INFERTILITY DUE TO UNSPECIFIED CAUSES

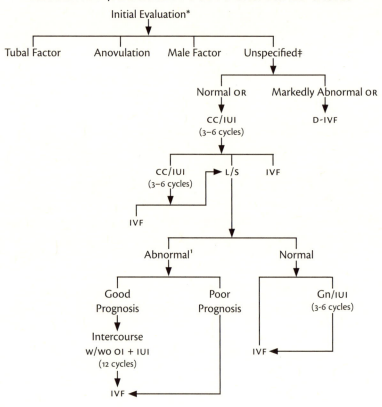

OR = ovarian reserve; D-IVF = donor oocyte *in vitro* fertilization;
CC = clomiphene citrate; IUI = intrauterine insemination; Gn = gonadotropins;
L/S = laparoscopy; IVF = *in vitro* fertilization (own eggs); w/wo = with or without;
OI = ovulation induction.

* Comprehensive history and physical examination, plus hysterosalpingogram
  (HSG) to evaluate fallopian tubes, confirmation of ovulation by history BBT.
  · serum progesterone or detection of LH surge, pelvic ultrasound, and semen
  analysis.

‡ Assumes normal HSG; semen analysis and documentation of ovulation.

¹ Includes pelvic adhesions and/or endometriosis.

Endnotes

1. P.C., R.G. Edwards, "Birth after reimplantation of a human embryo," Lancet 2:366, (1978).
2. For a fuller description of the initial work, see R. Edwards, P. Steptoe, *A Matter of Life—the Story of a Medical Breakthrough.* (London: Hutchinson and Co., Ltd., 1980).
3. Centers for Disease Control and Prevention. 2001 Assisted Reproductive Technology Success Rates. National Summary and Fertility Clinic Reports. U.S. Department of Health and Human Services, (Dec., 2003).
4. D. Navot, Z. Rosenwaks, E.J. Margolioth, "Prognostic assessment of female fecundity," Lancet 1:645–647, (1987).
5. Levi AJ, Raynault M.F., et al., "Reproductive outcome in patients with diminished ovarian reserve," *Fertility and Sterility* 76:666–669, (2001).
6. I.A.J. van Rooij, J.M.M. Bancsi, F.J.M. Broekmans, et al., "Women older than 40 years of age and those with elevated follicle-stimulating hormone levels differ in poor response rate and embryo quality in in vitro fertilization," *Fertility and Sterility* 29:482–488, (2003).
7. C.A. Gemzell, E. Diczfalusy, K.G. Tillinger, "Clinical effect of human pituitary follicle-stimulating hormone," *Journal of Clinical Endrcrinology and Metabolism* 18:1333, (1958).
8. See following section "Developments in the Laboratory."
9. B. Coroleu, O. Carreras, et al., "Embryo transfer under ultrasound guidance improves pregnancy rates after in vitro fertilization," *Human Reproduction*, 15:616–20, (2000).
10. G. Palermo, J.S. Devroey, A.C. Van Steirteghem, "Pregnancies after intracytoplasmic sperm injection of single spermatozoon in to an oocyte," *Lancet* 340:17–18, (1992).
11. M.G. Retzloff, M.D. Hornstein, "Is intracytoplasmic sperm injection safe?" *Fertility and Sterility* 80:851–859, (2003).
12. R.N. Asch, L.R. Ellsworth, J.P. Balmaceda, P.C. Wong, "Pregnancy after translaparoscopic gamete intrafallopian transfer," *Lancet* 2:134, (1984).
13. P. Devroey, P. Braekmans, J. Smitz, et al., "Pregnancy after translaparoscopic zygote intrafallopian transfer in a patient with anti-sperm antibodies," *Lancet* 1:1329, (1986).
14. A. Handyside, J.G. Lesko, J.J. Tarin, R.M.L. Winston, M.R. Huges, "Birth of a normal girl after in vitro fertilization and preimplantation genetic testing for cystic fibrosis," *New England Journal of Medicine* 327:905–909, (1992).
15. L. Gianaroli, M.C. Magli, A.P. Ferraretti, et al., "Preimplantation genetic diagnosis increases the implantation rate in human in vitro fertilization by avoiding the transfer of chromosomally abnormal embryos," *Fertility and Sterility* 68:1128–1131, (1997).
16. Although the word *mamzer* is traditionally translated as a bastard child, the

halakhic notion of a *mamzer* differs from the secular definition. The forbidden unions that create *mamzers* are explicitly defined halakhically as either incestuous relationships between certain family members (*"arayot"*), or as adulterous relationships between married Jewish women and Jewish men other than their husbands.

17. Special considerations exist for recruiting a donor when the recipient's husband is a *kohen*. In this case, a single Jewish woman who is known to have had intercourse with a non-Jew would also be unusable. Although it is not required that the potential donor be asked this question, if she volunteers such information then she should not be used as an egg donor for such a couple.

18. E.D. Clark, Z. Silverman, "Surrogate motherhood in the case of high-risk pregnancy," *Journal of Halacka and Contemporary Society.* 37:5–38, (1999).

19. Society for Reproductive Endocrinology and Infertility. Infertility Coverage for Benefit Managers: An Organized Approach to Diagnosing and Treating Infertility, (2003–2004).

Part v
Special Considerations for the Infertile Jewish Couple

Introduction

As we have seen in the case of *niddah* and *tahara*, infertile couples who are committed to halakha do not seek ways to circumvent their religious values; rather, they seek ways to reconcile treatment to the demands of halakha. But challenges in the delivery of fertility services to traditional Jewish couples do not stop with the laws governing marital relations. Many different forms of treatment require that care be given frequently within a short time frame, with examinations, consultations, and decisions made on a day-to-day basis. When Sabbath or other festival days occur in the midst of treatment, many problems potentially arise, as the opportunities for the couple to undergo any type of diagnostic study or treatment are restricted. For elective medical interventions there is no option of desecrating the holiness of the day.

Caregivers who are experienced in caring for Orthodox couples may tailor treatment protocols to minimize such conflicts. Still, most couples will not have the luxury of being treated by a staff that is familiar with Sabbath restrictions. In this section, the various timing conflicts that might arise during care are explored, along with some of the ways in which these conflicts might be avoided or resolved.

This section also explores one last accommodation, perhaps the most difficult of all, that should be available to Orthodox couples. The concept of a disinterested party—the *mashgiach*, or overseer—watching over the treatment process may seem foreign to many physicians, especially those who practice in areas where few Jewish couples seek care. However, rabbinical oversight is, for many couples, the *sine qua non* for undergoing assisted reproduction. Without such oversight, permission to treat is often withheld. In this section the rationale behind rabbinical oversight is described, and guidelines for establishing this type of program are presented. While the resources of different programs vary widely, it is helpful for all physicians who treat couples requesting oversight to understand the rationale for their request as well as the minimum standards required to fulfill their needs.

Gideon Weitzman

Fertility Treatment on the Sabbath and Festivals

The Importance of the Sabbath

Keeping Shabbat—the Jewish Sabbath—is one of the cardinal elements of Judaism, touching the very basis of faith.[1] By observing the laws of Shabbat every Jew bears witness that God both created the world and rules over it.[2] Just as God rested after He completed creating the world on the seventh day,[3] so the individual Jew rests on Shabbat, a gift lovingly given to him by God.[4] More than merely a remembrance of the act of creation, Shabbat is a weekly affirmation that it is the Holy One who ensures that the world continues to exist.[5] Shabbat is the weekly opportunity for the Jew to express his spirituality and to reaffirm his sacred obligation in the world.[6]

The observation of Shabbat is considered to be equivalent to observing all of the other mitzvot of the Torah.[7] The Rabbis promised that one who observes all of the laws of Shabbat properly will merit many gifts: He will have an unlimited portion,[8] his wishes will be granted[9] and he will be saved from slavery.[10] The Rabbis also declared that observing Shabbat will herald the messianic era.[11]

The opposite is also true. Someone who breaks the laws of Shabbat is liable to the most severe punishment. During the era of the *Beit HaMikdash*, the Jewish Temple, if one broke the laws of Shabbat unintentionally he had to bring a sin offering.[12] If one broke Shabbat in the presence of witnesses and after sufficient warning, he was liable to capital punishment. If the violation was intentional but witnesses were not present, he was punished with *karet*, being "cut off."[13] While one who transgresses Shabbat in our times cannot bring a sacrifice, nor is capital punishment employed, this does not decrease the severity of the offense. The Rabbis state that one who does not observe Shabbat is akin to one who practices idolatry.[14]

It is clear from the above that the observation of Shabbat is a basic and essential part of the observant Jew's life. The Rabbis directed that one should always prepare for Shabbat and, even throughout the week, should set aside special foods for this holy day.[15] Thus the Jew sees the week as flowing from Sabbath to Sabbath.[16]

The Jewish festivals, or *yamim tovim,* give the Jewish people a distinct nature and express their relationship with God.[17] As the festivals are dependent on the calendar, which is one of the unique expressions of the Jewish people as a nation, they differentiate between the Jew and the gentile.[18]

For the devout Jew, Shabbat and other festivals are not a burden. Rather, they are the pinnacle of his week and year. Their sanctity cannot be compromised. Many other considerations are pushed aside in order to observe Shabbat and the festivals. Even when the Jew is faced with business opportunities, Shabbat and the festivals take precedence. This is also true with certain types of elective medical treatment.

Laws of Shabbat and Festivals[19]

Shabbat is a day of rest and the Jew is commanded to rest on this day.[20] Rest is defined as refraining from *melakhah,* a unique concept roughly translated as "creative work," and not necessarily related to physical exertion or toil.[21] A *melakhah* is an action that changes the nature of items, such as cooking, which changes the nature of food, or building, which creates new structures. This is, however, a very general definition. One would need to study the laws of Shabbat in depth to understand even the basic rules of how certain actions came to be classified as *melakhah.* In the course of certain types of medical treatment, perfectly acceptable procedures may be prohibited during Shabbat and the festivals because they constitute a *melakhah.* We will examine these prohibitions as they relate to the treatment of infertility.

There are 39 categories of *melakhah,*[22] each derived from the types of work performed in the constructing of the Tabernacle in the desert.[23] Each category, called the *av melakhah,* also includes many derivatives, called *toladot.* For example, planting seeds is a *melakhah,* and a derivative may be watering plants, which also helps the plant grow.[24] Both the specific categories and their derivatives are forbidden by the Torah.[25]

In addition to the *melackhot* that constitute Torah prohibitions, there are a number of actions that are not prohibited by the Torah but nevertheless fall under the category of rabbinic prohibitions. In general, rabbinic prohibitions relate to actions that are similar or could be confused with actions prohibited by the Torah.[26] An example of these would be performing a forbidden act in an unusual way, such as a right-handed person writing with his left hand or writing with one's elbow or mouth instead of one's hand.[27] Another type of rabbinic prohibition relates to actions that might lead one to perform acts forbidden by the Torah.[28] The most famous of this type of prohibition is *muktzeh,* the restriction on moving items that have a forbidden use on Shabbat, such as a pen used for writing.[29] The Rabbis also prohibited any action that would diminish the special nature of the Shabbat day.[30] For example, one should not busy oneself with weekday activities[31] or undertake excessive work.[32]

Not only are Jews forbidden to perform these acts themselves, but they are also not allowed to ask a non-Jew to perform these acts for them.[33] This includes both Torah and rabbinic prohibitions.[34]

The laws of the festivals are identical to those of Shabbat with two exceptions. Cooking and derivatives of cooking are permitted on the festivals even though they are forbidden on Shabbat.[35] In addition, it is permitted to carry in the public domain on the festivals even though this is not allowed on Shabbat.[36]

Saving a Life

The Torah states "Keep My decrees and My laws, that when man does them he lives by them".[37] As the Torah equates the laws of the Torah with life, the Talmud deduces that the laws of the Torah can, and must, be suspended when life is threatened.[38] This applies also to the laws of Shabbat.[39] When life may be at risk it is allowed—indeed, commanded!—to suspend the laws of Shabbat to save life.[40] This is true even if the threat of life is not clear but is a remote possibility.[41] This is called *pikuach nefesh*, saving a soul, and it suspends all laws of Shabbat.[42] However, as we shall now see, the exact level at which the laws of Shabbat can be suspended depends on the level of medical severity.

Aches and Pains

If someone feels slightly ill on Shabbat but is not in danger, he cannot take any medicine nor can he ask a non-Jew to perform any work for him.[43] The rabbis were concerned that, were it permitted to take medicine, one would come to grind herbs and compounds to make powder for tablets.[44] As grinding is an *av melakhah* the rabbis prohibited taking any medicine.[45]

Disease without Threat to Life

There is also someone who is between the previous two categories. This is the person who is not in a life-threatening situation, but is actually ill, i.e. more than just feeling somewhat unwell. Such a person is termed *holeh she'ein bo sakanah*, a sick person who is in no danger. This category includes one who is ill in bed, or who has fever, or whose situation could become life-threatening if not treated, or who is in danger of losing an organ or the proper functioning of an organ. It also includes a post-partum woman.[46]

It is permitted to ask a non-Jew to perform tasks that entail a violation of Shabbat for such a sick person[47] if it is essential that they be done on Shabbat.[48] A Jew is permitted to break a rabbinic prohibition on Shabbat[49] on the condition that he performs the task in an unusual manner.[50] In the case of actual danger to organ, a Jew is permitted to violate a rabbinic prohibition, even without changing the usual way the act is performed.[51]

Halakhic Status of the Infertile Couple

How do we define the halakhic position of a couple experiencing infertility? They do not seem to fall into the category of the dangerously ill. Can we say that they are ill, or do they just feel some pain and discomfort, but are not sick?

The rabbis disagree about the exact status of such a couple. One possible source would be the Torah's description of the matriarch Rachel's pain as an infertile woman "Give me children, for if not I am dead."[52] From here the Talmud derives the notion that "one who is childless is as though he is dead."[53] However, even though the Talmud does refer to the infertile person as *like* the dead, this is more of a psychological definition than a medical one.[54] On the other hand, psychological pain is also recognized by the halakha.[55] Perhaps the psychological pain of an individual experiencing infertility renders such a person ill, by the definition of the Torah.

Some rabbis are of the opinion that the infertile couple are in the category of the slightly ill, as they are not actually suffering from a specific medical disease.[56] Others hold that they are considered ill, but that their lives are not in danger.[57] The majority of leading rabbis and *poskim* queried by this author hold the latter view, i.e. that the infertile couple can be defined halakhically as having a non-life-threatening condition.[58] In light of this it is permissible to undergo certain treatments by a non-Jew on Shabbat or festivals.

Diagnosis and Treatment on the Sabbath

Let us now examine the potential prohibitions connected with each stage and type of fertility treatment, and suggest alternate permissible methods of treatment.

MONITORING OVULATION

One of the initial forms of fertility "treatment" involves monitoring the occurrence and timing of ovulation. Such monitoring is generally important as a prerequisite to most forms of treatment, and improves the likelihood of conception. It is especially important in the case of an Orthodox woman with a relatively short menstrual cycle or a long menstrual flow, who may be ovulating before she immerses in the *mikvah*. In such a case, sexual relations will only be resumed after the *mikvah* and therefore after ovulation, effectively preventing pregnancy.[59] Confirming the time of ovulation is essential in the management of infertility in such circumstances.

All of the recognized methods for monitoring ovulation involve actions that are prohibited on Shabbat:

(1) *Basal Body Temperature* (BBT)—Due to the hormonal effects of ovulation, a woman's BBT (temperature while at rest) rises approximately 1° F at midcycle. Consistently measuring and recording temperature can therefore be used as a technique to detect ovulation. On Shabbat, this method can be problematic, as it involves measuring, which is a rabbinic prohibition.[60] However, measuring for the purpose of performing a mitzvah is permitted.[61] Therefore it is permitted to take one's temperature, even on Shabbat.[62] One

may only use a mercury thermometer, and not a digital, as using a digital thermometer is prohibited.[63] One is allowed to clean the thermometer prior to use but not to dip cotton wool in alcohol for this purpose.[64]

(2) *Home Ovulation-Prediction Test Kit*—This involves checking the level of luteinizing hormone (LH) in urine. The test is performed by dipping a chemically prepared stick that is sensitive to LH into the woman's urine. If there is a certain threshold level of LH indicating that ovulation is about to occur, a mark appears on the stick. This coloring would seem to be similar to the Shabbat prohibition against writing and coloring and would thus be forbidden. However, most authorities permit a woman to perform this type of test. This is because the type of coloring involved does not fit exactly into the category of permanent or necessary coloring that is forbidden on Shabbat.[65]

(3) *Ultrasound Scan*—This requires the use of electricity and is forbidden on Shabbat.[66]

(4) *Blood Test*—Blood testing to check various hormone levels is commonly done in the course of fertility therapy. Drawing blood is prohibited on Shabbat; therefore no blood tests should be done on Shabbat.[67]

The last two procedures are forbidden on Shabbat except in cases of actual danger.[68] In such a case it is preferable that they should be performed by a non-Jewish medical professional.

OTHER TESTS

Whenever testing can be performed during the week, it should be avoided on Shabbat. Such testing includes semen analysis, hysterosalpingogram, hysteroscopy, and laparoscopy. There is rarely a reason to perform any of these tests on Shabbat and it is therefore forbidden to do so.

HORMONE TREATMENTS

Until now we have discussed testing. In many cases the first treatment for infertility involves the oral administration of clomiphene citrate. Even though taking medication is prohibited on Shabbat,[69] most authorities do permit taking these drugs on Shabbat.[70] Additionally, one may tear the wrapping of the medication on Shabbat, but should be careful not to tear the letters.[71] In light of this, it is preferable whenever possible to prepare the tablets before Shabbat.

INJECTIONS

It is permitted for a non-seriously ill person to be given subcutaneous and intramuscular injections on Shabbat.[72] However, these injections do involve rabbinic prohibitions[73] and therefore it is preferable not to administer injections unless this is absolutely necessary on Shabbat. The injections used for ovulation induction may be subcutaneous or intramuscular and need to be administered every day. It is preferable to administer them before and after Shabbat where possible.[74] If this is impossible, it is preferable that a non-Jew should give the injection.[75] However, in a case where no other possibility exists, the injections may be given by a Jew on Shabbat. In such cases, it is preferable to affix the needle into the syringe before Shabbat and to cap the needle to preserve its sterility.[76] If this is not feasible, then it may be done on Shabbat.[77]

One may not use cotton wool dipped in alcohol to clean the site of the injection, as this entails squeezing, which is forbidden on Shabbat.[78] Instead one should use a pre-prepared alcohol swab of synthetic material.[79] Alternatively, one may pour alcohol directly onto the skin and then wipe off the excess with cotton wool.[80]

Chorionic gonadotropin (hCG) injections need to be given at a particular time in order to assure that ovulation occurs at an opportune point thirty-six hours later. In the case where the injection cannot be given before or after Shabbat, it may be administered on Shabbat. Again it is preferable that this should be done by a non-Jew, but when this is impossible then even a Jew may do so.[81] The same rules apply regarding fixing the needle in the syringe and cleaning the site of the injection. Receiving an injection on Yom Kippur appears to be permitted and is not considered in the category of eating.[82]

INTRAUTERINE INSEMINATION

Sperm preparation for intrauterine insemination involves a number of actions that are forbidden on Shabbat. The general running of a laboratory involves the use of electricity, including turning on the lights, using a microscope, etc. The use of a centrifuge for the processing and separation of sperm also requires electricity. As the use of electricity is forbidden on Shabbat,[83] it is preferable not to undergo such treatment on Shabbat. Therefore, all attempts should be made by the physician caring for the couple to ensure that they do not have to undergo an IUI on Shabbat or a festival.[84]

In the rare case where treatment must be performed on Shabbat, some authorities, who consider the infertile couple *holeh she'ein bo sakanah,* permit an IUI to be performed by non-Jewish medical staff.[85] In such a case, it is not necessary for the couple to request that the non-Jew perform the procedure in a way that would minimize the breach of Shabbat. The non-Jew can perform the action in his regular way. Other authorities, who maintain that the infertile couple is not in the category of ill people, prohibit such a procedure. Therefore, if such a case arises the couple must ask a competent halakhic authority how to proceed. It is preferable, of course, to get this halakhic advice before embarking on treatment, and to direct the physician in charge regarding the halakhic parameters. With careful planning, many halakhically problematic situations can be avoided, with the treatment being performed on a weekday. For example, physicians commonly perform an insemination on two consecutive days in order to improve the chances of a successful pregnancy. If one of the days is Shabbat, it may be sufficient to perform the procedure only on Friday, or on Friday and Sunday.[86] There is another, less direct, problem with undergoing an IUI on Shabbat. All fertility treatments that involve sperm entering and exiting the laboratory for use in treatment require close rabbinic supervision. Even if the insemination is performed on Shabbat, the supervisor must still be available to come to the laboratory. In places where the clinic is not near a residential Jewish area, this may create extremely grave, and even insurmountable, difficulties.

IN VITRO FERTILIZATION (IVF)

The laws regarding IVF are similar to those regarding insemination. The one important difference is in timing. In the course of in vitro fertilization, the hCG injection is administered exactly 35 hours prior to egg retrieval. Therefore, it should not be given on Thursday evening, as treatment would then be required on Shabbat. Likewise, it should be avoided in anticipation of a festival falling out on a weekday.[87]

According to the opinions that the infertile couple are considered as *holeh she'ein bo sakanah*, they can directly ask a non-Jew to perform biblically prohibited acts on Shabbat so long as they are necessary for IVF treatment. They can also ask a non-Jewish doctor to perform oocyte retrieval.[88] Likewise, the medical staff is permitted to check the embryos on Shabbat for signs of fertilization,[89] and a non-Jewish doctor is permitted to perform embryo transfer on Shabbat if this is absolutely necessary.[90] Again, care should be taken to ensure proper halakhic supervision of the entire process of IVF, from egg retrieval to fertilization to embryo transfer.

Traveling to the Hospital or Clinic on the Sabbath

In rare cases, such as in a case of impending ovarian hyperstimulation syndrome,[91] where delaying treatment is potentially life-threatening, a woman may travel to the hospital by car on Shabbat.[92] However, in regard to all other types of fertility treatment that may be permitted on Shabbat, many authorities do not permit traveling by car.[93] Therefore, it is preferable for the couple to stay within walking distance of the hospital or clinic over Shabbat or the festival whenever such situations arise.

Some rabbis hold that it is permitted for a non-Jew to drive a woman to hospital on Shabbat in order to undergo fertility treatment.[94] Even according to these opinions it is preferable to make this arrangement with the non-Jew before Shabbat. In addition, the non-Jew should open and close the door of the car if this causes the light to turn on and off.

Summary

The laws of Shabbat are intricate and form an integral part of the life of the halakhically committed Jew. However, in cases where life is threatened, these laws are suspended. Many halakhic authorities maintain that infertile couples are considered to be in the category of those who are dangerously ill, but whose lives are not in danger. It is permitted to ask a non-Jew to perform work on Shabbat for such a person even when a biblical prohibition is involved. Therefore, many authorities permit some fertility treatments on Shabbat and festivals, especially ongoing treatment that could not be deferred until after Shabbat.

Regarding treatment that could effectively be performed on any other day, it would be forbidden even to ask a non-Jewish doctor to perform such treatment. However, in the rare cases where there is no other possibility, some authorities permit treatment to be performed on Shabbat. Doing so may present additional practical difficulties, as the couple and the halakhic supervisor may need to be in close vicinity to the clinic over Shabbat or the festival.

Religiously observant Jews pray that, with the passage of time, God will direct man to find a cure for all ailments, including those of the infertile couple, and that these solutions will not require any compromise of the proper observance of Shabbat and the festivals.[95]

Endnotes

1. See *Hayei Adam*, Hilkhot Shabbat, Klal 1:1, *Arukh HaShulhan* Orach Hayim 242:3.
2. See *Mishnah Berurah,* introduction to vol. III.
3. See Genesis 2:2.

4. See Shabbat 10b.

5. Therefore the first time that the Torah records the Ten Commandments the reason given for keeping the Sabbath is that God rested on the seventh day (Exodus 20:11), whereas the second time the Torah gives the reason as a remembrance that God took the Jewish people out of Egypt (Deuteronomy 5:15). See the commentary of the Ramban Deuteronomy ad loc., which explains that the Sabbath contains two elements of faith: that of the creation of the world, and that of God's providence and continual connection with His people.

6. See Rav Kook's introduction to *Shabbat HaAretz*, (Jerusalem: Mossad HaRav Kook, 1985), p. 8, and my *Sparks of Light*, (New Jersey: Jason Aronson, Northvale, 1999), pp. 171–173.

7. *Yerushalmi Talmud*, Nedarim 3:9.

8. Shabbat 118a.

9. ibid. 118b.

10. ibid.

11. See Shabbat 118b, which says that if the Jewish people were to observe two consecutive Sabbath days, they would be immediately redeemed. However, compare with the statement of Rav Levi in the *Yerushalmi Talmud* (Ta'anit 1:1), which says that if the Jewish people were to observe one Sabbath, the son of David would immediately come. I attempt to explain the discrepancy between these two statements in my upcoming book on the festivals.

12. See Rambam, *Mishneh Torah*, Hilkhot Shabbat 1:1 with regards to the different levels of punishment for violation of the laws of the Sabbath.

13. *Karet* has been interpreted to mean that the offender will die childless (see Rashi on Shabbat 25b s.v. *karet*) or that he will die before his time (see Moed Katan 28a)

14. Hullin 5a and Rambam ibid. 30:15 and see *Arukh HaShulhan* 242:3, which explains that as the Sabbath is a symbol of belief in God's creation and providence over the world, one who violates Shabbat proves that he does not believe and therefore the Rabbis equated breaking the Sabbath with idolatry. This also explains the statement of Rav Hiya bar Abba and Rav Yohanan that one who observes the Sabbath is forgiven even idolatry (Shabbat 118b). If the Sabbath is the ultimate expression of faith, then it has the power to overcome the sin of idolatry. See also Beit Yosef on *Tur*, Orach Hayim 242 s.v. *afilu oved avodah zara,* which says that the Sabbath is considered to be equivalent to all of the other mitzvot of the Torah (see *Yerushalmi Talmud*, Nedarim 3:9) and that therefore one who breaks the Sabbath breaks all of the mitzvot of the Torah, in the same way that idolatry is a total contradiction of all of the mitzvot of the Torah.

15. See the opinion of Beit Shammai in Beitzah 16a, as opposed to the opinion of Beit Hillel, which says that one should trust that they will find suitable food for the Sabbath (see Rashi ad loc. s.v. *l'shem shamayim*).

16. See *Sefer Kuzari* 3:5, see also ibid. 3:10 that the Sabbath has been instrumental

in preserving the nature of Israel during the exile. This is reminiscent of the famous statement ascribed to Ahad Ha'Am that "more than the Jews have kept the Sabbath, the Sabbath has kept the Jews."

17. See *Arukh HaShulhan* 242:1.

18. For this reason the commandment to establish a calendar was the first mitzvah given to the Jewish people as a nation (Exodus 12:2 and see Rashi on Genesis 1:1) in order to set Israel apart through their distinct calendar. It is significant that this was commanded before they even left Egypt and it already set them apart from their Egyptian masters.

19. It will be clear that the intricate laws of the Sabbath cannot be explained in such an essay. The reader is directed toward one of the compendiums of laws of the Sabbath and the festivals, including a number of such volumes in English, e.g. *Shemirath Shabbath*, Rabbi Y. Neuwirth, (Feldheim Publishers). We will be using the Hebrew edition, *Shemirat Shabbat KeHilkhata*, as a source.

20. There are many positive commandments related to the Sabbath that give the day its sanctified nature. What concerns us here are only the prohibitions against work. However, this should not be construed as suggesting that the positive aspects of the day are any less important.

21. Exodus 20:10 and Deuteronomy 5:14.

22. *Mishnah*, Shabbat 7:2.

23. See Shabbat 49b and Tosafot on Baba Kama 2a s.v. *hakhey garsinan hakh d'havai b'mishkan*.

24. *Mishneh Torah* ibid. 8:2.

25. Baba Kama 2a and *Mishneh Torah*, Hilkhot Shabbat 7:7.

26. ibid. 21:1.

27. *Mishnah*, Shabbat 12:5, and *Mishneh Torah*, ibid. 11:14, which say that the Torah only forbade actions performed in the usual manner. See also Beitzah 13b, which limits the prohibition only to *melekhet mahshevet*.

28. *Mishneh Torah*, ibid. 21:1.

29. ibid. 24:13. An additional explanation is offered by Rambam, who sees the *muktzeh* prohibition as a mode of distinguishing the Sabbath as a special day for those who do not usually work. The Ra'avad sees *muktzeh* as being specifically related to the prohibition of carrying in the public domain.

30. *Mishneh Torah* ibid. 24:12. This class of prohibitions is based on the words of the prophet Isaiah 58:12, as explained by the Talmud, Shabbat 113a.

31. *Mishneh Torah* 21:3.

32. See for example ibid. 21:18.

33. *Shulhan Arukh*, Orach Hayim 307:2 and see *Shemirat Shabbat Kehilkhata* chap. 30, n. 2 on the reasons for this prohibition.

34. ibid. 5.

35. *Mishnah*, Megila 1:5 and see *Shulhan Arukh*, Orach Hayim 495:1 The prohibitions on the Sabbath and festivals are identical including both Torah and

rabbinic laws and the prohibitions against asking a non-Jew, see ibid. *Mishnah Berurah* note 1.

36. ibid. This leniency with regard to the festivals does not apply to Yom Kippur, which has the same restrictions as the Sabbath.

37. Leviticus 18:5.

38. See Yoma 85b and ibid. 82a which exclude three prohibitions from this injunction: idolatry, sexual immorality, and blood shed.

39. See ibid. 85b. The Talmud brings in a number of other sources that imply that the Sabbath can be suspended in the case of the threat of life and concludes with the verse from Leviticus. The Talmud then argues that all of the other sources can be overruled, with the exception of the latter source. The Talmud may bring the sources, even though they are overruled, as an attempt to find a source that particularly discusses Shabbat, since the exegesis from Leviticus is a general rule for all laws of the Torah. Eventually the claim is made that this source is the best, even though it is a general rule and Sabbath-specific.

40. See *Shulhan Arukh*, Orach Hayim 328:2.

41. See Yoma 85a and Tosafot s.v. *u'lefakeach* that this rule precludes even coming close to a threat of life.

42. We have not entered into the argument as to whether the laws of the Sabbath are temporarily suspended or whether they are eradicated completely. It could be argued that the *Shulhan Arukh* is of the opinion that the laws of the Sabbath evaporate in the face of the threat of life (see e.g. 328:12) whereas Rabbi Moshe Isserlis is of the opposite opinion (see the note of the Rema ad loc.)

43. *Shulhan Arukh*, Orach Hayim 328:1 and see Beit Yosef on *Tur* ad loc.

44. Shabbat 53b and Rashi ad loc. s.v. *Gezera mishum she'hikat semamemim* and see the wording of Rashi on Berakhot 36a s.v. *Lo y'areyno b'shemen.*

45. One of the 39 categories of work, see *Mishnah*, Shabbat 7:2.

46. See *Shemirat Shabbat Kehilkhata* chap. 33:1 for a full description of the conditions that are included in this category.

47. *Shulhan Arukh*, Orach Hayim 328:17 and see *Mishnah Berurah* ad loc. n. 47.

48. *Mishnah Berurah* ibid. n. 46, if it can wait until after Shabbat one should not even ask a non-Jew to perform such an act, unless there is some danger, in which case it should be performed immediately.

49. *Shemirat Shabbat Kehilkhata* 33:2

50. Which determines that the act is at most rabbinically prohibited as in order to be prohibited by the Torah an act must be performed in its usual manner, see Beitzah 13b and *Mishneh Torah*, Hilkhot Shabbat 1:9. In this case where the act is *de jure* a rabbinic prohibition the addition condition that one change the regular modus operandi creates a case of double rabbinic status rendering the act permitted in the case of a sick person.

51. See *Shemirat Shabbat Kehilkhata* ibid. Obviously the laws of treating a sick person and the degrees of defining a sick person are many and varied, one should consult with a halakhic authority in each particular case. The reader

is referred to *Shemirat Shabbat Kehilkhata* chap. 32–40 for a full account of these laws.

52. Genesis 30:1. This translation is based on the explanation of the Talmud; see both the Targum Onkelos and Targum Yonatan ben Uziel, which seem to me to be correct grammatically and in context. Despite this there are a number of editions that translate the final phrase in the future tense "I will die" or "let me die."

53. Nedarim 64b.

54. This is borne out by the following words of the Talmud that "Four are considered like the dead: a pauper, a person afflicted with *tzaraʿat*, a blind person, and one who is childless." Even though three of them are medical conditions, it appears that the Talmud refers to their psychological status and loneliness as opposed to their medical conditions, see Tosafot ad loc. s.v. *Arbaʿah hashuvim k'met*, and the version that appears in *Bereishit Rabba* 71:6, where the pauper is replaced with "One who loses his wealth," suggesting deep psychological pain. However, see the comment of the Maharal that the infertile person is dead in that they have no continuation after their own death (Gur Aryeh on Rashi, Genesis 30:1). Compare with Taʿanit 5b, which describes Yaʿakov as living through his offspring.

    Rabbi Yitzchak Zilberstein of Bnei Brak told me that the infertile couple are in the category of non-threatening illness and he used this as the source. He said that one could even argue that they are considered to be dangerously ill, as psychological stress can lead to serious disease. However, we can at minimum determine that they are *"holehi sheʾein bo sakanah"* and most treatment can be performed for them by a gentile. Rabbi Zilberstein told me that this is the opinion of his father-in-law, Rabbi Y. S. Elyashiv, one of the major Israeli *poskim*, as well. I also heard this opinion from Rav Zalman Nehemiah Goldberg, the son-in-law of the great Israeli *posek* Rabbi Shlomo Zalman Auerbach. He told me that his late father-in-law held this to be the halakha.

    However, see also the article by Rabbi Yigal Safran in *Techumim* XVII 335–339, "Tipulei Poriyut B'Shabbat" (Fertility treatment on the Sabbath) p. 336, where he states that it is clear that the infertile couple are not considered dangerously ill and that this statement from the Talmud only discusses a moral danger, and not a physical one.

55. See e.g. Tosafot on Shabbat 50b s.v. *Beshvil tzaʿaro* which defines psychological pain or stress as pain and therefore allows the removal of a scab even though this may transgress the prohibition of a man beautifying himself (Deutronomy 22:5). See also my article, "The halakhic approach to psychological pain" in *Kovetz HaTzionut HaDatit*, (2002), pp. 440–445.

56. Responsa *Beʾer Moshe* vol. 1:33. I also heard a similar opinion from Rabbi Yehoshua Yeshaya Neuwirth the author of *Shemirat Shabbat Kehilkhata*, who does not permit any fertility treatment on the Sabbath. He told me that even though he has told many couples to refrain from undergoing any type

of treatment on Shabbat, they have still eventually conceived. However, see *Nishmat Avraham* vol. IV sec. on Orach Hayim, p. 38, which brings Rabbi Neuwirth's opinion that it is permitted to treat a woman with a subfunctioning uterus on the Sabbath in order to help her conceive if this is totally essential.

Rabbi Dov Lior, the chief rabbi of Hebron, wrote to me that his original opinion was that the couple cannot be defined as ill, based on the definition that appears in the *Arukh HaShulhan*, Orach Hayim, 328:19. However, after consulting with two leading halakhic authorities, they suggested that the correct halakhic category was indeed *"Holeh she'ein bo sakanah."*

It is fascinating to note that the debate as to the nature of infertility as a disease has also been a subject for debate within the medical community as well. The reader is referred to a letter that appeared in *Fertility and Sterility*, (Aug., 2000), vol. 74 no. 2 p. 398, from Dr. Richard Dickey et al. entitled "Infertility is a symptom, not a disease." There they write,

> "The facts are that infertility and its frequent companion, anovulation, are not diseases; they are symptoms of underlying, sometimes serious diseases in one or both marital partners. One result of considering infertility and anovulation as diseases rather than as symptoms is that unnecessarily powerful and expensive treatments may be used to obtain an immediate pregnancy, whereas chronic disease that may affect lifelong health is overlooked."

In discussing this letter, a well-known fertility specialist commented to me that he would prefer the title "Infertility is a condition, not a disease." I believe that this distinction is far from pure semantics, but suggests a deep philosophical difference in approach to the reality of infertility and to the infertile couple. If infertility is a symptom of a disease, then the task of the doctor is to find the cause and treat the disease, not the infertility itself. If we view infertility as a condition, the treatment is causing pregnancy and birth.

This itself is the focus of much medical and public debate as to whether infertility specialists are sometimes too quick to offer IVF and other types of treatment instead of searching extensively for the root cause of the infertility. For a popular account of the situation in Israel, see the cover article of *The Jerusalem Report*, "IVF fever," (July 3, 2000).

57. See *Helkat Ya'akov*, Orach Hayim 150 in the new edition of this work published by the author's sons (Tel Aviv, 5752) originally published in vol. III, 23. However, in another responsa (Yoreh De'ah 62:6 [originally vol. II 6:8]) he claims that they have "at least" the status of feeling slightly ill.

58. Rabbi Mordekhai Eliyahu is of this opinion, as is Rabbi Ya'akov Ariel, the chief rabbi of Ramat Gan, and see notes 54 and 56 above. These opinions were given in personal communications.

59. See Allen J. Wilcox, Clarice R. Weinberg, Donna D. Baird, "Timing of sexual

intercourse in relation to ovulation," *New England Journal of Medicine*, (Dec. 7, 1995), 333:23 pp. 1517–1521. We could name this "religious infertility," as the cause is the religious requirement of refraining from sexual activity and contact for at least twelve days from the onset of menstruation.

60. *Shulhan Arukh*, Orach Hayim 323:1; the reason is that one may come to write, and that measuring is part of business (see Rambam, *Mishneh Torah*, Hilkhot Shabbat 23:13), or that the rabbis prohibited measuring, as it is a weekday activity. See *Mishnah Berurah* ibid. 8 and *Shemirat Shabbat Kehilkhata* 29:32 and n. 85.

61. See *Mishnah*, Shabbat 24:5, *Shulhan Arukh*, Orach Hayim 306:7.

62. See *Shemirat Shabbat Kehilkhata* 40:2, due to the opinion that the infertile woman is considered a "*hola she'ein ba sakanah.*" See *Iggrot Moshe*, Orach Hayim vol. 1:128 that measuring temperature is not a rabbinic prohibition but a "*humrah b'alma,*" a restrictive measure, and one is allowed to be lenient on the Sabbath, as it is considered to be for the purpose of a mitzvah.

63. Due to the prohibition of writing, see *Shemirat Shabbat Kehilkhata* 40:2 and *Birkat Banim* 10:16 also Rabbi Yigal Shafran op. cit. p. 339.

64. See *Shemirat Shabbat Kehilkhata* 40:2, a pre-prepared alcohol swab can be used for this purpose as long as it is not dripping with alcohol. However see *Birkat Banim* 10:25 n. 41, where he brings the opinion of Rabbi Yitzhak Zilberstein that these swabs are also forbidden. However, see ibid. for other opinions. Another problem with these swabs is that they come in closed wrappers often with writing on them. It is not permitted to tear the letters on the Sabbath. One should ideally open the wrapper before the Sabbath; however, if this was not done before the Sabbath, care should be exercised when opening the wrapper on the Sabbath itself to ensure that the letters are not ripped.

   It is pertinent to see the responsa *Tzitz Eliezer* XI 38 and XII 44:5, who permits measuring temperature specifically for the purpose of monitoring ovulation. (See also *Shemirat Shabbat Kehilkhata* ibid.) This is interesting in that we could argue that this measuring has no real purpose on the Sabbath, as it only really guides us regarding the timing of sexual intercourse. However, Rabbi Waldenberg permits taking temperature, as it alleviates the stress of the couple and this stress may disturb their required Sabbath tranquility.

65. See Responsa *Tzitz Eliezer* X 25:1 section 4. Several reasons to be lenient are presented there; the coloring is temporary, the coloring is unnecessary and only indicates the hormonal levels, and the coloring is less than the minimum quantity to be forbidden.

   See also *Shemirat Shabbat Kehilkhata* 33:20 and n. 83. Rabbi Neuwirth told me that he permits such a test and he heard this from Rabbi Elyashiv. See also *Birkat Banim* 10:11 and n. 16.

66. Rabbi Lior (in a personal communication with the author) permitted an ultrasound to be performed by a non-Jew, but it would appear that this can only be permitted in a case of real necessity. See following note.

67. Drawing blood trangresses the prohibition of extracting seeds from their natural habitat. See *Mishneh Berurah*, 328, n. 147. As the whole point of a blood test is to draw blood, this is biblically—not rabbinicly—prohibited.

68. Such as hyperstimulation. As there is often no real need to monitor ovulation but it is only permitted in order to alleviate stress from the infertile couple (see n. 64 above) we will cannot permit these last two methods when the previous methods are available. In addition the last two methods must be administered by a medical professional and usually require travelling to the clinic on the Sabbath which should be avoided whenever possible.

69. See note 44 above.

70. Responsa *Helkat Ya'akov* Orach Hayim 150 (see note 57 above) and Responsa *Be'er Moshe* I 33 ,who permits taking clomiphene to "boost" ovulation, as he holds that such a woman is not ill and therefore this tablet is not considered medication and was not forbidden by the Rabbis.

    As clomiphene citrate is taken as a course of treatment over a period of several days, it is permitted to take the tablets for someone who previously started this course of treatment (see *Birkat Banim* 10:3 and note 3 in the name of the Hazon Ish and others, and Rabbi Yigal Shafran ibid. p. 336).

    For a contrary opinion, see *Birkat Banim* ibid. n. 4, where Rabbi Moshe Feinstein and others permit taking this medication only in an unusual manner. I heard from Rabbi Avraham Shapiro, the previous chief rabbi of Israel, that the custom in Jerusalem was to eat tablets with a fork like food and in such a strange manner it was permitted.

71. *Shemirat Shabbat Kehilkhata* 33:4. Tearing the letters is considered erasing them, and this is forbidden on the Sabbath. However, see ibid. n. 29, where Rabbi Shlomo Zalman Auerbach permitted tearing letters in the case of a sick person, as this is not really considered erasing. One may rely on this only in a case where no other possibility exists, as there he permits it only in the case of a sick person and we have already seen that not all of the authorities agree on the halakhic status of the infertile couple.

72. *Shemirat Shabbat Kehilkhata* 32:58. With regard to intravenous injections, there are opinions that they are forbidden from the Torah as blood needs to be extracted prior to the injection, and this is prohibited on the Sabbath. They can only be used in the case of the dangerously ill patient. There are opinions that even intravenous injections are permitted from the Torah and therefore can be given to a non-seriously ill patient (see Responsa *Tzitz Eliezer* vol. VIII 15:12).

73. Such as taking medication on the Sabbath and the possibility that blood will be extracted, but as this is unlikely it is not forbidden by the Torah (as it is not considered a *psik reisha*). Even if the site of the injection does bleed, one could argue that it is not forbidden by the Torah as it is not part of the procedure, as opposed to a intravenous injection where the extraction of blood is an intrinsic part of the procedure. In the case of subcutaneous or

intramuscular injections, the drawing of blood is considered an unwanted consequence and is permitted, see *Birkat Banim* 10:19, n. 27.

74. *Birkat Banim* 10:18.

75. I heard this opinion from Rabbi Mordekhai Eliyahu. With regard to telling a non-Jew to perform such a task on the Sabbath for a Jew, see *Shemirat Shabbat Kehilkhata* 30:11 based on *Shulhan Arukh*, Orach Hayim 328:17, and the gloss of the *Mishnah Berurah* ad loc.

76. *Shemirat Shabbat Kehilkhata* 33:9 and *Birkat Banim* 10:19.

77. ibid. See also Responsa *Tzitz Eliezer* vol. xv 17 who permits this if the syringe is disposed of immediately after the injection, however see note 43 in *Shemirat Shabbat Kehilkhata* in the name of the Hazon Ish, that even if the syringe is discarded it is still forbidden.

78. *Shemirat Shabbat Kehilkhata* 33:10.

79. ibid. and see note 64 above, also *Birkat Banim* 10:25 note 41 in the name of Rabbi Yitzhak Zilberstein that such swabs are also forbidden on the Sabbath, and see contrary opinions ibid.

80. ibid. One should be careful in this case that the cotton wool should not become so wet as to emit water when lightly squeezed. Several pieces of cotton wool should be used in order to prevent this.

81. See *Techumim* xvii p. 338, and the reference to *Birkat Banim* 10:9 note 13, where it appears that Rabbi Zilberstein does not allow hcg injections to be administered on the Sabbath. In my own discussions with Rabbi Zilberstein, he related to the infertile couple as non-seriously ill due to their psychological stress and anguish (see note 54 above) and thus it appears that subcutaneous injections where no Torah prohibitions are involved may be performed even by a Jew even in the absence of subjective psychological pain.

82. This can be deduced from the fact that even one who is not seriously ill can swallow bitter tablets for his health (*Shemirat Shabbat Kehilkhata* 39:8). This is because only eating that has some satisfaction is forbidden on Yom Kippur from the Torah (see Rambam, *Mishneh Torah*, Hilkhot Shvitat Asor 2:5 and *Mikraei Kodesh*, Rabbi Moshe Harari, 9:39 and note 143, Jerusalem, 5754). Injections are not in this category and therefore are permitted.

   However, see Responsa *Tzitz Eliezer*, vol. x 25:22, who does not permit the oral taking of even bitter medicines on Yom Kippur. Even according to the latter opinion we could still argue that injections would be permitted, albeit it is appropriate to avoid this when at all possible.

83. See *Shemirat Shabbat Kehilkhata* 13:1 and note 1 in the name of the Hazon Ish.

84. See Rabbi Shafran, *Techumim* xvii p. 339, who points out that in Israel laboratories are generally closed on the Sabbath in the same way that most labs are closed in the us or the uk on Sunday. Doctors time treatment to be convenient with their laboratories schedules, and so the case of an iui falling on the Sabbath should be rare with foresight and careful planning.

   This is different from injections on the Sabbath and festivals, as they are part of an ongoing course of treatment that includes the Sabbath, an IUI is a procedure performed on one (or two) specific day(s). It is generally accepted that one can continue a course of medicine if started before the Sabbath. See *Birkat Banim* 10:3 and note 3 in the name of the Hazon Ish and others, also *Orhot Rabbeinu Kehilat Yaakov* I 214 pp. 155–156 in the name of the Hazon Ish, and *Shemirat Shabbat Kehilkhata* 34:17 and note 76. This is based on Rambam, *Mishneh Torah*, Hilkhot Shabbat 2:2 and *Shulhan Arukh*, Orach Hayim 328:11.

However, in *Iggrot Moshe*, Orach Hayim vol. III:53, Rabbi Moshe Feinstein discusses a person who is not ill but is taking medicine, and would usually be forbidden to take such medication on the Sabbath. The question was raised as to whether one can be lenient when it involves a course of medicine over a period of ten days. Rabbi Feinstein only allows this in extreme circumstances where the discontinuation of the medicine will lead to serious anguish and even a nervous breakdown. Rabbi Feinstein himself comments there that this is a rare occurrence and in other cases it is forbidden. See also Responsa *Beer Moshe* vol. I, 33:7 where he brings a proof that one cannot continue a course of medicine even if started several days before the Sabbath. "Therefore one sees a proof from the Talmud, and all of the poskim, that this opinion which is accepted by the masses has no halakhic basis; rather it is clearly stated to the contrary in the Talmud."

As previously discussed in the case of the infertile couple, there is ground to consider them as ill and therefore they are permitted to take medicine on the Sabbath.

85. See *Shemirat Shabbat Kehilkhata* 38:4–13 and ibid. 30:14 n. 46, which establishes that for a rabbinic prohibition it is permissible to tell a non-Jew directly to perform the action on the Sabbath and the operation does not need to be done in an irregular manner.

86. This is dependent on the actual time of ovulation.

87. ibid. 338.

88. The woman is not considered as assisting the doctor in this procedure, as she is totally passive. The Talmud (Beitzah 22a) discusses a case where a non-Jew applies ointment to an eye on the Sabbath. The Talmud forbids this and the reason given is that the Jew assists the non-Jew by opening and closing his eye. Rabbi Moshe Isserlis permits slight assistance (gloss of the Rema on *Shulhan Arukh*, Orach Hayim 328:17 and see *Mishnah Berurah* ad loc. n. 61, who disagrees). However, in this case the woman has received either local or general anesthetic and does not assist at all.

89. The checking itself does not involve any the Sabbath prohibitions and the non-Jew is permitted to turn on the light and the like for his own benefit.

90. This is not usually the case and the couple should alert the staff to this consideration before embarking on treatment. Where necessary, a day 2 or day 4 transfer would be the treatment of choice.

91. See J. Schenker, D. Weinstein, "Ovarian hyperstimulation syndrome: A current survey," *Fertility and Sterility* 30:255–268, (1978).
92. This is obvious; see *Shemirat Shabbat Kehilkhata* 32:36 and see ibid. 40:50–73 with regard to the specific laws and considerations when traveling to a hospital or for the needs of a dangerous sick person on the Sabbath.
93. This includes even many *poskim* who are of the opinion that the infertile couple can be considered as ill. I heard this opinion from Rabbi Mordekhai Eliyahu, Rabbi Dov Lior, and Rabbi Yitzhak Zilberstein. The latter also raised the point that psychologically it is difficult to tell a person to travel by car on the Sabbath unless it is for *pikuach nefesh*, therefore, this is something that should be avoided where possible.
94. In the same way that it is permitted to ask the non-Jew to perform any other forbidden action on the Sabbath even when a Torah prohibition is involved. I heard this opinion from Rabbi Ya'akov Ariel, Rabbi Ephrayim Greenblatt, and Rabbi Zalman Nechemiah Goldberg.
95. We have not discussed here the halakhic status of the unborn fetus and the laws of breaking of the Sabbath to save it. See *Shemirat Shabbat Kehilkhata* 36:2, where Rabbi Neuwirth permits transgressing the Sabbath to save the unborn fetus even when this fetus is less than forty days old, and see ibid. 32 n. 13 based on the end of the *Biur Halakha* on *Shulhan Arukh* 330:7 s.v. *O safek*. However, see Responsa *Teshuvot V'Hanhagot* 11 182, where Rabbi Sternboch presents the opinion that one can only break the Sabbath to save a fetus less than forty days old in a case where the danger is certain and not when there is only a *safek*, a possibility of danger. Therefore, he did not allow a husband to drive his wife to the hospital in a case where his wife's menstrual period was several days late and the husband raised some concern about the health of the possible fetus. However, in this case there are two uncertainties: 1) it is unclear whether the woman is actually pregnant, 2) the danger is not clear. But in a case of only one *safek*, such as a case where the wife is definitely in the early stages of pregnancy but the danger is not certain, it is not clear whether he would permit the husband to drive to the hospital on the Sabbath.

Rabbi Avrohom Friedlander

Rabbinical Supervision during Fertility Therapy

T he discipline of reproductive medicine and its many fertility-enhancing techniques are subject to a variety of regulations by governing health authorities. Their job is to ascertain that those who practice medicine are sufficiently skilled to practice their craft safely and with acceptable outcomes. The concern of the rabbis with regard to fertility therapy is not, therefore, to add an additional layer of bureaucratic oversight. Nor can any degree of rabbinical supervision absolutely prevent the misdeeds of an unscrupulous practitioner. The concept of rabbinical supervision in the lab is mainly to prevent human error. Even with stringent safeguards, it has happened from time to time, as reported by the media, that mistakes in embryology laboratories have occurred. While such mistakes have wreaked havoc on the lives of unsuspecting patients, the halakhic implications of such a mistake for an observant Jewish couple would go beyond psychological and social readjustments. Secular courts have the authority to assign and revise parental relationships. Halakha, on the other hand, can only discover them.

The uncertain lineage and possible forbidden relationships that might occur as a result of an error in the laboratory would pose potentially insurmountable problems.

These concerns notwithstanding, couples who follow the precepts of halakha need not be prevented from having proper treatment for infertility, including the use of assisted reproductive techniques, where indicated. In such situations, the rabbis decreed that all of the procedures performed for the purpose of diagnosing and treating infertility must be subject to the strict and exacting supervision of the masters of Torah or their appointees. The couple has an obligation to stay in constant touch with their *posek*, their personal rabbi or *dayan*, in every step they take in medical care. All aspects of the problem should be brought to the rabbi and it is up to him to rule on the permissibility of each aspect of care. Both the couple and their caregivers must stand beneath the watchful and strict supervision of the *morei halakha* (halakhic decisors), to be certain that treatment is given only according to the rulings of the rabbinical authorities of our generation.

Basic Halakhic Problems

The matter of fertility therapy is intimately related to the subject of sperm procurement. This evokes the prohibition of *hoza'at zera levatalah*, bringing forth seed in vain, which is a complex and extremely serious issue that is handled delicately by all halakhic authorities.

Before the husband undergoes evaluation by semen analysis, he must ascertain with complete clarity that his wife does not have a fertility impairment. Even if this is ascertained, it is customary to wait for a certain period of time after marriage before the husband begins such an evaluation. The exact period of time that must pass is a matter of controversy among the authorities. Some say that a full ten years are required, some say five, some say only two, and some say even less than that. Therefore each couple must ask their own *posek*, who must settle between the different opinions. Only upon the advice of a competent rabbi with specific knowledge of fertility issues should the couple begin with the examinations and treatments that require production of semen for the purpose of artificial reproduction.

Once it has been determined that there is no choice but to examine sperm from the husband, one must begin with the least problematic test. The postcoital test (PCT) does not require the production of semen specifically for examination. Instead, natural relations may take place. The sperm are examined upon removal from the woman's vagina within hours after intercourse has occurred. The PCT is permissible when needed without any concern of transgression. Occasionally, it may be preferable for intercourse to take place in the physician's office, so that the semen specimen is available immediately. Although some hold that one may not have intercourse in a physician's office, many rabbis are lenient about this as long as there is a special room for this purpose set aside in the physician's office and that modesty is preserved.

If there is a problem indicated in the sperm examined by PCT and a semen specimen must be analyzed, there are various halakhic opinions about the advantages and disadvantages of the different forms of production (see "Male Infertility: Halakhic Considerations"). Which is the right way is a decision that is left to the halakhic decisor. Those who permit the procuring of semen by one of these methods for the purposes of examination also permit doing so for the purpose of insemination. Some authorities have in fact permitted the examination of the semen only in conjunction with insemination of the wife.

There are some women who have an atypical menstrual cycle that causes infertility only because they observe *taharat hamishpa'ha*. That is, there is no real barrier to conception, except that they must be exposed to sperm before the time that they can immerse in a *mikvah* and end their *niddah* status. The most common example of such a problem is a woman who has a short cycle and who, by the time she can immerse and be purified, is already past the time of her ovulation. There is an argument among *poskim* whether it is permissible to perform artificial insemination while such a woman is a *niddah*. Some hold this is permissible while others hold it is not. Still others argue that the insemination should be done during the clean days, (See "General Aspects of Female Infertility") after the woman has immersed (but is still a *niddah*) so that at least the biblical prohibition of *niddah* is not violated. However, one should not do so without the instruction of a reliable authority.

Halakhic Problems during Fertility Therapy

Other halakhic questions often arise in the midst of therapy for infertility. These may be serious issues that require the instruction of an expert authority. Such questions include the following:

1. Does a woman become a *niddah* because of the performance of a specific procedure, e.g. intrauterine insemination or egg retrieval?
2. What should be done if egg retrieval becomes necessary on the Sabbath?
3. Are insemination, in vitro fertilization of the egg, or transfer of the embryo to the woman permissible on the Sabbath? Does it matter if the physician who performs these procedures is Jewish?
4. Is one permitted to dispose of excess sperm that are not used for the purpose of in vitro fertilization, or excess eggs that have already been fertilized? If they are to be left with the physician, how would one be assured that they will not be used on behalf of others? In a situation where the couple have divorced, how will one be assured that such material will not be used with a different partner?
5. In the case where a multifetal pregnancy results from treatment, and it is beyond the woman's ability to safely carry and deliver all the fetuses, is it permissible to abort one or more fetuses in order to protect the health of the mother and the other fetuses?
6. Is it permissible to use the eggs of one woman to initiate pregnancy in another?
7. Is it permissible to transfer the wife's egg, already fertilized by the husband, to a surrogate carrier?
8. Is sex selection permissible? May one use preimplantation genetic diag-

nosis with IVF in order to create embryos that are specifically male or female and select those of the desired gender for transfer?

All of the above subjects require halakhic instruction prior to implementation. It is therefore best for the couple to try to anticipate the problems that may arise during their care, and to discuss them frankly with their physician and their rabbi. Although it is impossible to anticipate every halakhic impediment that might occur, it certainly is incumbent upon observant couples to make their best effort to avoid them whenever possible. For example, each couple should inform their physician, prior to beginning an ovulation induction, that the timing of therapy should be arranged to best assure that insemination, egg retrieval and/or embryo transfer do not occur on Sabbath or festivals.

Procedures Requiring Rabbinical Supervision

Every couple must clearly understand the halakhic issues regarding their particular situation and proposed treatment. Discussions between their rabbinical authority and their treating physician may be necessary to clarify certain aspects of care. Once it has been determined that they should proceed with a treatment, it becomes equally important to ascertain that all aspects of therapy taking place in the treatment rooms and laboratories belonging to the physician are under rabbinical oversight.

Rabbinical supervision, or *hashga'ha,* is required for the following procedures and circumstances:

A. Semen analysis
B. Sperm washing
C. Sperm freezing for the purposes of using in the near or distant future
D. Egg retrieval for the purpose of IVF
E. In vitro insemination of the oocyte
F. Intracytoplasmic sperm injection
G. Embryo transfer

H. Cryopreservation of sperm or embryos

I. Washing of sperm in preparation for intrauterine insemination (IUI)

J. When necessary, retrieval of sperm from the husband by artificial means, e.g. by a procedure such as electroejaculation (EEJ), testicular biopsy or aspiration (TESE), or microsurgical epididymal aspiration (MESA)

Rationale for Rabbinical Supervision

The major reason that persistent rabbinical supervision is required is to prevent the mixing of gametes—sperm, egg, or embryos—between couples. Both intentional and accidental misuses of material from one couple for another have been reported in the news, and many *poskim* have understandably voiced their concern. Most agree that it is halakhically forbidden to perform any of the aforementioned treatments without ongoing *hashga'ha* (supervision). For example, Rabbi Shlomo Zalman Auerbach, one of the great *poskim* of our generation, permits artificial insemination, but does so specifically on the condition that a system of *hashga'ha* be in place to assure that only sperm from the husband are used. At the conclusion of his responsum, he muses: "But if this *heter* becomes widespread, one would be concerned that those who are less exacting would have insemination without *hashga'ha*. Still, it is not for us to disallow permitted acts, and therefore there is no use preventing good people from doing what is permissible on account of those who are simple-minded."[1]

Along similar lines, Rabbi Eliezer Waldenberg concurs that "it is necessary to observe with both eyes open so that no mixing will occur, God forbid, of the sperm from one man with that of another, as any lapse in this oversight process can turn the lives of the couple upside down, and bring destruction where there should have been joy."[2]

Other major rabbinical authorities have also stipulated that there be *hashga'ha* over all laboratory procedures involving gametes, both to prevent mistakes as well as to guard against intentional misuse. Unfortunately, the reality of our experience with procedures such as artificial insemination demonstrates that the concerns of the *poskim* are not out of place. All couples who require reproductive therapy involving laboratory procedures should therefore be aware that expert and complete rabbinical supervision is probably required by Jewish law, and that compromise or leniency in this area is problematic.

However, there are different schools of thought about the requirement for *hashga'ha*. For example, some rely on the strength of science to assure that gamete switching does not occur. According to this viewpoint, the availability of DNA testing, and its accuracy in clarifying genetic parenthood, is a sufficient incentive to lab workers to be meticulous and honest in their processing of gametes. A related viewpoint relies on the authority of the law to prosecute those who are negligent or abusive, seeing the legal ramifications as sufficient to prevent breaches of propriety from occurring. Others have allowed couples to depend on the promises or protocols of the specialists (whether their physicians, or the hospital), or to arrange that a specific, devout laboratory worker be the supervisor. However, all of these views, in my opinion, overlook an essential point regarding *hashga'ha* in the fertility clinic: the issues involved are no less important than matters of *kashrut* and *niddah*—are perhaps more so—and it therefore must take place under the most stringent criteria. This means that couples undergoing treatment must investigate and know the *hashga'ha* as well as the rabbi that stands behind it. He should be an expert, a *baal semacha* not less than the rabbis on whom they depend for other important personal matters.

The Supervisor

For reasons of *tzini'ut*, it is preferable that the rabbinical supervisor be a woman. As a *mashgiha*, she works directly under the authority of the rabbi in charge, acting as his emissary to the laboratory. The *mashgiha* should be a person known to the community as a

God-fearing person who would avoid sin. She should also be of an age where it is appropriate that she be dealing with such crucial matters, and capable of taking on such serious responsibility. In addition, she should have a sufficient yeshiva background to know the laws concerning the minimal standards of supervision required, for example, for *kashrut*.

It is preferable that the supervisor be known as a reliable person, capable of keeping a secret. Her past should be free of any complaints of having done anything irresponsible or unethical in the context of her work. Certainly, her past should be free of any financial improprieties. She should also be known as a person who defers to the opinions of those above her.

The supervisor is called upon in many different situations, sometimes on short notice and often under trying circumstances. She should therefore be energetic, motivated, able to function well under pressure and, most importantly, capable of adjusting to various situations. Because she must work with many different personalities in the laboratory in addition to her intimate interaction with the patients, she should be a person with some natural ability to get along with other people and a gentleness of manner.

Suggested Oath of Secrecy

Date _____

I, _____ obligate myself, in the service of [rabbi or institution], [the fertility clinics/hospital], and the requesting couples, to guard their secrecy and to maintain appropriate discretion. I will not speak with any person about anything that is known about the couples or the work of the laboratory. It is understood by me that this is a basic condition for all my work in this regard.

_____
Signature

Practical Aspects of Rabbinical Supervision

The process of supervision should be arranged with the leaders of the practice providing the fertility care. These include the scientists who work in the laboratories as well as the physicians. There should be clear agreement on all aspects of the supervisory process. It is crucial that the rabbi in charge have direct access to all parties so that communication about the process can be ongoing. As proper *hashga'ha* involves extended periods of interaction, it is important that feedback between supervisors and technicians be frequent, open, and productive. The value of a cooperative working relationship cannot be overstated!

It is important to emphasize that the process of *hashga'ha* is built on trust and good will from both sides. The clinic staff must understand that halakhic supervision is required not because they are suspect of any malintent, but rather to completely prevent and dispel any suspicion of human error that might occur in the midst of treatment. Furthermore, and above even the issue of trust, it must be understood that supervision is something that is required by halakha. It is this process of rabbinical oversight that in effect opens up the possibilities of assisted reproduction for observant Jewish couples. By allowing proper *hashga'ha* to occur on their premises, medical personnel show their sensitivity to the needs of couples who are interested in such services.

The religious supervisors, for their part, must understand that they are guests in a process that has enormous complexity, which often extends beyond what occurs in the laboratory. What is more, confidentiality issues prevent the discussion of clinical circumstances with them. They must therefore limit the scope of their involvement solely to what is required of them by halakha.

In any case of a problem, a doubt or even the hint of a doubt, it is incumbent upon the rabbinical supervisor to report the occurrence to the director of the clinic and to inform him or her of the need to investigate the matter. In case of a halakhic question, the supervisor must report to the rabbi in charge of the *hashga'ha* process.

The following principles relate directly to the performance of rabbinical supervision:

1) The foundation of supervision is the *certain knowledge*, throughout the entire process, of exactly what is happening with the sperm, eggs, and/or embryos. The supervisor must therefore be present at every step of the laboratory procedure, i.e. from the moment the sperm is submitted until the procedure on the couple is finished. Every treatment involving sperm or eggs needs to be under the watchful eye of the supervisor. The *mashgiha* must stay in the lab the entire time, even when equipment is closed or not working for whatever reason, unless the sperm, eggs, or embryos are locked away and only she can open the lock.

2) The *mashgiha* must check all materials that are used or that come into contact with the sperm, eggs, and/or embryos. This includes all culture media, especially when a new bottle is opened. Each day, and periodically throughout the supervision process, sample inspections must be done under a microscope. As a practical matter, one must ask the technologist in a nice manner, to put a little of the media on a slide in order to view it under the microscope.

3) Supervision of these various laboratory procedures does not imply halakhic approval of the specific treatment. For example, the fact that supervision of a semen analysis is done does not mean that semen analysis is allowable for any specific couple. It is recommended that, for any treatments that involve halakhically unresolved issues (such as donor egg and the like), supervisory services should be given only when the couple has obtained a clear *pesak din*, or halakhic decision, from their personal rabbinic authority.

4) Because of the very emotional nature of infertility and the ethical and religious needs for secrecy, it is the obligation of every supervisor to act with complete discretion. Nothing relating to the couples who have been treated may ever be divulged, including the very fact that the couple has been treated.

5) As a representative of the supervising rabbi, the *mashgiha* must maintain good relations with the clinic staff. This includes discretion, maintenance of confidentiality, and consistent promptness.

PROCEDURE FOR SUPERVISING INSEMINATION WITH HUSBAND'S SPERM

1) Before commencing this work, the supervisor examines all of the materials that are used in the various processes with the laboratory microscope.

2) The supervisor identifies the specimen and the couple signs that the specimen that has been submitted is that of the husband.

3) The supervisor must confirm that the test tube in which the sperm are placed is marked with an identifier that is accepted in the lab. It is important to understand that halakhic supervision is an *addition*, not a replacement, to the normal safety precautions that are a part of standard laboratory procedure. The supervisor must ensure that all the laboratory's usual steps for preventing human error are still performed when there is halakhic supervision.

4) The supervisor accompanies the sperm from the moment it is submitted by the couple until the moment it is inseminated into the wife. It is sufficient to hand the washed sperm suspension to the wife so that she may keep it with her until it is used by the physician or nurse for insemination.

5) It must be confirmed that all of the sperm are inseminated to the woman. The leftover from the process should be handled with supervision, so that it is not put to any other use, even for the purpose of research.

SUPERVISION DURING IVF

1) All steps required for insemination, as listed above, are also to be followed for IVF.

2) In addition, the *mashgiha* confirms that the test tubes and petri dishes containing the sperm and egg are marked with the names of the couple, as well as an additional identifying mark.

3) The supervisor is present at the egg retrieval, or observes the process of the retrieval through the window between the laboratory and the operating room. She must see the entire procedure, in all of its details, without anything being hidden.

4) At the time that the supervisor is busy with supervising the egg retrieval, the sperm specimen should be sealed with a double seal in an agreed-upon location. In halakha, this is known as "a seal within a seal." If the supervision of the egg retrieval is done through the lab window, it is allowable to have the tubes with the sperm within eyeshot of the supervisor.

5) A special place needs to be reserved in the incubator where the fertilized eggs can be locked by the supervisor with a private key, or with another method of locking that will have been agreed upon with the clinic staff. In some clinics, there are special incubators and freezing tanks designated for the sole use of couples whose IVF is being done under *hashga'ha*.

6) A supervisor that needs to leave the laboratory *even for just a few seconds* must lock up the sperm/eggs under the principle of "seal within a seal," and may only then leave.

7) Petri dishes can be opened only while she is present.

8) The process of embryo transfer must be done with the presence of the supervisor.

9) Cryopreservation of sperm or embryos must occur under supervision. Once frozen, the material must be sealed with the rabbi's insignia and transferred to a place where there is permanent supervision, i.e. a locked tank that can only be opened by the rabbi or his designated *mashgiha*.

10) Whenever there is a departure from any of the above procedures, the supervisor must notify the rabbi in charge in order to determine what action needs to be taken. For halakhic reasons, departure from proper supervision may indicate the need to discard the sperm and eggs.

The Sabbath

In the event that there arises a critical medical need to check embryos on Shabbat, the supervisor must be informed prior to Shabbat with regard to the hour the checking will be done. By special arrangement, she will arrive on time to open the incubator and will accompany the entire process until the embryos are returned to the incubator. Carrying out *hashga'ha* on Shabbat may involve many halakhically complicated issues and must therefore always be done in close consultation with the supervising rabbi.

Endnotes

1.   *Nishmat Avraham*, vol. III, p. 7
2.   *Tzitz Eliezer*, vol. IX, 51:4, chap. 6

Part VI
Ethical Issues

Introduction

The decision to engage in artificial procreation is a difficult one for any couple to make. The medical instructions and procedures that need to be followed are exhaustive, the time commitment involved is substantial, and the process can be prohibitively expensive. Still more difficult, for many couples, is coming to terms with having a child through a reproductive process that is distinctly separate from their intimate relationship. Indeed, they may need to work with an entire team of doctors, nurses, and scientists in order to be successful, exposing every detail of their reproductive functioning. Far from being a natural outcome of a healthy, loving relationship, the baby they plan for will grow out of a calculated and precise clinical plan.

Within the halakhic community there is no objection to harnessing scientific knowledge to improve the human condition. The biblical juxtaposition of the command "be fruitful and multiply" with "fill the earth and conquer it" suggests that man may intervene in and manipulate nature for the betterment of life. This consideration is the basis for the general halakhic acceptance of modern technology, including medical advances. In principle, therefore, the idea of procreating through the use of a medical procedure should be one that is acceptable to halakha. Nevertheless, the halakhically committed couple who looks to in vitro fertilization or any of the other assisted reproductive technologies must be concerned with the specifics of the procedure. That is, is there halakhic objection to any one of the steps required? A positive finding in this regard would render the procedure impermissible.

In the early days of assisted reproduction, when all that was available was in vitro fertilization using gametes from husband and wife, the issues were straightforward. Halakhic concerns were limited to methods for procuring sperm and eggs and of establishing parental identity. Although the latter concern led some noted halakhic authorities to disapprove of the procedure, many also allowed it. Today, the array of procedures that falls under the rubric of assisted reproduction has grown considerably, and so have the halakhic questions. While many (if not most) are still controversial and unsettled, the material that follows is meant to acquaint the reader with the basis for the ongoing halakhic discussion.

Richard V. Grazi and Joel B. Wolowelsky

New Ethical Issues

Introduction*

Assisted Reproductive Technology (ART) has enriched the lives of millions of couples who, just a few short decades ago, would have been childless. There is no denying that the Jewish tradition considers this an unqualified and welcome blessing. Sickness, whether in the form of a physical aliment or barrenness, is a challenge to humankind to be overcome. *"Ve'rapo yirape*—he shall surely heal," says the Bible (Exodus 21:19), from which the Rabbis learned the permissibility and duty of the physician to heal. But healing is not a goal unto itself. It must be approached ethically—and for the religious Jew, this means conformity with the values, goals, and constraints of the halakha, traditional Jewish law and ethics.

While ART has provided new opportunities, it also presents new ethical challenges. In this chapter we outline the major recent

---

* The purpose of this chapter is to generally acquaint the reader with these ethical issues and not to explore them fully. References to the specific halakhic sources have therefore been omitted in most cases.

halakhic deliberations on the subject. Our aim is not to provide a comprehensive citation of all the recent discussions, but rather to familiarize the reader with the overriding issues. Detailed references to contemporary sources can be found in such volumes as the recent *Encyclopedia of Halakha and Medicine*.

The major sources for a discussion of Jewish ethics consist of the Bible, the Mishnah and Talmud, and universally accepted codifications such as Maimonides' *Mishneh Torah* or the later *Shulhan Arukh*. Rulings on contemporary issues cannot be promulgated by any central authority, there being no formal hierarchal structure to the various contemporary rabbinic authorities and courts. Positions on contemporary issues are developed by circulation of responsa to questions posed to various rabbinic authorities. Collegial review and community acceptance eventually allow for specific opinions to emerge as dominant. Yet even when one view surfaces as authoritative, individual rabbis or layman will often defer to their local authority, whose position is considered decisive.

Because fertility treatment is a fast-changing and intensely personal and private area of life, most observant people, let alone general members of the Jewish community, have little exposure to the ethical issues until they have to address them with some degree of urgency. Infertile couples look for direct religious guidance as they set off on unchartered courses, and this often brings them to their rabbi with a request for advice. The rabbi, in turn, is sometimes put in a situation of tracing a course he himself has not yet traveled. Reproductive technology is moving at such a fast pace that "general practitioners"—be they gynecologists, *rashei yeshiva*, or congregational rabbis—have difficulty keeping up with the literature, let alone forming judgments about it.

Compounding the problem is the general discomfort religious authorities feel in addressing the issue. Doctors always "play God" to some extent, but it is the Torah that permits them to preserve and maintain health. However, creating life is qualitatively different from preserving life, and it demands a degree of humility that many religious authorities have found lacking in the medical community. Some *poskim* see doctors as cavalierly harvesting eggs, manipulating genes, creating a host of involved "parents"—gestational, genetic, surrogate—all to satisfy the needs of an "unfulfilled" childless couple. This often seems to bespeak an arrogant assumption that it is man and not God who is the ultimate creator.

There is some truth to this, but it is terribly exaggerated. Rabbis would have a greater appreciation for the ethics of the doctor—and doctors would have a greater appreciation for rabbis—if there were more continuous interchange between them. The responsibility for creating such mutual respect lies with both the doctor and rabbi, and requires continuous hard work from both groups.

In any event, a *posek* must deal not only with theory but also with individual couples who have their own specific personal and psychological needs. And, as Rabbi Aharon Lichtenstein has noted,

> A sensitive *posek* recognizes both the gravity of the personal circumstances and the seriousness of the halakhic factors.... He might stretch the halakhic limits of leniency where serious domestic tragedy looms, or hold firm to the strict interpretation of the law when, as he reads the situation, the pressure for leniency stems from frivolous attitudes and reflects a debased moral compass.

It is therefore not surprising that, on an individual level, *poskim* often have been forthcoming with leniencies that may appear to be at odds with public positions issued by senior halakhic authorities. Indeed, it is not surprising that many of their lenient decisions are made in consultation with those very same authorities. This is not the least bit hypocritical. On a public level, halakhists have an obligation to resist the tide of moral permissiveness that informs too much of the drive to obtain fertility at any cost. But on a private level, it is the individual situation that must be addressed, not the global issues. These lenient decisions are often circulated to only a small group of scholars lest they be exploited by those whose "pressure for leniency stems from frivolous attitudes [reflecting] a debased moral compass." This means that the person who relies only on the relatively few public statements available will have a myopic view of the halakhic options open to an infertile couple. Being aware of the true full range of halakhic options available—including the serious reasons calling for stringencies in some cases—is the first duty of the rabbinic counselor.

Just as the rabbi must understand the halakhic intricacies involved, he must also be aware of the underlying family dynamics at play. Indeed, the most important initial advice that the rabbi might offer is that there is rarely a fertility problem that needs immediate medical attention.

General Issues in Consultation

Most people can quote the biblical injunction "to be fruitful and multiply" (Genesis 1:28). However, it is important to understand that this is not a command to be actualized at all cost. Indeed, most halakhists maintain that the only obligation incumbent on a man is to engage in regular sexual activity with his wife, rather than to seek any outside assistance in overcoming infertility. Furthermore, a woman is not obligated at all in this commandment (most probably because having a child involves significant physical risks). Of course, the lack of a biblical obligation does not put aside the universal natural desire to have a child. Nevertheless it explains the hesitation of many halakhists to suggest any form of "unnatural" ART, especially when it might be seen as "compromising" natural sexual relations or requiring otherwise prohibited activity (such as masturbation by a man).

Despite the tremendous pressure in the religious community to have children as quickly as possible, barring a known medical condition, it is inappropriate to seek professional advice until the couple has had regular sexual relations for at least twelve months. (If the wife is of advanced age, a six-month period is more appropriate.) Not only is such advice unnecessary, it may be detrimental, as the tension associated with the medical evaluation of infertility can create its own psychological problems. During this period, however, many couples may seek rabbinical guidance. Though *tzini'ut* considerations generally discourage a frank exchange about the couple's intimate life, such open communication is required in any halakhic discussion. Rabbis should be aware that even when the proper approach might well be to refer the couple to a competent doctor or therapist, this initial encounter with a religious authority figure may well influence any possible future counseling and therefore demands a thoughtful, responsible reaction.

In making a suggestion to seek medical treatment, the rabbi should be careful to point out that a halakhically committed couple should raise with the doctor a number of changes in the standard medical protocol. The first is the medical work-up of the husband. Normally, the first course of action would be to check the quality of the husband's sperm. This involves a relatively inexpensive and non-invasive test but it usually involves masturbation, coitus interruptus, or other techniques which raise the problem of *hash'hatat zera*. It therefore should be put off until the wife has been thoroughly examined and there is some medical indication that the infertility might be due to a problem with the husband's sperm. The second problem is that of *niddah*, the halakhic statutes that govern when a married couple can have sexual relations. The doctor should be given a working knowledge of *hilkhot niddah*, and be informed how it impacts on the couple's sex life and how various treatments influence the *niddah* status of the wife. Some standard fertility treatments can invoke *niddah* status, frustrating all attempts to achieve pregnancy. It is unfair to place on the couple the burden of educating the doctor on this issue, and the rabbi, as part of his general pastoral duties, should have a professional relationship with doctors treating his congregants. These two issues have been dealt with in some detail in other chapters of this volume ("Male Infertility: Halakhic Considerations," and "Diagnostic Procedures in the Female Patient.")

In general, one should be aware that religious counselors and professional therapists have very different, yet legitimate, agendas in their respective discussions with childless couples. The latter's job is to help the couple come to terms with their situation and explore the family-dynamic consequences of the various options open to them, including remaining childless or adopting. Religious counselors, on the other hand, have an obligation to help the individuals grow in their religious convictions and observances. These respective objectives are certainly not inherently contradictory, but they should be understood and sorted out. Of course, any therapist to whom the couple is referred should have a thorough understanding (if not commitment to) the halakhic values that guide the couple's lives. It is to be hoped that in a mutually respectful relationship between the religious and professional counselors, the couple will find all their needs addressed.

Multifetal Pregnancy Reduction

The technique of ovulation induction that is commonly used during fertility treatment may involve a serious ethical issue. Previous chapters have described circumstances under which ovulatory stimulants might be used, both for standard ovulation induction and in preparation for in vitro fertilization. Even in experienced hands, this therapy will commonly result in a pregnancy of twins or triplets. Occasionally, a more dangerous multifetal pregnancy, involving four or even more fetuses, may result. This type of "high order" multifetal pregnancy can seriously compromise the future health of all the fetuses and even the mother.

A woman protects herself, so to speak, from the dangers and strains of a multifetal pregnancy by delivering before term. The more fetuses she is carrying, the greater the probability of an early delivery; the earlier the delivery, the greater the probability of the fetuses being compromised physically or intellectually. The ethical issue is complicated by the fact that we are dealing with probabilities and not medical certainties.

It is possible to eliminate much of the danger by reducing the pregnancy to a safer level. In the very early stages of the pregnancy, a long needle is inserted into the woman's uterus, and one by one the "excess" fetuses are "reduced." There is a small danger of stimulating a total miscarriage, but in most cases the result is a normal pregnancy of twins or triplets. (It is interesting to note that the specialists who perform this service will almost never agree to a reduction simply to make the pregnancy more comfortable for the mother. They are in the business of helping pregnancies proceed, not in aborting healthy gestations.)

The moral difficulties in the procedure are reflected in the various names it has acquired: selective abortion, multifetal pregnancy reduction, MPR. It is in many ways a subset of the general "lifeboat" ethical problems in which members of an otherwise doomed group must be "sacrificed" so that the rest can survive. (Here though, the fetuses are not necessarily doomed to death, but more often are *in danger* of a life compromised by serious physical and intellectual difficulties.)

There is a spectrum of views in traditional Judaism concerning abortion. All agree that abortion is moral to save the life of the mother, and all agree that abortion on demand for the simple convenience of the mother is anathema. But there is a strong position allowing abortion for "serious" considerations, especially when the resulting pregnancy will impact on the mental health of the mother who must cope with a seriously compromised child. (Thus some halakhists will allow the abortion of a Tay-Sachs baby.) Most—but not all—authorities who have addressed the issue allow a reduction in the case of a high order multifetal pregnancy.

Status of the Child

In deciding on which ART they will feel comfortable adopting, religious couples have yet another consideration in addition to whether or not it conforms to the requirements of the halakha. Aside from questions of a procedure's conformity or lack of conformity to halakha, the religious couple must consider another serious issue when deciding which ART they will adopt: Some variations of ART can affect the religious status of the child. Such a compromise is not merely a technicality; it can have an impact on the children's eventual ability to marry freely within the Jewish community. There are many ways that ART can influence the halakhic status of a child, and many opinions regarding such influence.

Some halakhists feel that a child conceived through "artificial" means loses his or her halakhic filial relationship with the genetic parents. Some limit this to IVF procedures while others include even children born through artificial insemination with the husband's sperm. However, the majority of contemporary authorities reject this view, maintaining that the same parent-child relationships exist as would have been created through a natural conception.

There is much halakhic leniency in allowing artificial insemination with the husband's sperm. But there is an accompanying fear—driven by sensational though rare media stories—that doctors are so intent on demonstrating professional success that they will substitute or add foreign, potent sperm to the insemination. Most doctors would take umbrage at such a suggestion because the vast majority of professionals are ethical people, well aware that such deception violates the professional standards of medicine (not to mention the malpractice liability to which it would expose them). Nonetheless, assurances should be made and a review of the technical procedures conducted. Some hospitals have instituted rabbinic supervision of their labs upon request, much as caterers with impeccable reputations hire rabbinic supervisors to supervise the *kashrut* standards of their establishments (see "Rabbinical Supervision in the Laboratory.")

Much more complicated is the issue of donor sperm, which involves not only technical halakhic concerns, but core issues of personal identity. Couples sometimes think that donor insemination (DI) is preferable to adoption because at least one of the parents (the mother) is the genetic parent. But, at the least, this carries with it the possibility of jealousy when tensions that arise in any household emerge. This is one reason why even those halakhists who are willing to see the procedure as technically allowable are most reluctant to recommend it.

When the Ethics Committee of the American Fertility Society approved procedures involving donor gametes, it recorded a dissent on the involvement of third-party donors which noted five major objections: (1) The procedure severs procreation from the marital union, violating the exclusive nature of the marriage covenant. (2) It brings into the world a child with no bond of origin, thereby blurring the child's genealogy and potentially compromising the child's self-identity. (3) It encourages adultery by creating an environment wherein insemination of a wife by the sperm of another man is considered morally acceptable. (4) It marks a subtle but unmistakable move toward eugenics. (5) It tends to absolutize sterility as a disvalue and childbearing as a value, thus distorting and threatening the value of marriage and family. Virtually all halakhists—including those who are willing to allow donor gametes under certain conditions—share these reservations to some extent or another.

The two ends of the halakhic spectrum regarding adultery as a component of donor insemination are defined by the respective opinions of Rabbi Yoel Teitelbaum and Rabbi Moshe Feinstein, two late leading American *poskim*. Rabbi Teitelbaum (known popularly as the Satmar Rebbe) argues that the halakhic definition of adultery is the deliberate introduction of a third party's sperm into the vagina of a married woman. He therefore condemns DI as morally repugnant and concludes that a wife who undergoes such a procedure is an adulteress. The concurrence of the husband is no more relevant than it would be in the case of sexual relations between a married woman and a man not her husband. Following through on the logic of his definition, he argues that the person who mechanically introduces the sperm specimen is also guilty of adultery.

Rabbi Teitelbaum's position is summarily rejected by Rabbi Feinstein. Rabbinic authorities cite two sources in refuting the charge of adultery. The first is the case of Ben Sira, the grandson of Jeremiah the prophet, whose daughter, according to tradition, was impregnated by her father's sperm while bathing in a pool into which her father had previously ejaculated. Ben Sira is considered legitimate. (For more detail, see "A Brief History of Fertility Therapy.") The second is a ruling by the medievalist Rabbi Peretz ben Elijah of Corbeil which sets out what has become the dominant current rabbinic view:

> A woman may lie on her husband's sheets but should be careful not to lie on sheets upon which another man slept lest she become impregnated from his sperm.... [However, in the event that she does,] as there is no forbidden intercourse, the child is completely legitimate even from the sperm of another.... We are concerned about the sperm of another man [only] because the child may [unknowingly] eventually marry his [half-] sister.

Rabbi Feinstein argues from this source that regardless of whether or not the case described is possible, it is clear that adultery is not considered the basis of the concern that a woman be impregnated accidentally. In his view, physical sexual contact is part of the definition of adultery, and absent such contact the wife cannot be charged with promiscuity (nor can the child be branded illegitimate). He cautions, however, that the fidelity required in marriage commands that donor insemination is prohibited without the husband's consent.

Others, however, have argued that even if the charge of adultery cannot be sustained, the source's ruling cannot be extended to permit donor insemination. A woman may not lie on the sheets upon which another man slept despite the far-fetched and unintended possibility that she be impregnated; *a fortiori* she may not allow insemination by a person other than her husband even if she cannot technically be charged with adultery. Rabbi Eliezer Yehuda Waldenberg, a member of Israel's High Rabbinic Court, argues that even if technical halakhic objections cannot be marshaled to oppose DI, the procedure runs counter to basic halakhic values which stress genealogy and family integrity. He cautions that whether or not the charge of adultery is technically sustainable, DI without the husband's consent is grounds for divorce.

While Rabbi Feinstein was adamant in his position that DI violates no technical halakha, he was equally resolute in his position that such a procedure was only a course of last resort. He was careful to caution that he would permit the procedure only in the extreme instance where the wife is under severe mental stress and the individual circumstances have been reviewed by a competent halakhic authority.

The extent to which the lenient position is accepted is not adequately reflected in the written literature. Anyone who has had a close dialogue with halakhists and *rashei yeshiva* who deal with the problem knows that on a private level many *poskim* are willing to entertain this possibility when it can be seen as a therapy for a distraught couple. They are unwilling to do so publicly because it can accelerate current norms which impact negatively on the sanctity of the marriage institution. Even most—but not all—of those who prohibit donor insemination as a clear halakhic violation concede that charges of adultery cannot be maintained against the wife if her husband consented to the procedure, and that the child is free from illegitimate status. (Also, by his consent the husband assumes financial responsibility for raising the child; insemination without his consent constitutes grounds for divorce.) Certainly donor insemination should not be considered without a thorough thrashing-out of the personal issues involved.

Most authorities who reluctantly allow donor insemination prefer that the donor be a non-Jew. Halakhically, there is no filial relationship between a Jewish child and its non-Jewish genetic father. This avoids potential problems of the child unknowingly marrying his or her half-sibling by the same donor father. If the donor is Jewish, it is necessary to maintain clear records so that there will be no impediment to the child eventually marrying. A minority prefer that the donor be the husband's brother, as there is closer genetic affiliation and little danger of the child marrying a close relative. It is clear that serious rabbinic and psychological counseling must accompany any decision here.

The likelihood of concealment of the use of donor sperm creates additional complications. While in the case of adoption, at least some members of the surrounding community are aware of the circumstances, there is a real possibility of keeping donor insemination a secret, provided the couple has not shared this information with anyone at the time of conception. (Indeed, many doctors advise their patients, "Tell no one!") This creates three additional technical problems that must be considered, even if sperm from a gentile are used. The first is that of *halitza*. If a man dies childless, his surviving brother must release the widow through a *halitza* ceremony before she can remarry. With donor insemination, the husband is in actuality childless, and his widow would have to reveal the facts to her surviving brother-in-law should she wish to remarry. The second is that of priestly status. A son born of donor sperm would be unrelated to the husband and would not inherit his status as a *kohen* (priest) or *Levi* (Levite). (Rabbi Shlomo Zalman Auerbach maintains that in the case of insemination from a non-Jewish donor, the child takes on the status of the mother, becoming a *kohen* or *Levi* if his maternal grandfather has that status.) In these cases, it would be almost impossible to keep the facts a secret as they would become known through the regular services in the synagogue, such as *aliyot*. The third possible complication is that of inheritance. The child cannot legally inherit from the deceased husband because there is no familial bond between them. This can be addressed easily by preparing a halakhic will.

A more recent phenomenon has been the insemination of single women who have come to the conclusion that for one reason or another they will not marry before their biological clock makes it impossible for them to have a child of their own. There has been little formal discussion of this phenomenon in halakhic literature. From a technical perspective insemination of a single woman is less complicated halakhically than donor insemination of a married woman. There are no possible charges of adultery or illegitimacy, and gentile sperm obviates other concerns, such as the child unknowingly eventually marrying a half-sibling. Yet even those allowing donor insemination for a distraught couple refuse to extend it to a single woman, because they see it as undermining the norm of a family consisting of a father and mother. No doubt there will be more extensive halakhic discussion of this phenomenon as it becomes more widespread in the general community.

Even more complicated is the matter of donor ova. Here the major consideration is not so much the halakhic prohibitions involved (the charge of adultery is not really heard), but the halakhic consequence—most significantly, whether it is the gestational or genetic mother who is the halakhic mother. On a "gut level," many people feel that if a woman carries a donor egg she is certainly the mother. On the other hand, when dealing with a surrogacy situation—where the wife cannot carry her own genetic child—there is sometimes the tendency to consider the surrogate as a "fetus-sitter" who has no relationship to the child. At this stage, most would hold that both the genetic and gestational mothers be considered the halakhic mother, at least for the purpose of forbidding the child from marrying first-degree relatives.

The situation is much more complicated if either the donor or the surrogate is not Jewish, as the Jewish status of the child is then called into question. Some hold that the child is Jewish, others that it is a non-Jew who needs conversion (and who would then be halakhically unrelated to any of its parents), while yet others hold that it requires some form of conversion but nonetheless remains related to its genetic parents.

It is not until the child is ready to marry that his or her status will have to be established before a religious authority, and it is therefore important to maintain good records as to the religious identity of the donor or surrogate. If everyone is Jewish, it is necessary to have sufficient information on file regarding the donor or surrogate to be able to establish that the child is not marrying a first-degree relative. (It would be beneficial if some authoritative rabbinic organization would undertake such a registry.) In Israel, the rabbinate seems ready to give its unenthusiastic consent to a secular law that would allow surrogacy if the surrogate is Jewish and single (so that no charge of adultery can be brought against her), and is officially recognized as the child's mother who gives the child up for adoption to the genetic parents. This whole issue has not been thoroughly explored in the halakhic literature.

Gender Selection

As technology increases, additional ethical issues have emerged. Among them is determining the gender of the child. The general thinking in the medical community is that such a procedure is unacceptable for "social reasons" (that is, when the parents simply prefer to have a boy or girl for "their own reason") but acceptable for "medical reasons" (as when there is fear of a sex-linked genetic disease). Traditional Judaism does not accept this position, and indeed the Talmud quotes various "folk" advice for ensuring one gender or the other for one's potential child. What concerns the halakhah is the method for ensuring the desired gender.

Anything that does not interfere with normal marital sexual activity (such as position, timing, foods, etc.) is acceptable—but generally not effective. Sperm sorting into X and Y components is more effective, but involve two problems: first, it does not guarantee the desired gender; second, it involves masturbation, which might be permitted for effecting a pregnancy (in the case of artificial insemination with the husband's sperm when the count is low) but not necessarily to effect a pregnancy of a desired gender.

The sure standard for gender selection is IVF with preimplantation genetic diagnosis, where only that embryo of the desired gender is implanted. This involves great expense and radical interference with natural relationships. This brings us back to Rabbi Lichtenstein's comment at the opening of this chapter: The ethical motivation of the parents plays a role in the *posek*'s decision. A case where the couple carries a sex-linked gene for a serious illness and wants to avoid either having to grapple with the question of aborting a fetus carrying the illness or carrying a sick child to term is clearly very different from a situation where a family wants a child who will conform to their preconceived notion of gender order or balance. Then again, this is not the same as a couple who have five children of one gender and who will consider a sixth only if it is of the other gender. There has not been extensive discussion of this question in the contemporary literature.

Posthumous Reproduction

There are two main circumstances that bring us to the question of posthumous reproduction. The first involves a couple who have been undergoing fertility therapy and have cryopreserved the husband's frozen sperm or the couple's fertilized embryo for future use. If the husband dies before the pregnancy is affected, the widow might want to give birth to her deceased husband's child. To some extent, this is but an instance of the question of insemination of a single woman, although here it is hard to argue that this undermines the notion of family values. There are, however, two other questions to be considered: imposing fatherhood on a dead person and the status of the child.

Halakhists and secular authorities agree that it would be unethical to impose fatherhood on the deceased without clear expression of his desires before death. Agencies that store frozen sperm or embryos now require that formal instructions be filed at the time of cryopreservation to be sure that the man has an opportunity to make his wishes known.

Halakhists and secular authorities also agree that any child born in such a situation would not be related to his or her dead genetic father. Their reasoning is similar: there must be legal finality to such situations. Estates must be settled and relationships finalized—and in halakhic discussions the "childlessness" of the deceased, must be determined to know whether *halitza* is necessary. (It is interesting to note that, in the secular arena, some court challenges have resulted in a softening of this position to the extent that child benefits are allowed. Also, in halakhic cases, it is doubtful if marriage would be allowed between such a child and his or her paternal half-sibling.)

A relatively new dimension to this issue has emerged with the ability to procure semen from a brain-dead individual—say, one killed in an accident. Hospital administrators have been faced with an increasing number of such requests, and the courts have been required to intercede. Halakhists and secular authorities agree that such posthumous paternity cannot be imposed on the deceased without a clear indication of his wishes.

Future Issues

It is impossible to foresee all the new ethical issues that will emerge as new technologies yield new possible procedures. It seems, for example, that cloning will eventually be a real possibility and, when it emerges, halakhists will certainly discuss it in great detail. At first glance, it would seem that it should present less ethical difficulty than, say, donor insemination. Transferring the husband's cell nucleus to the wife's egg and implanting it in her uterus seems more acceptable than involving a third person in the procedure. The "artificial" nature of it all will eventually fade as the procedure becomes more common—just as IVF did. Of course, proving it to be a safe procedure is the *sine qua non* for establishing it—or any other procedure—to be ethically acceptable. But whatever the future may bring, the approach will be the same, balancing the excitement of new possibilities for helping suffering couples with an understanding of the subtle ethical problems that may lie hidden below the surface. For this we need a continuing interchange between halakhists, scientists and clinicians, as God, man, woman and doctor join to fulfill the blessing of "be fruitful and multiply."

Joel B. Wolowelsky and Richard V. Grazi

Future Directions

This book has focused on the day-to-day problems encountered by infertile couples and those who care for them. Most infertility is just that—a decrease in natural fertility. It is not, generally, absolute sterility. The essential components for creating a pregnancy—some sperm, some eggs, a womb—exist, albeit in an impaired state, and are naturally accessible to most infertile couples. Rarer situations do exist, however, in which any of these components, and sometimes two or three, will be missing. In such cases, novel approaches such as donor gametes or gestational surrogacy may be considered. As mentioned earlier, there is as yet no unanimity on the halakhic permissibility of these techniques.

It is likely that scientist and physicians of the future will develop new techniques to cure even the most severe forms of infertility. While it is impossible, of course, to predict what advances lay over the horizon, it is worthwhile addressing some techniques that are in their early developmental stages, if only to begin addressing the potential halakhic hurdles.

Cloning

The dramatic announcement in February 1997 that a sheep ("Dolly") had been cloned using a non-embryonic cell set off a choir of condemnation, echoing fears of scientists about to go too far. Virtually every politician, religious thinker and scientist who spoke out on the subject—including the scientist himself who had cloned Dolly—condemned the possibility of cloning humans as unethical and repugnant. Leon Kass summarized the objections as follows:

> People are repelled by many aspects of human cloning. They recoil from the prospect of mass production of human beings, with large clones of look-alikes, compromised in their individuality; the idea of father-son or mother-daughter twins; the bizarre prospects of a woman giving birth to and rearing a genetic copy of herself, her spouse, or even her deceased father or mother; the grotesqueness of conceiving a child as an exact replacement of another who has died; the utilitarian creation of embryonic genetic duplicates of oneself, to be frozen away or created when necessary, in case of need for homologous tissues or organs for transplantation; the narcissism of those who clone themselves and the arrogance of those who think they know who deserves to be cloned or which genotype any child-to-be should be thrilled to receive; the Frankensteinian hubris to create human life and increasingly to control its destiny; man playing God.[1]
>
> *The New Republic*
> *June 2, 1997*

Yet some of Kass' objections could just as easily apply to many less dramatic techniques of the new reproductive technologies, such as egg donation for postmenopausal women or embryo donation, with which many religious and secular ethicists are quite comfortable. This does not mean that we should now embrace cloning of humans. On the contrary, it might force us to reconsider previously held positions. It simply means that any discussion on the ethics of cloning must factor out and identify the issues that are unique to cloning.

Objections regarding the dehumanization of the child are clearly not new. Healthy parents see their children as individuals who are ends in themselves, not entities created to fulfill some other end. However, long before the new reproductive technologies, parents had children to "replace" a deceased child. They dressed him or her in the dead sibling's clothes, sometimes used the same name or a close variation, planned out similar educational or career plans, and so on. The unhealthy and unethical aspect of this "replacement" lies not in the fact that the new child is not an exact genetic duplicate. Healthy parents of identical twins have long realized that their children are identical only in their genetic codes.

Let us take the following case to try to see if we really object to creating genetically identical humans. We have no moral difficulty with an infertile couple using in vitro fertilization with their own gametes to establish a pregnancy. But a transferred embryo does not always implant, so it has become routine for doctors to harvest many eggs from the wife—using various ovarian stimulants—and fertilize all of them with the husband's sperm. These artificially created fraternal twins or triplets are welcome to most of us. Moreover, if the harvesting produces more embryos than can safely be transferred to her uterus, there seems to be little objection to freezing them so that future pregnancies may be established without the additional risks associated with ovarian stimulation and egg retrieval.

But suppose only one egg can be harvested and the doctor suggests dividing the fertilized egg at the four cell stage so that more than one embryo can be implanted. All of the motivations are identical; the additional technological intervention—cloning—is introduced only to solve a practical medical problem, the same way couples turn to IVF when artificial insemination will not overcome their inability to conceive. Would healthy parents relate to their artificially created identical twins any differently than would parents who have such children without any medical intervention?

TYPES OF CLONING

In order to sort through the halakhic debate on cloning, it is useful to first explain exactly what cloning is and what it is not. There are essentially three types of cloning:

Embryonic cloning—This refers to extraction of a blastomere, the earliest identifiable cell of the newly fertilized embryo, and its insertion into an embryonic shell that has been emptied of its blastomeres. Since every blastomere is totipotent—meaning that it retains the capacity to grow into all the structures necessary to produce an entire human being—the donor embryo remains unaffected by its missing blastomere and, once that blastomere has begun to divide within its new shell, the newly cloned embryo which it forms is exactly like the original. This technique is a way of making identical genetic copies of offspring, and is used extensively in research and industry. Its potential use to alleviate human infertility is the scenario described above.

Reproductive cloning—This technique uses adult, somatic cells to produce the clone. Nearly all cells of the body are somatic cells, each containing the exact, complete set (diploid) of genetic information, in the form of DNA. They are distinguished from germ cells—eggs and sperm—which have only half of a set (haploid) of DNA and are, therefore, the building blocks for sexual reproduction. Somatic cells also differ from embryonic cells, formed when male and female germ cells meet, in that somatic cells have already undergone a process called differentiation. This means that, although they all started out from a single parent cell, by the process of cell division they have taken on new characteristics, i.e. becoming different in both structure and function. Differentiation is achieved by the cell turning on or off different segments of its DNA. Somatic cell cloning is more difficult and problematic than embryonic cloning, because it involves the use of adult, differentiated cells. To produce the clone, the scientist must first coax the cell to undergo a process of de-differentiation, essentially causing it to turn on all of its genetic instructions and revert to its original, totipotent state. The nucleus of the totipotent, somatic cell—now with a full set of DNA instructions that exactly resembles the cell donor—can then replace the nucleus of an egg to produce a functional clone. An electrical pulse causes the membrane of the "clonor" nucleus to fuse with the "clonee" egg cytoplasm, and a cloned embryo results. If the embryo is successfully implanted, the resultant offspring will be an identical physical copy of the genetic parent, regardless of who gestates and delivers it. This was the technique used to produce Dolly, the lamb.

Stem cell cloning—This technique refers to the cloning of stem cells, which are primitive, precursor cells that give rise to individual organs. There are two types of stem cells: those that are produced during early embryonic development—called embryonic stem cells—and those that are produced during later life—called adult stem cells. All stem cells are somatic cells and carry a full complement of DNA. However, stem cells differ from other somatic cells because, by definition, they are relatively undifferentiated. There is currently great interest in stem cells because scientists are fairly certain that, as technology progresses, they will be able to clone stem cells in the laboratory and have them grow into a variety of tissues and organs. Those organs will then be available to replace diseased organs and cure a vast number of illnesses. Adult stem cell cloning has generated no ethical debate, as the process involves only cells that are derived from adult tissues. Embryonic stem cells, on the other hand, must be derived from early human embryos, a process that results in the destruction of the embryo. Because the completely undifferentiated embryonic stem cells can potentially be derived from a somatic cell clone, their potential for organ replacement is enormous. However, some in our society believe that embryos must be treated as full human beings; they object to the use of embryonic stem cells as being destructive to human life.

Although there has been intense public debate on stem cell cloning, the sensational media coverage of cloning has focused on reproductive cloning. This technique will potentially allow the production of exact copies of people, truly the fodder of science fiction.

But this imaginative presentation of cloning is not exactly accurate. Although a cloned individual would clearly *appear* identical to its parent, it would not be identical in other ways. For although a person's genetic endowment is responsible for much, genes do not account for the sum total of the person. The physical and psychological environments that nurture every individual determine, to a large extent, the direction of his or her genetic endowment. These environmental conditions differ even among identical twins ("nature's clones"). In the true sense, therefore, no two individuals will ever be exactly alike, even if they are clones. Even the DNA content of clones will differ somewhat, because only the nuclear DNA will be cloned. Another type of DNA, called mitochondrial DNA, will be inherited from the donor of the egg cell. (At present, the function of mitochondrial DNA is unclear.)

TWO HALAKHIC APPROACHES

In addressing the topic of cloning, Prof. Abraham S. Abraham has pointed out that the default position of halakha is permissive.[2] As a general rule, there is no need to find a halakhic source in order to render something permissible, as not everything that is *mutar* (permissable) is explicitly stated in the Torah. On the contrary, all things that are not specifically prohibited are assumed to be permitted. Moreover, although the halakha is dependent on precedent, there are many situations for which no halakhic precedent exists, and cloning seems to be one of them. In the absence of a specific *issur* (prohibition), therefore, it would seem that all forms of cloning would be allowable.

On the other hand, Prof. Abraham argues, not everything that is prohibited is stated in the Torah either. There are certain things beyond what we find in *taryag mitzvot* (the 613 commandments) that are prohibited by force of reason. For example, Adam was only given one commandment, to serve God. Murder was not specifically prohibited. Yet Cain was guilty of transgressing the word of God because murder is prohibited by the *force of reason*. Likewise, the people of Sodom were punished because they did not give charity. Ammon and Moab were excluded from *klal Yisrael* because they were not hospitable to the children of Israel. Rabbi Nissim Gaon, in his introduction to tractate *Berakhot*, maintains that the halakhic obligation to follow naturally derived mitzvot is equal to the obligation to follow the mitzvot clearly stated in the Torah. In his *Moreh Nevukhim*, Maimonides puts forth the precept of reward for doing something good according to the dictates of reason, and punishment for doing something evil according to the dictates of reason. The deed need not be specifically permitted or prohibited by the Torah. As an example, Maimonides brings the case of someone who grafts together two species. Such a person, he states, behaves as if God did not complete His creation, and has transgressed.

Prof. Abraham speaks authoritatively in the name of Rabbi Shlomo Zalman Auerbach, with whom he learned for many years. But Rabbi Auerbach did not issue a ruling on cloning, as he died before it became a possibility. Prof. Abraham maintains that he has discussed the issue with Rabbi Yosef Elyashiv three times, and that each time Rabbi Elyashiv prohibited human reproductive cloning for all of the reasons stated above. According to this view, the cloned individual is a new *beriah*, a new creation not intended by God's plan. Using cloning to achieve a pregnancy is impermissible—*hadash assur min haTorah!*[3] In the case of a child born from cloning, its halakhic status as a *human* would be doubtful, as it was not created in the way God intended people to procreate. The cloning of animals and stem cells for the purposes of therapeutic cloning is, on the other hand, permissible according to the precept of *Ve'rapo yirape* ("He shall surely heal"; Exodus 21:19).

A completely opposite conclusion is reached by Michael Broyde.[4] In his treatise on human cloning, he systematically reviews the pertinent halakhic issues. With regard to assisted conception in general, the normative position is permissive in regards to its conclusion that (a) there is a parental relationship to the offspring created by in vitro fertilization, (b) there is therefore no prohibition of *hash'hatat zera* and (c) a mitzvah is fulfilled, if not *peru u'revu* then *lashevet yitzrah*. Against this background, reproduction via cloning poses no great difficulty. In one aspect, in fact, it is less problematic than routine IVF, as it involves no issue whatsoever of *hash'hatat zera*. Regarding the viewpoint that the cloned individual is a new *beriah* Broyde, basing himself on the *Yerushalmi Talmud, Niddah* 3:2, points to the *prima facie* evidence that, by virtue of its gestation in utero and birth to a human mother, the child must be human.

As with any IVF pregnancy, the halakhic mother of a clone is no doubt the gestational/birth mother. Determining halakhic paternity in the case of a male clonor is intuitive. If halakha sees a natural genetic father as one who contributes half of the child's DNA, then one who contributes his entire DNA to a child born would certainly lay claim to halakhic paternity. By the same logic as in standard IVF, he would then fulfill the mitzvah of *peru u'revu*. The case of a woman clonor would be more problematic. She cannot be the halakhic mother, as someone else has laid claim to that title. Perhaps, as Rabbi J. David Bleich has suggested in the case of egg donation,[5] this is a case where two halakhic mothers are present. (Alternatively, this situation may invoke the case of a female father!) In any event, because the woman has no mitzvah to fulfill, cloning of a woman would at best be considered a *hesed* (kindness). According to this viewpoint, then, cloning a person would be halakhically neutral and, under certain circumstances, it may even be a mitzvah.

Broyde draws inspiration for his viewpoint from the words of Rabbi Judah Luria, known as the Maharal of Prague, who explained the power of human creativity as follows:

> The creativity of people is greater than nature. When God created in the six days of creation the laws of nature, the simple and complex, and finished creating the world, there remained additional power to create anew, just like people can create new animal species through interspecies breeding....[6] People bring to fruition things that are not found in nature; nonetheless, since these are activities that occur through nature, it is as if it entered the world to be created....[7]

It is unlikely that there will be a reconciliation of these opposing views, as it is not only differing halakhic analysis that divides them.

Rather, they are basing themselves on radically different under-
standings of man's place in God's plan. As with other reproductive
technologies, the acceptance of human cloning will depend on
which view emerges, over time, as dominant among *poskim*. The
need to bring this issue to closure is not pressing, however, as
somatic cell cloning technology is still in its infancy.

POTENTIAL APPLICATIONS OF CLONING

The groundwork for using true reproductive cloning in humans
has not yet been laid. However, were all the scientific and medical
obstacles to be solved, there are a variety of potential applications
in humans. The obvious first use of this technique would be in the
treatment of reproductive failure.

Currently, even with the use of the most advanced form of
reproductive technologies, there remain situations where male and
female infertility are not treatable. For example, gonadal failure
is not uncommon in both men and women. This may occur as
a result of genetic disease (e.g. Klinefelter's Syndrome in males
and Turner's Syndrome in females), ionizing radiation, or surgery.
Other cases are unexplained (e.g. Sertoli Cell Syndrome in males
and Premature Ovarian Failure in women [see "Evaluation and
Treatment of Male Infertility" and "General Aspects of Female
Infertility" respectively]). In all of these cases, there exists no source
of (haploid) germ cells with which to begin fertilization and embryonic development, precluding treatment. Cloning would allow the
use of (diploid) somatic cells for embryonic development, albeit
without true fertilization. In the case where the male is affected,
the wife's egg could be used to host the husband's somatic cell DNA.
Halakhic paternity would not appear to be in question. In the case
where the female is affected, a host egg from which the nucleus has
been extracted would need to be used. Still, as the birth mother in
this situation she would likely be considered the halakhic mother,
and, as the egg donor in this case supplies no nuclear DNA, there
would not be the complication of two halakhic mothers. (Those
who oppose egg donation on the grounds of uncertain lineage may
have less difficulty in this situation.) Because the mitzvah of *peru*

u'revu falls on the husband, it would be his somatic cell that would be chosen for cloning more commonly than the wife's.

Justifying the use of cloning technology to create new individuals would seem limited to the situations described above. Even then, however, there are serious questions that must be addressed before proceeding with full human cloning. And here, it must be said, not all agonadal individuals are alike. Specifically, if there is a known genetic etiology to the gonadal failure and the individual harboring that gene is to be cloned, is it fair to propagate that genetic problem in the next generation? Does this not increase the future need for cloning? Or is life as an agonadal human clone infinitely more valuable than no life at all? Unfortunately, the ethical discussion cannot take place without also addressing the cold facts of a society's limited resources. Who will pay for all of this? Or can only the rich be cloned?

The Human Genome Project, recently completed, will no doubt increase the power of reproductive technologies, including human cloning. Still, sequencing genes is different from understanding them. Gene therapy is presently more of a concept than a reality. Eventually, however, it is likely that inserting, removing, or modifying genes will be a standard part of medical practice.

Using genetic manipulation to cure illnesses is likely halakhically neutral and perhaps a mitzvah. Halakhic difficulties might arise, however, when the genetic manipulation occurs in the germ cell line and, as such, is transmitted across generations. The same difficulty would arise if a somatic cell were genetically altered and then used for cloning. Still, although the potential impact of such therapies is obviously more profound than standard medical therapy, it is not clear why they would be halakhically problematic as long as a specific genetic disease was being eliminated. Indeed, withholding such therapy, were it available, would seem halakhically questionable. On the other hand, the use of such procedures on healthy people or embryos in order to alter physical, mental or other characteristics that may render them more "desirable," would be a frivolous intervention and therefore, in all likelihood, prohibited.

434

Cytoplasmic Transfer

The current halakhic debate about the use of gamete donors— whether egg or sperm—is unlikely to be resolved. For reasons already stated, it is possible that cloning may ultimately provide an alternate solution for agonadal individuals. But gamete dona- tion as currently applied is not used only in agonadal individuals. Indeed, the vast majority of donor egg recipients are women in the perimenopausal phase of life, who have eggs, albeit ones not capable of successful fertilization and implantation. For them, an interesting technique has been described which uses donor eggs but permits the recipient to bear her own genetic child. This technique is called "cytoplasmic transfer."

The theory behind cytoplasmic transfer is that the defect in older eggs is not located in the nucleus of the egg, where the DNA resides, but rather in the cytoplasm of the egg. The cytoplasm is the site of all of the cellular organelles which provide the energy needed for fertilization and development. In cytoplasmic transfer, standard IVF is done with the sperm and eggs of the husband and wife, except that a small volume of cytoplasm is removed from the eggs of a young donor and transferred to the cytoplasm of the wife's eggs. Some women who repeatedly failed IVF, presumably because of the aging of their eggs, have been able to conceive suc- cessfully using this technique.[8] Halakhically, maternal status does not appear to be affected by cytoplasmic transfer, but it should be noted that such children have been shown to carry DNA from two women, nuclear DNA from the genetic/gestational mother, and some mitochondrial DNA from the cytoplasm donor.

Nuclear Transfer

It is well known that the live birth rate in women drops precipitously with increasing maternal age and that this decline is accompanied by an increase in the incidences of miscarriage and fetal genetic anomalies. Most of these genetic anomalies involve aneuploidy, a condition where an abnormal number of chromosomes is present in the embryo or fetus. Similarly timed declines in clinical pregnancy and implantation rates are also observed when IVF statistics are examined. Increases in oocyte and embryo aneuploidy as well as decreases in oocyte and embryo number, vitality and quality appear to account for these declines. Studies have shown that the susceptibility of the aging oocyte to abnormalities in genetic development is a result of cytoplasmic factors.

It has been reported that the nucleus of the human egg can be removed from its surrounding cytoplasm and inserted into the cytoplasm of a second egg.[9] By subjecting the hybrid cell to a small electrical pulse—"electrofusion"—the membranes fuse to form one single, reconstructed cell. Using this technique, nuclear material was extracted from the eggs of older women and "reconstructed" using the nuclear free cytoplasm of the eggs from younger donors. Researchers using this technique have been able to achieve maturation, fertilization, and cleavage of these eggs. Although research on this technology has been subjected to a moratorium in the United States, it is ongoing in other countries.

With nuclear transfer, the resultant embryo would receive its genetic instructions from the nuclear material within the older egg of the wife as well as from the sperm of her husband. Conception and birth would proceed normally. The resultant offspring would be the genetic offspring of the wife's egg (save for the mitochondrial DNA) and the husband's sperm. In contrast to egg donation, the technique would allow older women and those with poor egg quality to be the genetic as well as the gestational mother. The question is whether nuclear transfer would solve the halakhic dilemmas of egg donation. Would the concern of those *poskim* who hold that the egg donor may be, at least in part, the halakhic mother, disappear? How much genetic material must one donate in order to be the halakhic mother? Does mitochondrial DNA count? Should nuclear transfer become applicable in humans, these questions would need to be addressed by halakhic authorities.

Oocyte Cryopreservation

Most established IVF clinics offer embryo cryopreservation as a routine service of the embryology laboratory. However, many of the legal, ethical, and religious dilemmas created by freezing human embryos might be avoided by cryopreserving oocytes (eggs) instead. This technology would also benefit young women who face serious illnesses requiring chemotherapy or radiation.

While the oocytes of several other species of mammals have been successfully frozen and thawed, the technology enabling the reliable freezing and thawing of unfertilized human oocytes is only now becoming a reality. In 1997, Dr. Eleonora Porcu described the first child born from a frozen and thawed egg.[10] Recent advances in understanding the inherent problems with egg freezing and the development of more sophisticated techniques to freeze them have finally begun to pay off in additional pregnancies and births.

The great advantage of this technique is that it does not require the egg to be fertilized prior to preservation. This means that when single women face the prospect of requiring medical treatment that is expected to be toxic to their eggs, they retain the option of having their eggs extracted and frozen prior to their treatment. Likewise, single women who must, for health reasons, undergo surgical removal of their ovaries have the option of pre-surgical egg extraction and storage. This is very much akin to the option already available to men for many years, i.e. sperm freezing. Were the problems of egg freezing to be completely resolved and the pregnancies to become routine, a great benefit would be the ability to establish egg banks for use with egg donation, much as sperm donation is currently practiced. (The lack of reliable pregnancies from frozen oocytes with the current technology necessitates the use of freshly removed eggs from donors, a far more complicated process.)

An alternative to egg freezing, which often is simpler and more effective, has been described by Oktay and colleagues.[11] Using this technique, whole pieces of ovarian tissue containing large numbers of eggs can be cryopreserved. Recently, the first pregnancy has been reported using thawed and retransplanted tissue. There is no reason to believe that this success cannot be duplicated. This technique would be especially useful to young girls facing the prospect of chemotherapy for cancer. In them, the process of egg retrieval and freezing is technically difficult, but removing part or all of an ovary for storage is not. In addition, the technique of ovarian tissue freezing requires no hormonal pretreatment, or any of the other delays that are associated with egg freezing.

Once these techniques are perfected, of course, it can be anticipated that they will find other uses. In addition to simplifying the process of egg banking, the technique would be attractive to legions of younger women who, confronting their own aging, might want to "insure" their prospects for future fertility by having their eggs stored while they are still young. Will the halakha sanction such procedures? Is there a difference if the procedure is carried out because of a compassionate need, say, for a young girl with cancer, as opposed to a thirty-something single professional too busy at the moment to worry about marriage?

Were many women to avail themselves of egg freezing, another problem that would undoubtedly arise would be the prospect of how to dispose of this material in the event that the "owner" dies. As mentioned in the preceding chapter, halakha has already had to confront the problem of children being fathered posthumously with frozen sperm. But there the problem is more straightforward, as only one party can claim halakhic fatherhood. Motherhood, by contrast, has two separate components, conception and parturition (birth). How would halakha establish maternity in the case of eggs that have been used posthumously to create children?

Future options such as those provided by oocyte freezing will clearly change the spectrum of clinical and ethical dilemmas faced by fertility specialists. For couples—and single women—facing serious illness, they will be seen as nothing short of a blessing that preserves their ability to reproduce.

Looking Forward

When the Wright Brothers unlocked the secret of flight some one hundred years ago, their flying machine was no doubt greeted with some degree of skepticism by a world unprepared for men to fly. How must Wilbur Wright have looked to New Yorkers in 1909 as he flew his first flight around Manhattan Island! Today, of course, we hop the globe routinely, enjoying the great benefits of a fully matured science of flight. One should view the accomplishments of Steptoe and Edwards in 1978 as the "first flight," so to speak. Their introduction of in vitro fertilization to the world was only the beginning of an era in which fertility could truly be assisted in the scientific laboratory. In that perspective, it is most likely that we stand today about where flight was during that 1909 flight around Manhattan, with our current techniques akin to the biplane. With respect to the science of fertility therapy, what will be the equivalent of space flight, and of landing on another planet? Only time will tell. It is important for infertile couples to retain the hope that scientific advances relevant to them will come soon. Jewish couples who live within the guidelines of halakha must add to that hope the belief that, as God reveals His wonders through scientists and physicians, so will He reveal a consistent and productive way for observant couples to avail themselves of the developing technologies.

Endnotes

1. Leon R. Kass, *The New Republic*, (June 2, 1997).
2. Personal communication.
3. This pun is attributed to the Hatam Sofer. See *Mishpatei Uziel* 4 Hoshen Mishpat 6; *Tzitz Eliezer* 7:30; *Mishnah Halakhot* 12:181, 12:265 and 13:197.
4. M. Broyde, "Cloning people: A Jewish law analysis of the issues," *Connecticut Law Review*, 30:2, (1998).
5. J.D. Bleich, "In vitro fertilization: Questions of maternal identity and conversion," *Tradition* 25(4):82–102.
6. Concerning the prohibition on interspecies mixing, the Maharal explains, "There are those who are aghast of [sic] the interbreeding of two species. Certainly, this is contrary to Torah, which God gave the Jews, which prohibits

interspecies mixing. Nonetheless, Adam (the First Person) did this. Indeed, the world was created with many species that are prohibited to be eaten. Interspecies breeding was not prohibited because of prohibited sexuality or immorality.... Rather it is because [Jews] should not combine the various species together, as this is the way of Torah. As we already noted, the ways of the Torah, and the [permissible] ways of the world are distinct.... Just like the mule has within it to be created [but was not created by God]...but was left to people to create it. Even those forms of creativity which Jewish law prohibits for Jews, is not definitionally bad. Some are simply prohibited to Jews." Yehudah Luria of Prague (Maharal MePrague), *Bi'Ur Hagolah*, (Jerusalem, 5731), pp. 38–39.

7. Yehudah Luria of Prague (Maharal MePrague), *Bi'Ur Hagolah* , (Jerusalem, 5731), pp. 38–39.

8. J.A. Barritt, S. Willadsen, C. Brenner, J. Cohen, "Epigenetic and experimental modifications in early mammalian development: Part II. Cytoplasmic transfer in assisted reproduction," *Human Reproduction Update*, 7(4):428–435, (2001).

9. J. Zhang, et al., "In vitro maturation of human preovulatory oocytes reconstructed by germinal vesicle transfer," *Fertility and Sterility* 71:726–731, (1999).

10. E. Porcu, R. Fabbri, et al., "Birth of a healthy female after intracytoplasmic sperm injection of cryopreserved human oocytes," *Fertility and Sterility* 68:724–726, (1997).

11. K. Oktay, et al., "Ovarian tissue cryopreservation and transplantation: preliminary findings and implications for cancer patients," *Human Reproduction Update* 7(6):526–534, (2001).

Part VII
Resources

A Glossary of Medical
Acronyms and Terms

ACROSOME: The enzymes in a sperm's head that allows it to make a hole in the coating around an egg, penetrate, and fertilize the egg.

ADHESION: Scar tissue. Commonly occurs as a result of infection, endometriosis, or trauma, including surgery. Adhesions that occur in the pelvic cavity, fallopian tubes, or inside the uterus can interfere with transport of the egg and implantation of the embryo in the uterus.

ADNEXA: The region of the pelvis that includes the ovary, fallopian tube, and surrounding ligaments.

AMENORRHEA: The absence of menstruation. *Primary amenorrhea* defines a woman who has never menstruated. *Secondary amenorrhea* defines a woman who has menstruated at one time, but who has not had a period for six months or more.

ANOVULATION: The absence of ovulation. The failure of the ovary or ovarian follicle to develop and discharge eggs.

ANDROGENS: Male sex hormones such as testosterone and DHEAS.

ANDROLOGIST: A physician or scientist who performs laboratory evaluations of male fertility. May hold a PhD degree instead of an MD. Usually affiliated with a fertility treatment center and working with in vitro fertilization.

ANEUPLOIDY: Condition of having an abnormal number of chromosomes. A common cause of miscarriage is aneuploidy of the embryo.

ANTAGON®: A variant (analog) of gonadotropin releasing hormone (GnRHa) that causes suppression of gonadotropin (LH and FSH) secretion. Suppression occurs immediately with use.

ANTISPERM ANTIBODIES: Antibodies are produced by the immune system to fight off foreign substances, like bacteria. Antisperm antibodies attach themselves to sperm and inhibit their movement and ability to fertilize.

ARTIFICIAL INSEMINATION (AI): The placment of sperm into the vagina, uterus, or fallopian tubes through artificial means, usually by injection through a catheter or cannula. This term is often modified depending upon whether the procedure involves use of sperm from the husband (Artificial Insemination by Husband; AIH) or from a donor (Artificial Insemination by Donor; AID*). Intrauterine insemination (IUI) is the most common type of insemination performed and involves placement of sperm directly into the uterus. Common indications for IUI are low sperm counts, poor

---

* In the medical community, the term AID has largely been replaced by TDI, Therapeutic Donor Insemination, or simply DI, Donor Insemination.

motility, and to bypass hostile cervical mucus. *There are numerous halakhic issues pertaining to* AIH *and* AID. *Although most rabbinical authorities allow* AIH, *length of infertility,* niddah *status and method of semen production must all be considered. The use of donors for insemination is controversial.*

ASHERMAN'S SYNDROME: A condition where the uterine walls adhere to one another. Usually caused by uterine inflammation.

ASSISTED HATCHING (AH): A micromanipulation technique used in conjunction with in vitro fertilization. A small hole is created in the shell surrounding the embryo (zona pellucida) prior to transfer to the uterus. This may facilitate hatching of the embryo from its shell and increase the chance of implantation.

ASSISTED REPRODUCTIVE TECHNOLOGY (ART): A general term for several procedures employed to bring about conception without sexual intercourse, using a laboratory dish to incubate sperm, eggs, and embryos. Includes IVF, GIFT, and ZIFT. *Although most halakhic authorities allow the use of* ART, *there is no blanket approval for their use. Every case of infertility must be considered on its own merits prior to approving the use of* ART. *Certain conditions during* ART *may also be imposed.*

AZOSPERMIA: Absence of sperm in the ejaculate. This can result either from a lack of sperm production (non-obstructive azospermia) or from an inability of the sperm to reach the ejaculate (obstructive azospermia). *Obstructive azospermia* involves the obstruction in either the upper or lower male reproductive tract (epididymis, vas deferens, seminal vesicles or ejaculatory ducts). Sperm production may be normal (this can be verified through testicular biopsy), but the obstruction prevents the sperm from being ejaculated. Some causes of obstructive azospermia are vasectomy, congenital absence of the vas deferens, scarring from past infections, and hernia operations. *Non-obstructive azospermia* on the other hand, involves severely impaired or non-existent sperm production. Sperm found and extracted directly from the testicles may be used in conjunction with in vitro fertilization. *Diagnosing the cause of azospermia often requires testicular biopsy, which raises the problem of* pitzuah daka. *Azospermia that is non-obstructive may be absolute and therefore not amenable to any treatment, including* ART. *The only option for parenting may be the use of donor insemination, which is halakhically controversial.*

BASAL BODY TEMPERATURE (BBT): A woman's body temperature when taken at its lowest point, usually in the morning before getting out of bed. Charting BBT is one method of confirming ovulation.

BETA hCG TEST: A blood test used to detect very early pregnancies and to evaluate embryonic development. A beta test usually refers to a quantitative test of hCG level in which units of hCG are measured. It may also refer to a qualitative (yes/no) test that detects the presence of hCG level above a certain concentration.

BICORNUATE UTERUS: A congenital malformation of the uterus where the upper portion (horn) is duplicated.

BLASTOCYST: An embryo five or six days after fertilization. At this point the embryo has two different cell types and a central cavity. The surface cells (trophectoderm) will become the placenta, and the inner cell mass will become the fetus. A healthy blastocyst should hatch from the zona pellucida by the end of the sixth day. Within about 24 hours after hatching, it begins implanting into the lining of the uterus.

BLASTOCYST TRANSFER: Allowing in vitro fertilized embryos to reach the blastocyst stage before transferring them to the uterus.

BLASTOMERE: One of several identical cells in the early embryo, produced during early division (cleavage).

BRAVELLE®: Medication consisting of follicle stimulating hormone

(FSH), extracted and purified from human urine. Used for ovulation induction. Similar to Fertinex®.

BROMOCRIPTINE (PARLODEL®): An oral medication used to reduce high prolactin levels, including those produced by pituitary tumors. Common side effects include dizziness and upset stomach. It is helpful to start with low doses in order to limit these symptoms. Parlodel is equally effective when the tablet is used vaginally.

BUSERELIN: A long-acting gonadotropin releasing hormone analog (GnRHa) available in Europe as a nasal spray and used to suppress the function of the ovaries. May be used as a treatment for endometriosis, fibroid tumors, PMS, and hirsutism and also in conjunction with ovulation induction.

CAPACITATION: A change in sperm that occurs as it travels through the female reproductive tract. Capacitation enables the sperm to penetrate the egg.

CERVICAL STENOSIS: Blockage of the cervical canal. May result from a congenital defect or be acquired as a result of previous inflammation.

CERVICAL MUCUS: A viscous fluid plugging the opening of the cervix. Most of the time this thick mucus plug prevents sperm and bacteria from entering the womb. At midcycle, following ovulation, under the influence of estrogen, the mucus becomes thin, watery, and stringy to allow sperm to pass into the womb.

CHEMICAL PREGNANCY: A pregnancy where hCG levels are detected, but the pregnancy is lost before a gestational sac is seen on an ultrasound examination. This is the earliest form of pregnancy loss—often occurring before a woman misses her period—and not usually considered by physicians to be a true miscarriage.

447

CHLAMYDIA: A bacteria which is sexually transmitted and can lead to pelvic inflammatory disease (PID).

CHOCOLATE CYST: A cyst in the ovary that is filled with old blood. These cysts occur when endometriosis implants in an ovary and, over time, bleeds enough each month to form a blood filled sac, or endometrioma. (Over time, the blood takes on a characteristic chocolate color and consistency.) Frequently, patients with large endometriomas do not have any symptoms. If the cyst ruptures or the ovary containing the cyst twists, emergency surgery may be necessary. Management is usually by laparoscopic surgery.

CHROMOTUBATION: Usually done in conjunction with a diagnostic laparoscopy. It involves injecting colored liquid through the cervix and uterus and examining the ends of the fallopian tubes for spillage of dye. Spillage of dye indicates patent (open) tubes. Obstructed tubes will not transmit dye into the pelvis.

CHROMOSOME: The structure in the cell that carries genetic material (genes; DNA); the genetic messengers of inheritance. Normal human beings have forty-six chromosomes, twenty-three originating from the egg and twenty-three originating from the sperm.

CLEAVAGE: The series of cell divisions, or one of the cell divisions, of the fertilized egg that results in the formation of a multicellular embryo.

CLOMIPHENE CITRATE (CLOMID®, SEROPHENE®): A drug that stimulates ovulation through the release of gonadotropins from the pituitary gland.

CLOMIPHENE CITRATE CHALLENGE TEST (CCCT): This test entails the oral administration of 100 milligrams of clomiphene citrate on menstrual cycle days 5–9. Blood levels of FSH are measured on cycle day 3 and again on cycle day 10. Elevated blood levels of FSH on either day are associated with very low potential for pregnancy.

CONGENITAL ADRENAL HYPERPLASIA (CAH): Syndrome characterized by elevated androgens originating from the adrenal gland. Results in suppression of the pituitary gland and interference with sperm production in men and ovulation in women. Girls with CAH may have ambiguous genitalia from the excess production of male hormone. Certain forms of CAH may cause inadequate male hormone levels, resulting in ambiguous genitalia in genetic boys.

CONTROLLED OVARIAN HYPERSTIMULATION (COH): The use of fertility medications to stimulate the growth of multiple follicles for ovulation, generally in preparation for in vitro fertilization. Also called "Superovulation."

CORPUS LUTEUM: Translates literally to "yellow body." It is formed from the egg follicle after the egg is released, and produces progesterone, which causes the lining of the uterus (endometrium) to prepare for implantation of a fertilized egg.

CRYOPRESERVATION: Freezing and then storing tissue. Often used for sperm and embryos. More recently, unfertilized eggs and ovarian tissue have been cryopreserved. *Although it is feasible to freeze sperm and eggs for future use, individuals who are unmarried have no halakhic obligation to procreate; their use of these techniques is therefore halakhically problematic. Many authorities require that procurement and storage of cryospreserved material be performed under rabbinical supervision.*

CRYPTORCHIDISM: Failure of one or both testicles to descend into the scrotum.

CYTOPLASMIC TRANSFER: A variant of in vitro fertilization. The egg and sperm from the recipient couple are combined with some cellular fluid from a donor's egg. Currently of interest as a possible means to improve the outcome of in vitro fertilization in women with poor quality eggs. *Because cytoplasmic transfer involves the transfer of foreign genetic material—mitochondrial DNA—to the recipient, this technique raises most of the same controversial issues as standard egg donation.*

DANAZOL®: A synthetic estrogen used to treat edometriosis. Suppresses LH and FSH production by the pituitary and estrogen by the ovary. Produces a state of amenorrhea, during which implants of endometriosis may atrophy. Side effects with prolonged use include oily skin, acne, weight gain, abnormal hair growth, deepening of the voice and muscle cramps.

DIETHYLSTILBESTEROL (DES): A synthetic estrogen prescribed to women in the 1950s, 1960s and early 1970s to prevent miscarriage. Many male and female fetuses exposed in utero to this drug developed reproductive problems, including blockage of the vas deferens, uterine abnormalities, cervical deformities, miscarriages, and unexplained infertility. In 1971 the Federal Drug Administration banned the use of DES in the United States.

DILATION & CURETTAGE (D&C): A procedure used to dilate (expand) the cervical canal and remove the contents of the uterus. The procedure may be used to diagnose or treat the cause of abnormal bleeding. It is also used to terminate an or abnormal unwanted pregnancy.

DONOR EGG: Eggs donated by one woman to another.

DONOR INSEMINATION: Artificial insemination with donor sperm. (See ARTIFICIAL INSEMINATION)

DOSTINEX® (CABERGOLINE): An oral medication used to reduce high prolactin levels, including those produced by pituitary tumors.

Side effects are less common than with bromocryptine and pills are taken twice weekly instead of daily.

DYSMENORRHEA: Painful menstruation.

DYSPAREUNIA: Difficult or painful coitus.

ECTOPIC PREGNANCY: A pregnancy outside of the uterus, usually in the fallopian tube. Such a pregnancy cannot be sustained. Rupture of the tube is a medical emergency and may lead to loss of function. With early diagnosis of ectopic pregnancy, conservative measures to preserve tubal function are now available.

EGG DONOR: A women who contracts to donate eggs to an infertile couple for use in conjunction with in vitro fertilization. *The use of donated eggs to establish a pregnancy is a matter of halakhic controversy. Those authorities allowing the use of egg donors may favor particular characteristics of the egg donor, e.g. Jew, gentile, unmarried.*

EGG RETRIEVAL: The removal of eggs from the ovaries. A required part of many forms of assisted reproduction, including in vitro fertilization (IVF), gamete intrafallopian transfer (GIFT) and zygote intrafallopian transfer (ZIFT). For IVF and ZIFT, ultrasound is used to guide a needle through the vagina and into the ovary. During GIFT, eggs are retrieved by laparoscopy. *Undergoing egg retrieval on the Sabbath or festivals is problematic. Proper timing of therapy can avoid this problem.*

EJACULATE: The semen and sperm released at orgasm, or the act of releasing semen at orgasm. *Halakha recognizes that the emission of sperm need not always be for the purpose of procreation; however, under normal circumstances ejaculation should occur naturally and in conjunction with sexual intercourse. Ejaculation and examining of the ejaculate for fertility purposes has been extensively addressed by rabbinic authorities.*

ELECTROEJACULATION (EEJ): A controlled electric stimulation used to induce ejaculation in a man. Used when the nerves that control ejaculation are damaged, as in paraplegia. May also be used in psychogenic conditions causing inability to ejaculate. In such cases the procedure must be done under general anesthesia. *Instances exist where a healthy man must produce a semen specimen for evaluation or treatment, but cannot do so with sexual intercourse. In such cases, some rabbis prefer the use of EEJ to masturbation.*

EMBRYO: The early product of conception; the undifferentiated beginnings of a baby; the conceptus. *The embryo, while deserving of respect as a potential human being, has no halakhic status prior to implantation. Spare embryos produced as a result of ART may be discarded.*

EMBRYO TOXIC FACTOR: The immune response of a woman against her own fetus. May result in repeated pregnancy loss.

EMBRYO TOXICITY ASSAY (ETA): A combination of two procedures. The first involves maternal cell (lymphocyte) culture, aimed at stimulating the lymphocytes using components of the human embryo (trophoblast) cell line, and the second is an embryo culture. These procedures are used to determine if the patient's lymphocytes secrete anything toxic to the embryo (the test utilizes two-cell stage mouse embryos). Women who have been sensitized in the course of their earlier pregnancies, or by any other mode, could mount an immune response against their own fetus in the following pregnancy and end up losing it, either in the implantation process or later in the first trimester.

EMBRYO TRANSFER (ET): Placing an egg fertilized outside the womb into a woman's uterus or fallopian tube.

EMBRYOLOGIST: A scientist who specializes in embryo development and manipulation.

ENDOCRINE SYSTEM: System of glands including the hypothalamus, pituitary, thyroid, adrenals, and testicles or ovaries.

ENDOMETRIAL BIOPSY (EMB): A test used to detect defects in the luteal phase of the menstrual cycle. A small tissue sample of the uterine lining is removed and examined microscopically. Characteristics of the uterine lining and the cycle are considered in determining whether the ovary is appropriately secreting its hormones. *The performance of endometrial biopsy invariably results in uterine bleeding. A halakhic authority should be consulted to determine if a state of* niddah *results.*

ENDOMETRIOMA: A solitary, non-neoplastic mass containing endometrial tissue and blood. See CHOCOLATE CYST.

ENDOMETRIOSIS: Growth of endometrial tissue outside the uterus. The tissue may attach itself to the reproductive organs in the pelvis or to other organs in the abdominal cavity. Each month the endometrial tissue bleeds with the onset of menses. The resultant irritation may cause adhesions to form. Endometriosis may also interfere with ovulation and implantation of the embryo.

ENDOMETRIUM: Medical term for the lining of the uterus, which is built up to sustain pregnancy and shed through menstruation if pregnancy does not occur.

EPIDIDYMIS: A coiled, tubular organ attached to and lying on the testicle. Within this organ the developing sperm complete their maturation and develop their powerful swimming capabilities. The matured sperm leave the epididymis through the vas deferens.

ESTRADIOL (E2): The principal form of estrogen produced by the ovary. Responsible for formation of the female secondary sex characteristics such as breasts; supports the development of the uterine lining. At midcycle the high estrogen level triggers the release of luteinizing hormone (LH) from the pituitary gland. The "LH surge" is necessary for the release of the ovum from the follicle. LH in men stimulates the testicle to produce testosterone. Fat cells in obese men and women can manufacture estrogen, which suppresses normal pituitary function and interferes with normal fertility. The blood test to monitor estradiol is the E2-Rapid Assay. Women on injectable fertility drugs have routine E2 testing in conjunction with serial transvaginal sonograms (TVS). *Frequent E2 and TVS monitoring must accompany ovulation induction, especially in conjunction with ART, and are often performed on a daily basis. One must be careful, when planning a cycle of treatment, to make sure that such monitoring will not be required on Sabbath or a festival.*

ESTROGEN: The female sex hormone. First recognized around 1915, estrogen is responsible for the development of the secondary feminine sex characteristics, which include breasts and rounded hips. Together with progesterone, another female hormone secreted by the ovaries, estrogen regulates the changes that occur with each monthly period and prepares the uterus for pregnancy.

FALLOPIAN TUBE: Duct through which the egg travels to the uterus after it has been released from the follicle. Sperm also travel through the tube for some time following intercourse which occurs around the time of ovulation. The fallopian tube is the site at which fertilization usually occurs. The fallopian tube is divided anatomically into several regions: closest to the uterus and within the uterine wall is the "interstitial" portion; moving outward is the "isthmus," the "ampulla," and then the "infundibular" portion. The "fimbria" are located at the very end of the tube, adjacent to the ovary.

FALLOPOSCOPY: The visual examination of the inside of the fallopian tube. A small flexible catheter is inserted through the cervical canal, uterine cavity and finally into the fallopian tube. A tiny, flexible fiber optic endoscope is threaded through the catheter into the fallopian tube. A camera at the end of the falloposcope transfers images of the inside of the tube to a video monitor so that the surgeon can thoroughly visualize and examine the inside of the tube. If problems are found, surgical repairs can be made at the same time. This procedure has not gained wide use in the United States.

FERNING: A pattern characteristic of dried cervical mucus viewed on a microscope slide. When the fern leaf pattern appears, it signifies that the mucus has been thinned and prepared by estrogen for the passage of sperm. Lack of ferning signifies that at the time of the test the mucus is impenetrable to sperm.

FERTILITY SPECIALIST: A physician with special training and experience in the treatment of reproductive disorders. Usually refers to physicians certified by the American Board of Obstetrics and Gynecology as specialists in Reproductive Endocrinology and Infertility. Physicians with such certification are called Reproductive Endocrinologists (RES).

FERTILITY TREATMENT: Any method or procedure used to enhance fertility or increase the likelihood of pregnancy. Includes medical and surgical interventions, such as ovulation induction, microsurgery to repair damaged fallopian tubes, and varicocele repair. The goal of every fertility treatment is either to help a woman conceive or to help a man father a child.

FERTINEX®: Follicle stimulating hormone (FSH) derived from human urine, highly purified and used to stimulate follicular growth, which can be injected subcutaneously. Similar to Bravelle®.

FETUS: A term used to refer to a developing baby during the period of gestation between eight weeks and term.

FIBROID (MYOMA; LEIOMYOMA): A benign tumor of the uterine muscle and connective tissue.

FIMBRIA: The finger-like projections at the end of the fallopian tube nearest the ovary. These projections capture the egg as it is released from the follicle and deliver it into the fallopian tube.

FIMBRIOPLASTY: Plastic or reconstructive surgery to repair fimbria that are damaged and interfere with capture of the egg by the fallopian tube.

FOLLICLE: Fluid-filled cyst in the ovary in which the egg matures prior to its release at ovulation.

FOLLICLE STIMULATING HORMONE (FSH): A pituitary hormone that stimulates spermatogenesis in men and follicular development in women. In men FSH stimulates the Sertoli cells in the testicles and supports sperm production. In women FSH stimulates egg maturation and growth of the ovarian follicle. Elevated FSH levels are indicative of poorly functioning testicles or ovaries.

FOLLICULAR FLUID: The fluid inside the follicle that cushions and nourishes the egg.

FOLLICULAR PHASE: The preovulatory portion of a woman's cycle during which a follicle develops and high levels of estrogen cause the lining of the uterus to proliferate. Normally takes between 12 and 14 days.

FOLLISTIM®: Medication consisting of highly purified follicle stimulating hormone (FSH), produced using recombinant DNA technology. Used in ovulation induction and controlled ovarian hyperstimulation. Similar to Gonal f®.

FROZEN EMBRYO TRANSFER (FET): A procedure where frozen embryos are thawed and then placed into the uterus.

GAMETE: A reproductive cell; sperm in men, the egg in women.

GAMETE INTRAFALLOPIAN TRANSFER (GIFT): A technique that may be used in lieu of in vitro fertilization for women with patent (clear, open) fallopian tubes. After egg retrieval the eggs and sperm are combined and immediately injected into the woman's fallopian tubes, where fertilization may occur *in vivo.* The procedure is carried out through laparoscopy. *In earlier days of ART, some rabbis preferred GIFT to IVF because fertilization occurred in the natural environment of the fallopian tube. In addition, pregnancy rates with GIFT were somewhat higher than those with IVF. IVF as currently practiced yields pregnancy rates superior to those with GIFT, and is also more useful than GIFT for many indications. The dominant halakhic view is that IVF and GIFT are equally permissible.*

GERM CELL: Cells from which sperm are produced in men and eggs are produced in women. Healthy testicular tissue continues to produce germ cell throughout a man's reproductive life; women have a finite supply of germ cells, which they lose at the rate of about one thousand per menstrual cycle, although usually only one egg ovulates during each cycle.

GERM CELL APLASIA (SERTOLI CELL ONLY): An inherited condition in which the testicles have no germ cells. Since men having this condition have normal Leydig cells, they develop normal secondary sexual characteristics, such as muscular build and facial hair. May also be caused by exposure to toxins or radiation. See AZOSPERMIA. *The only option for parenting in this situation is the use of donor insemination, which is halakhically controversial.*

GESTATIONAL HOST: A woman who contracts to carry a pregnancy for someone else. The host gives birth to, but is not the biological mother of, the baby being carried. *Using a gestational host invokes numerous halakhic issues, including the question of who is the halakhic mother. The guidance of a rabbinical authority with special expertise in reproductive halakha should be sought.*

GONADOTROPIN RELEASING HORMONE (GnRH): The hormone that controls the production and release of gonadotropins (FSH and LH) from the pituitary gland. Pulsatile secretion from the hypothalamus occurs every sixty to ninety minutes.

GONADOTROPINS: Hormones that control reproductive function: follicle stimulating hormone (FSH) and luteinizing hormone (LH).

GONAL F®: Medication consisting of highly purified follicle stimulating hormone (FSH), produced using recombinant DNA technology. Used in ovulation induction and controlled ovarian hyperstimulation. Similar to Follistim®.

HAMSTER TEST: A test of the ability of sperm to penetrate a hamster egg which has been stripped of its zona pellucida (outer membrane). Also called Sperm Penetration Assay (SPA).

HIRSUTISM: The overabundance of body hair, such as a mustache or pubic hair growing upward toward the navel, found in women with excess androgens.

HORMONE: A substance produced by an endocrine gland that travels through the bloodstream to a specific organ, which it influences.

HOST UTERUS: Also called a "gestational host." A couple's embryo is transferred to another woman who carries the pregnancy to term and returns the baby to the genetic parents immediately after birth. *Using a gestational host invokes numerous halakhic issues. The guidance of a rabbinical authority with special expertise in reproductive halakha should be sought.*

HOSTILE MUCUS: Cervical mucus that impedes the natural progress of sperm through the cervical canal. *The most straightforward* *way of overcoming infertility that results from hostile cervical mucus is intrauterine insemination. If this is not permitted halakhically, then alternative, medical measures are occasionally successful in changing the characteristics of the cervical mucus.*

HUMAN CHORIONIC GONADOTROPIN (hCG):* The hormone produced in early pregnancy that keeps the corpus luteum producing progesterone. Used via injection to trigger ovulation after some fertility treatments. Also used in men to stimulate testosterone production.

HUMAN MENOPAUSAL GONADOTROPIN (hMG, REPRONEX®, PERGONAL®, HUMEGON®): Combination of hormones FSH and LH that is extracted from the urine of post-menopausal women. Used in ovulation induction and controlled ovarian hyperstimulation.

HUMEGON®: Combination of hormones FSH and LH that is extracted from the urine of post-menopausal women. Used in ovulation induction and controlled ovarian hyperstimulation. Similar to Pergonal®. No longer used in the United States.

HYPERPROLACTINEMIA: Excessive prolactin levels, which may impair fertility.

HYPERSTIMULATION (OVARIAN HYPERSTIMULATION SYNDROME/OHSS): An uncommon but potentially life-threatening side effect of ovulation induction with injectable fertility medications such as hMG and FSH. The ovaries produce an overabundance of eggs, causing hormone levels to rise. After ovulation, the ovaries may enlarge and cause fluid to collect in the abdominal cavity, causing pain and bloating. Dehydration is common, and increases the danger of blood clotting (thrombosis). Twisting of the ovary or

---

* Gonadotropin exists in similar but distinct forms in different species. The small h in the abbreviation indicates specifically human CG.

rupture of a cyst may occur. Symptoms include sudden weight gain and abdominal pain. Careful monitoring of a woman's response to these fertility medications by ultrasound scans and hormone testing is used to prevent or limit the occurrence of OHSS.

HYPOTHALAMUS: A part of the brain that acts as the hormonal regulation center, located adjacent to and above the pituitary gland. In both the man and the woman this tissue secretes GnRH every sixty to ninety minutes. The pulsatile GnRH enables the pituitary gland to secrete LH and FSH, which stimulate the gonads.

HYSTEROSALPINGOGRAM (HSG): An x-ray of the pelvic organs in which a radio-opaque dye is injected through the cervix into the uterus and fallopian tubes. This test checks for malformations of the uterus and/or blockage of the fallopian tubes.

HYSTEROSCOPY: Procedure in which a fiberoptic telescope is placed through the cervical canal and into the uterine cavity in order to detect and repair abnormalities.

IDIOPATHIC (UNEXPLAINED) INFERTILITY: Infertility for which no cause can be found even after substantial testing.

IMMATURE OOCYTE RETRIEVAL (IOR): A procedure in which immature eggs are aspirated from the ovaries and treated in the laboratory to bring them to maturity. At maturity they are mixed with sperm and the resulting embryos are transferred into the uterus.

IMMATURE SPERM (GERMINAL CELL): A sperm that has not matured and gained the ability to swim. In the presence of illness or infection such sperm may appear in the semen in large numbers.

IMMUNE SYSTEM: The body's defense mechanism against any injury or invasion by a foreign substance or organism.

IMMUNOBEAD BINDING TEST (IBT): Used to detect antisperm antibodies (ASA).

IMPLANTATION: The embedding of the embryo into tissue so it can establish contact with the mother's blood supply for nourishment. Implantation usually occurs in the lining of the uterus approximately five days after ovulation; in an ectopic pregnancy implantation occurs outside of the uterus.

IMPOTENCE: The inability of a man to achieve or maintain an erection and to ejaculate due to physical or emotional problems, or a combination thereof. This is not the same thing as being sterile.

INCOMPETENT CERVIX: A cervix that opens up prematurely during pregnancy, which may cause the loss of the fetus. Cervical cerclage is a procedure in which a stitch is placed around the cervix to prevent its opening prematurely. It is removed when the pregnancy reaches term.

INFERTILITY: The inability to conceive after a year of unprotected intercourse in women under 35, or after six months in women over 35, or the inability to carry a pregnancy to term. Includes problems such as anovulation, tubal blockage, low sperm count. *The occurrence of infertility does not necessarily imply halakhic permission to treat. Although the halakha generally takes a positive position toward medical intervention, including for the purposes of alleviating infertility, the proper approach to diagnosis and treatment varies according to different halakhic authorities.*

INTRACERVICAL INSEMINATION: Artificial insemination where the sperm are placed into the cervical canal. Most often used when the sperm counts are normal, as with donor sperm or in psychogenic infertility.

INTRACYTOPLASMIC SPERM INJECTION (ICSI): A procedure in

which a single sperm is injected into the egg to enable fertilization with very low sperm counts or with non-motile sperm.

INTRAMUSCULAR (IM): An IM medication is given by needle into the muscle. Contrast with a medication that is given by a needle, for example, into the skin (intradermal) or just below the skin (subcutaneous) or into a vein (intravenous).

INTRAUTERINE INSEMINATION (IUI): A relatively "low-tech" fertility-enhancing procedure in which washed sperm are placed directly into the uterus, bypassing the cervix and approaching nearer to the fallopian tubes, where fertilization occurs. Used to overcome hostile cervical mucus and to compensate for sperm count and motility problems. *There are many potential halakhic pitfalls during the performance of IUI. These include timing during the cycle, sperm procurement, rabbinical oversight in the laboratory, post-procedure bleeding, and more. It is useful for observant couples undergoing IUI to have discussed all of these concerns with their* posek *prior to commencing therapy.*

IN VITRO FERTILIZATION (IVF): Literally means "in glass." Fertilization which takes place outside the body in a small glass dish. The actual Petri dishes that are used during IVF today are made of plastic. *IVF is widely accepted by halakhic authorities. However, many potential halakhic conflicts exist. It is useful for observant couples undergoing IVF to have discussed all of these concerns with their* posek *prior to commencing therapy.*

KARYOTYPE: The chromosomal characteristics of a cell.

KRUGER MORPHOLOGY: A grading system, first described by Tineas Kruger, used to microscopically describe the structure of human spermatozoa. The Kruger criteria include exact requirements for sperm head length and width, as well as other criteria for measuring the acrosome, midpiece, and tail. Also called "strict morphology," the test correlates better than standard morphology criteria in predicting the outcome of in vitro fertilization.

LAPAROSCOPE: A thin telescope that can be inserted through an incision in the abdominal wall for viewing the internal organs; the instrument used to perform a laparoscopy. Commonly used to diagnose and treat a number of fertility problems including endometriosis, pelvic adhesions, and various forms of tubal damage. Also used in some ART procedures such as GIFT and ZIFT.

LAPAROSCOPY: Examination of the pelvic region using a small telescope called a laparoscope.

LEYDIG CELL: The testicular cell that produces the male hormone testosterone. The Leydig cell is stimulated by LH from the pituitary gland.

LOW RESPONDER: A woman who does not produce many egg follicles when treated with fertility medications. Such women usually have a relatively low number of eggs within their ovaries.

LUPRON®: A variant (analog) of gonadotropin releasing hormone (GnRHa) that causes suppression of gonadotropin (LH and FSH) secretion. Suppression occurs after a brief period of stimulation.

LUTEAL PHASE: Postovulatory phase of a woman's cycle. Characterized by control by the corpus luteum, which secretes progesterone to prepare the uterine lining for implantation of the embryo.

LUTEAL PHASE DEFECT (OR DEFICIENCY; LPD): Inadequate function of the corpus luteum that may prevent a fertilized egg from implanting in the uterus, leading to infertility or early pregnancy loss.

LUTEINIZED UNRUPTURED FOLLICLE SYNDROME (LUFS):

Failure of a follicle to release the egg even though a corpus luteum has formed.

LUTEINIZING HORMONE (LH): The pituitary hormone that stimulates the manufacture of sex hormones in both men and women. In women the sharp spike in LH secretion causes ovulation.

LUTEINIZING HORMONE SURGE (LH SURGE): The intense release of luteinizing hormone (LH) from the pituitary gland that occurs when an egg reaches maturity in the ovary. This hormonal surge brings about a series of changes in the egg follicle that leads to release of the egg. Ovulation predictor kits (OPK) detect the sudden increase of LH, signaling that ovulation will occur within 24–36 hours.

MAGNETIC RESONANCE IMAGING (MRI): A procedure using a magnet linked to a computer to create detailed pictures of areas inside the body.

MATURATION ARREST: A testicular condition in which at one stage of sperm production all sperm development halts throughout all testicular tubules. May result in OLIGPSPERMIA or AZOSPERMIA.

MEIOSIS: The cell division, peculiar to reproductive cells, which allows genetic material to divide in half. Each of the two new cells produced by meiosis contains 23 chromosomes. Spermatids (immature sperm) and ova (eggs) are produced by meiosis. When they combine (fertilize) normally, the resulting embryo has a normal complement of 46 chromosomes.

MENARCHE: The time when a girl first menstruates.

MENOPAUSE: The time a woman stops menstruating.

MENORRHAGIA: Heavy or prolonged menstrual flow. *This usually confers the state of* niddah. *When prolonged, the woman may retain* her niddah *status for weeks or even months. Careful examination by a physician or nurse is required to determine the source of bleeding. It is often helpful for the examiner to confer with a halakhic authority competent in the area of* niddah *in order to properly advise the woman.*

METHOTREXATE: An anticancer drug that is an analog of folic acid and an antimetabolite. Used to treat molar pregnancies. Often used as an alternative to surgery for ectopic pregnancies that have been diagnosed prior to rupture.

METRODIN®: Medication consisting of follicle stimulating hormone (FSH), extracted and purified from human urine. Was used for ovulation induction. No longer in production in the United States.

MICROSURGICAL EPIDIDYMAL SPERM ASPIRATION (MESA): Using microsurgery to remove sperm from the epididymis for use with in vitro fertilization, often with ICSI. *Any procedure performed on the male external genitalia raises the issues of* pitzuah daka *and* kerut shifhah. *Although generally permissible, there are numerous halakhic considerations that should precede performance of* MESA.

MISSED ABORTION: The fetus fails to develop or dies in the uterus, but there is no bleeding or cramping. A D&C is usually done to remove the conception and prevent complications.

MITOSIS: The division of a cell into two identical cells, each containing the original genetic complement of chromosomes.

MORPHOLOGY: The study of shapes; here for semen analysis. The higher the percentage of misshapen sperm, the less likely fertilization will take place.

MOTILITY: The ability of sperm to swim. Poor motility means the sperm have a difficult time swimming toward their goal, i.e. the egg.

MYOMECTOMY: Surgical removal of a uterine fibroid.

NON-OBSTRUCTIVE AZOSPERMIA: Severely impaired or nonexistent sperm production. See AZOSPERMIA.

NUCLEAR TRANSFER: A micromanipulation procedure used to exchange genetic material between oocytes. Requires electrofusion to stimulate fusion of the cell membranes. Exchange of nuclear material from one egg to another has implications for the possible treatment of infertility due to female aging.

OBSTRUCTIVE AZOSPERMIA: Failure of sperm to be emitted in the semen as a result of blockage in the male reproductive tract. Sperm production may be normal but the sperm remain trapped inside the epididymis. See AZOSPERMIA. *This condition may be overcome with surgical repair or by the use of ART with sperm retrieved from the testicle or epididymis. When feasible and logical, surgical repair may be halakhically preferable to ART.*

OLIGOMENORRHEA: Infrequent menstrual periods.

OLIGOSPERMIA: Having few sperm.

OOCYTE: Egg cell

OVARIAN FAILURE: The failure of the ovary to respond to FSH stimulation from the pituitary gland because of the complete loss of eggs. Diagnosed by elevated FSH levels in the blood. Ovarian failure may be natural, as with normal menopause, or premature (POF), as a result of genetic abnormalities, surgery, or unexplained factors. *When there are no eggs, the only option for pregnancy is with the use of egg donation. The use of donated eggs to establish a pregnancy is a matter of halakhic controversy.*

OVARIAN CYST: A fluid-filled sac inside the ovary. An ovarian cyst may be found in conjunction with ovulation disorders, tumors of the ovary, and endometriosis.

OVARIAN DRILLING: During a laparoscopy, an electrosurgery needle or laser fiber is used to destroy egg follicles in each ovary. This procedure may help reduce androgen levels and restore normal ovulation in some women with polycystic ovary syndrome (PCOS).

OVARIAN HYPERSTIMULATION SYNDROME: See HYPERSTIMULATION.

OVULATION: The release of the egg (ovum) from the ovarian follicle.

OVULATION INDUCTION: Medical treatment performed to initiate ovulation. See also, BRAVELLE®, CLOMIPHENE CITRATE, FERTINEX®, FOLLISTIM®, GONAL-F®, HUMEGON®, METRODIN®, PERGONAL®, REPRONEX®.

OVULATION PREDICTOR KIT (OPK): A test kit a woman can use at home to predict forthcoming ovulation; based on a surge of luteinizing hormone (LH).

OVULATORY DYSFUNCTION: A problem existing in the ovary where either the developmental process of the follicle is abnormal or the egg is not released from the follicle.

OVUM: The egg; the reproductive cell from the ovary; the female gamete; the sex cell that brings the woman's genetic information to the new embryo.

PARLODEL®: See BROMOCRIPTINE.

PATENT: The condition of being open, as with tubes that form part of the reproductive organs. An HSG, for example, is done to see if the fallopian tubes are patent.

PELVIC INFLAMMATORY DISEASE (PID): An infection of any of the pelvic organs that, if left untreated, may result in infertility. Usually, but not always, caused by a sexually transmitted disease.

PERCUTANEOUS EPIDIDYMAL SPERM ASPIRATION (PESA): A procedure whereby a small needle is passed through the skin of the scrotum directly into the head of the epididymis and fluid is aspirated. Any sperm found may be used in conjunction with in vitro fertilization and ICSI. *Any procedure performed on the male external genitalia raises the issues of* pitzuah daka *and* kerut shifhah. *Although generally permissible, there are numerous halakhic considerations that precede performance of* PESA.

PERGONAL® (**HMG**): Follicle stimulating hormone (FSH) and luteinizing hormone (LH) recovered from the urine of postmenopausal women. Used to stimulate follicular growth in some fertility treatments. Similar to Humegon®. No longer in production in the United States.

PITUITARY GLAND: Sometimes called the master gland; the gland that is stimulated by the hypothalamus and controls all hormonal functions. Located at the base of the brain just below the hypothalamus, this gland controls many major hormonal factories throughout the body including the gonads, the adrenal glands, and the thyroid gland.

POLAR BODY: The discarded genetic material resulting from female germ cell division.

---

* There are no actual cysts in the polycystic ovary. The term refers to the appearance of the small egg follicles when viewed under a microscope. Surgical intervention is usually not required.

POLYCYSTIC OVARY SYNDROME (PCOS; "STEIN-LEVENTHAL SYNDROME"): A condition found in women who do not ovulate, characterized by excessive production of androgens (male sex hormones) and the presence of many small egg follicles in the ovaries.* Typical symptoms of PCOS include excessive weight gain, acne, excessive hair growth, menstrual irregularity and infertility.

POLYP: A growth or tumor, usually benign, on an internal surface such as the uterine wall. *Uterine polyps may be a source of intermittent bleeding or menorrhagia. Such bleeding may confer on a woman a state of prolonged or even perpetual* niddah. *Removal of the polyp in such cases may obviate the halakhic dilemma.*

POLYSPERMY: More than one sperm entering and fertilizing an egg. The resultant embryo is nonviable. If implantation occurs, miscarriage inevitably occurs.

POSTCOITAL TEST (PCT): An examination of the woman's cervical mucus after intercourse. Determines the presence of sperm and if they are able to move within the mucus. *The significance and worth of performing postcoital testing is debated among fertility specialists, many of whom have abandoned it altogether. The worth and significance of performing this procedure for observant Jewish couples, however, is clear. Most rabbis prefer that postcoital testing be done prior to semen analysis because of the many halakhic problems surrounding the latter test. While the results of the PCT cannot supplant those of the traditional semen analysis for assessing male fertility, in some cases the result of the PCT is suggestive enough to point in a certain direction. For example, when an accurately timed PCT repeatedly shows no sperm, sexual dysfunction and/or a problem with sperm production must be considered.*

PREIMPLANTATION GENETIC DIAGNOSIS (PGD): A method of assessing the genetic composition of embryos prior to transfer to the uterus. Used in conjunction with in vitro fertilization. *PGD is used mainly to prevent the transmission of genetic diseases to the offspring. For couples already undergoing in vitro fertilization for infertility, there are virtually no halakhic issues. Couples without infertility but who are carriers for genetic diseases face the dilemma of pregnancy and miscarriage or abortion, or undergoing IVF with PGD. This matter requires rabbinical consultation. Other than to select out a sex-linked recessive gene, the use of PGD for gender selection is generally not permissible halakhically.*

PREMATURE OVARIAN FAILURE (POF): The cessation of menses before age 40. Diagnosed by the finding of high levels of gonado-tropins and low levels of estrogen. The ovary may intermittently produce mature follicles. See OVARIAN FAILURE.

PRIMARY INFERTILITY: Refers to a woman or couple with infertility who has never before conceived. Popular usage has been extended to include those who have conceived but not had a live birth.

PROGESTERONE: The hormone produced by the corpus luteum of the ovary during the second half of a woman's cycle. Responsible for preparing the lining of the uterus to allow implantation of a fertilized egg. Many forms of progesterone are used to support early pregnancy during reproductive therapy.

PROGESTERONE WITHDRAWAL: A diagnostic procedure used to analyze menstrual irregularity and amenorrhea; uterine bleeding that occurs within two weeks after taking progesterone; a procedure used to demonstrate the presence or absence of estrogen and to demonstrate the ability of the uterus and reproductive tract to bleed. Prior to ovulation induction therapy, progesterone withdrawal may be used to induce a menstrual period.

PROGESTIN: Synthetic hormone that mimics the effect of proges-terone.

PROLACTIN: The hormone that stimulates the production of milk in breast-feeding women. Excessive prolactin levels when not breast-feeding may result in infertility.

PROVERA®: A type of Progestin in common use, especially for the induction of progesterone withdrawal bleeding.

PYOSPERMIA: The presence of white cells in the semen; indicates possible infection and/or inflammation.

RECOMBINANT FOLLICLE STIMULATING HORMONE (r-FSH, rh-FSH): Genetically engineered follicle stimulating hormone, as contrasted with FSH extracted from the urine of post menopausal women. Synthesized in vitro by cells into which genes encoding for FSH subunits have been inserted. Brand names are Gonal-F® and Follistim®.

RECURRENT PREGNANCY LOSS (RPL): Repeated miscarriages. Testing can be done to try to determine the cause of such losses. If an underlying condition is found, the woman may need to be treated for the problem before a pregnancy can be carried to term.

REPRODUCTIVE ENDOCRINOLOGIST: An obstetrician/gynecologist (OBGYN) with special training and certification in the treatment of hormonal disorders and infertility. All reproductive endocrinologists are considered "fertility specialists." However, not all physicians who refer to themselves as "fertility specialists" are certified reproductive endocrinologists.

REPRODUCTIVE SURGEON: An obstetrician/gynecologist or urologist who specializes in the surgical correction of anatomical disorders that affect reproductive function.

REPRONEX®: Medication consisting of follicle stimulating hormone (FSH) and luteinizing hormone (LH), extracted and purified from human urine. Used for ovulation induction. Similar to Pergonal® but can be injected subcutaneously.

RETROGRADE EJACULATION: A male fertility problem characterized by sperm emission into the bladder instead of out of the penis; usually due to a failure in the sphincter muscle at the base of the bladder. *There are fewer halakhic problems with specimen production because there is no emission during ejaculation. Sperm may be retrieved from the bladder and used for insemination or in vitro fertilization, each of which entails numerous halakhic considerations.*

SALPINGECTOMY: Surgical removal of the fallopian tube.

SALPINGITIS: An inflammation of one or both fallopian tubes, usually a result of infection. May result in tubal damage and female infertility.

SALPINGOSTOMY: A surgical procedure used to repair a fallopian tube blocked at its end, in which an incision is created to allow future entry of the egg. This term is also commonly used to describe the surgical procedure used to remove a tubal pregnancy (more properly termed salpingotomy).

SECONDARY INFERTILITY: The inability of a couple who has successfully achieved pregnancy to achieve another. This strict medical definition includes couples for whom the pregnancy did not go to term. The common vernacular, however, refers to a couple who has at least one biological child but is unable to conceive another.

SEPTATE UTERUS: A congenital abnormality in which the uterine cavity is divided into two halves by the presence of a fibrous band of tissue. May cause recurrent pregnancy loss.

SEMEN: The ejaculated fluid from the male containing sperm and secretion from the testicles, prostate, and seminal vesicles. *The halakha does not distinguish between semen and sperm. Both are interchangeably referred to as zera. In halakhic parlance the semen is considered in some fashion to be alive; hence the prohibition of needlessly spilling the seed.*

SEMEN ANALYSIS: A laboratory test used to assess semen quality: measures sperm quantity, concentration, morphology (form), and motility (movement). In addition, it measures semen (fluid) volume and whether or not white blood cells, which would indicate an infection, are present. *The predictive value, cost, and level of invasiveness (none) of the semen analysis makes it one of the first tests normally performed in the clinical evaluation of infertility. For the observant Jewish couple, the order of testing may need to be changed because of halakhic problems relating to the production of semen for analysis.*

SEROPHENE®: Brand name for CLOMIPHENE CITRATE.

SONOGRAM (ULTRASOUND): Use of high-frequency sound waves for creating an image of internal body parts. Used to detect and count follicle growth (and disappearance) in many fertility treatments. Also used to detect and monitor pregnancy. During fertility treatments, nearly all sonograms are performed using a special probe inserted through the vagina (transvaginal sonogram; TVS). *The performance of TVS is akin to a bimanual exam, and can never confer the state of niddah. Cervical bleeding that may occur as a result of TVS does not render a woman niddah.*

SONOHYSTEROGRAM: A sonogram in which saline is injected into the uterus. Used to check for uterine abnormalities such as polyps or fibroids. It has some similarity to a hysterosalpingogram, but does not require radio-opaque dye injection or radiation exposure. Is not used to demonstrate tubal patency and anatomy.

SPERM: The microscopic cell that carries the male's genetic information to the female's egg; the male reproductive cell; the male gamete.

SPERM BANK: A place where sperm are kept frozen in liquid nitrogen for later use in artificial insemination. The sperm bank may store material from intimate partners as well as from anonymous donors.

SPERM COUNT: The number of sperm in the ejaculate. Also called sperm concentration; given as the number of sperm per milliliter.

SPERM WASHING: Laboratory techniques for separating sperm from semen, and separating motile sperm from non-motile sperm, for use with intrauterine insemination or other forms of assisted reproduction. *With all types of sperm washing there is loss of motile sperm along with the immotile sperm and seminal fluid. Halakha does not consider this to be "wasting" of the seed, as it is an unintentional byproduct* (psolet) *of the washing procedure.**

SPINNBARKEIT: The inherent ability of cervical mucus to stretch; the stringy quality of cervical mucus that only occurs at midcycle under the influence of estrogen.

SPONTANEOUS ABORTION: An unplanned end to a pregnancy during the first 20 weeks. *The halakha requires men who are not from the Levite tribe to perform* pidyon haben, *the redemption of the first product of the womb* (peter rehem) *if it is male. The delivery must be natural (vaginal) and there must have been no preceding births. A spontaneous abortion that occurs prior to 40 days after conception, when fetal parts become recognizable, is not considered a birth for purposes of* pidyon haben.

STERILITY: An irreversible condition that prevents conception.

SUPEROVULATION: Stimulation of multiple ovulations with fertility drugs; also known as controlled ovarian hyperstimulation (COH). Used mainly in preparation for assisted reproduction.

---

*   Personal communication, Prof. Abraham S. Abraham.

SURROGATE MOTHER: A woman who is artificially inseminated and carries to term a baby that will be adopted and raised by its genetic father and his partner. The term is usually used for a woman who is the genetic mother of the baby she is carrying, as contrasted with a gestational host, who carries a fetus that is not genetically hers. *As the biological mother of the egg as well as the birth mother is the same woman, the halakhic mother can only be the surrogate as well.*

TERATOGEN: Any substance capable of causing malformations in a developing embryo or fetus.

TESTICULAR BIOPSY: A minor surgical procedure used to take a small sample of testicular tissue for microscopic examination. This test is used to distinguish obstructive from non-obstructive causes of azospermia. *Any procedure performed on the male genitalia raises the issues of* pitzuah daka *and* kerut shifhah. *Although generally permissible, there are numerous halakhic considerations that precede performance of testicular biopsy.*

TESTICULAR FAILURE: *Primary Testicular Failure* refers to a congenital, developmental, or genetic error resulting in a testicular malformation that prevents sperm production. *Secondary Testicular Failure* refers to acquired testicular damage, such as might result, for example, from drugs, prolonged exposure to toxic substances, or a varicocele.

TESTICULAR SPERM ASPIRATION (TESA): A needle biopsy of the testicle used to obtain small amounts of sperm. A small incision is made in the scrotal skin and a needle is used to aspirate sperm from the testicle. Usually does not result in enough sperm to freeze for later use. *Any procedure performed on the male genitalia raises the issues of* pitzuah daka *and* kerut shifhah. *Although generally permissible, there are numerous halakhic considerations that precede performance of TESA.*

TESTICULAR SPERM EXTRACTION (TESE): An open biopsy done through a skin incision where seminiferous tubules from the testicle are removed. After transfer to a culture medium, sperm are released from within the tubules and are extracted from the surrounding testicular tissue. It is possible to get enough sperm to freeze for future use. *Any procedure performed on the male genitalia raises the issues of* pitzuah daka *and* kerut shifhah. *Although generally permissible, there are numerous halakhic considerations that precede performance of* TESE.

TESTOSTERONE: The male hormone responsible for the formation of secondary sex characteristics and for supporting the sex drive. Testosterone is also necessary for spermatogenesis.

THYROID GLAND: The endocrine gland in the front of the neck that produces thyroid hormones to regulate the body's metabolism.

TRANSVAGINAL ULTRASOUND (TVS): An ultrasound examination performed by means of inserting a probe into the vagina. This type of ultrasound is common for viewing follicle growth. Used in early pregnancy to produce images that are superior to those that can be obtained by conventional sonograms done over the abdomen.

TUBAL EMBRYO TRANSFER (TET): The placement of an embryo inside the fallopian tube after in vitro fertilization. The process is meant to mimic the natural process of a fertilized embryo traveling down the tube and implanting in the uterus.

TUBAL PATENCY: Open and unobstructed fallopian tubes.

TUBOPLASTY: Plastic* or reconstructive surgery of the fallopian tubes in order to correct a blockage that has resulted in infertility.

ULTRASOUND: See SONOGRAM.

---

* This term has led some to believe that damaged tubes can be removed and plastic replacements inserted. This is obviously not possible.

UNICORNUATE UTERUS: A congenital abnormality in which the uterus is "one sided" and smaller than usual.

UROLOGIST: A physician/surgeon specializing in disorders of the urinary tract and male reproductive tract.

VAGINISMUS: A spasm of the muscles of the vagina, making penetration during sexual intercourse either impossible or very painful. Can be caused by physical or psychological conditions.

VARICOCELE: Varicose veins in the scrotum. The resulting swollen vessels surrounding the testicles create a pool of stagnant blood, which elevates the scrotal temperature and impairs sperm production. A common cause of male infertility.

VASECTOMY: The surgical separation of both vas deferens. A procedure used for birth control/sterilization. *Halakha strictly prohibits vasectomy.*

VASECTOMY REVERSAL: Surgical repair of previous vasectomy in order to restore fertility. *There are also halakhic issues that pertain to this procedure. Men who have undergone vasectomy may require reversal to rescind their status of* pitzuah daka.

VENEREAL DISEASE: Any infection that is sexually transmitted, such as chlamydia, gonorrhea, and syphilis. Many of these diseases will interfere with future fertility and some may cause severe illness if neglected.

X CHROMOSOME: The genetic information in the cell that transmits the information necessary to make a female. All eggs contain one X chromosome, and half of all sperm carry an X chromosome. When two X chromosomes combine, the baby will be a girl.

Y CHROMOSOME: The genetic material that transmits the information necessary to make a male. The Y chromosome can be found in one-half of the man's sperm cells. When an X and a Y chromosome combine, the baby will be a boy.

ZONA PELLUCIDA: Shell membrane surrounding the oocyte (egg).

ZYGOTE: A fertilized egg that has not yet divided.

ZYGOTE INTRAFALLOPIAN TRANSFER: An ART in which eggs are removed from a woman's ovaries, fertilized with the man's sperm in a laboratory dish, and the resulting zygotes are transferred into the woman's fallopian tubes using laparoscopy.

Material in this chapter was adapted from information provided by The International Council on Infertility Information Dissemination, Inc., www.inciid.org.

Acronyms

AI	artificial insemination
AIH	artificial insemination by husband
AID	artificial insemination by donor
AH	assisted hatching
ART	assisted reproductive technologies
ASA	antisperm antibodies
BBT	basal body temperature
CAH	congenital adrenal hyperplasia
CCCT	clomiphene citrate challenge test
COH	controlled ovarian hyperstimulation
DE	donor egg
DI	donor insemination
E2	estradiol
EEJ	electroejaculation
EMB	endometrial biopsy
ETA	embryo toxicity assay
ET	embryo transfer
FET	frozen embryo transfer
FSH	follicle stimulating hormone
GIFT	gamete intrafallopian transfer
GnRH	gonadotropin releasing hormone

GNRHA gonadotropin releasing hormone analog/agonist/
       antagonist
HCG   human chorionic gonadotropin
HSG   hysterosalpingogram
ICSI   intracytoplasmic sperm injection
IUI   intrauterine insemination
IVF   in vitro fertilization
LH   luteinizing hormone
LPD   luteal phase defect
MESA   microsurgical epididymal sperm aspiration
OHSS   ovarian hyperstimulation syndrome
OPK   ovulation predictor kit
P4   progesterone
PESA   percutaneous epididymal sperm aspiration
PCOS   polycystic ovary syndrome
PCT   postcoital test
PID   pelvic inflammatory disease
PGD   preimplantation genetic diagnosis
POF   premature ovarian failure
RE   reproductive endocrinologist
RPL   recurrent pregnancy loss
TDI   therapeutic donor insemination
TESA   testicular sperm aspiration
TESE   testicular sperm extraction
TET   tubal embryo transfer
TVS   transvaginal sonogram
ZIFT   zygote intrafallopian transfer

Glossary of Halakhic Terms

Aharonim: Rabbis who lived in the past few centuries (after approximately the sixteenth century).

Aliya; aliyot, pl.: As part of the ceremony of the public Torah reading in the synagogue, various men are called up (given an *aliya*) to recite blessings on the Torah. A *kohen* is generally given the first *aliya* and a Levite is given the second.

Amoraim: Rabbis who lived from the year 200 to 500 CE.

Arayot: Specific biblical sexual prohibitions (see Leviticus 18).

Assur; issur: Religiously prohibited; decree regarding something religiously prohibited.

Beitzim: May refer to the testicles or ovaries.

Betulim: The hymen. Tearing the hymen during the first intercourse begins a state of *niddah*. This is the only exception to the rule that only uterine bleeding causes *niddah*.

Biah: Sexual intercourse.

Dayan: Halakhic decisor, or judge, in a rabbinic court.

Gemilut hasadim: Acts of loving-kindness.

Halakha; halakhot, pl.: Jewish law.

Halitza: The ritual whereby a man releases the wife of a deceased, childless, brother from levirate marriage.

Hashga'ha: Monitored by a religious authority.

Haredi: Lit. "one who trembles." Rigorously Orthodox person; often refers to members of Hasidic sects.

Hazal: Acronym for *hakhameinu zikhronam levrakha*, "our sages of blessed memory."

Hesed: A "kindness"; a righteous deed, usually above that which has been commanded; contrasted with "mitzvah," which is a deed that has been commanded.

Heter: Religiously permissible.

Hotza'at zera levatala: Wasting the seed. Usually refers to the prohibition against masturbation.

Kaddish: Prayer for the dead.

Kashrut: Jewish dietary laws.

Ketubah: A contract holding the husband monetarily responsible to his wife in case of divorce or his death.

Kohen; kohanim, pl.: A priest, or of the priestly class.

Kohen gadol: The high priest.

Lashevet yitzrah: Based on the words of Isaiah 45:18, refers to the rabbinic command to continue having children beyond one boy and one girl.

Makkah: A "wound"; bleeding from an injury, which is contrasted to natural menstrual bleeding, and does not impose a state of *niddah*.

Mamzer: Commonly translated as "illegitimate," actually refers to the offspring of a relationship of *arayot*. Such a child may not marry most Jews.

Mashgiach; mashgiha, f.: An overseer for halakhic purposes.

Melakha: Actions that are biblically forbidden on Shabbat.

Mikvah: Ritual pool used for purification, in which a woman immerses herself at the end of her *niddah* period.

Mishnah: Ancient Jewish text based on statements by scholars who lived during the second temple period until the year 200 CE, collected and edited by Rabbi Yehuda HaNasi; earliest compilation of Jewish oral law.

Mishneh Torah: Lit. "Review of the Torah"; the name of Maimonides' twelfth-century comprehensive code of Jewish law. The first systematic codification of the entire corpus of Jewish law ever written.

Mitzvah; mitzvot, pl.: Any of the collection of 613 commandments or precepts in the Bible and additional ones of rabbinic origin that relate chiefly to the religious and moral conduct of Jews.

Moreh halakha: A Jewish scholar who renders halakhic decisions.

Muktzeh: Objects that are prohibited to casually move on Shabbat.

Mutar: Permissible according to Jewish law.

Niddah: A state of ritual impurity imposed by menstrual bleeding, involving many complex rules. During the period of *niddah*, a husband and wife are forbidden physical contact.

Peru u'revu: The biblical commandment to procreate.

Pesak din; pesak halakha: A halakhic decision.

Peter rehem: Lit. "the opener of the womb." First born of the mother.

Petzuah daka: A man who has been permanently wounded in the testicle(s). There are halakhic restrictions regarding whom such a man may marry.

Pikuach nefesh: Cases when a person's life is in danger, and one may violate a biblical prohibition.

Posek; poskim, pl.: Jewish scholars who render halakhic decisions.

Rambam: Rabbi Moses ben Maimon (1135–1204), also known as Maimonides. Perhaps the most influential of medieval rabbis and Jewish philosophers. Was also physician to the sultan of Egypt.

Ramban: Rabbi Moses ben Nahman Gerondi, (1194–1270), also known as Nahmanides. Highly influential commentator on the Torah and Talmud.

Rashi: Rabbi Solomon ben Isaac (or: Shlomo Yitzhaki; 1040–1105), a great French rabbinical scholar. Best known for his lucid commentaries on the Bible and Babylonian Talmud.

Rif: Rabbi Joseph Alfassi (1013–1103). An eminent Talmudist and halakhist.

Rishon; Rishonim, pl.: Rabbis from the Middle Ages.

Rosh: Rabbi Asher. A significant *Rishon*.

Rosh Yeshiva; rashei yeshivot, pl.: A rabbi who stands at the head of a rabbinic academy; a dean of a yeshiva.

Shabbat: The Jewish Sabbath.

Shalom bayit: Circumstances that would create peace in the home.

Shiddukh: A couple who meet through an arrangement by a third party.

Shiva: Seven-day period of mourning.

Shulhan Arukh: The definitive Code of Jewish Law, compiled by Rabbi Yosef Karo.

Sukkah: Temporary dwelling erected during the holiday of Sukkot.

Tahara: Ritual purity.

Taharat hamishpa'ha: Lit. "family purity." An area of Jewish law that relates to marriage, sexuality and women's health.

Tannaim: The compilers of the Mishnah, or rabbis who lived in the Mishnaic era.

Tzini'ut: Behavior based on a code of ethics that emphasizes modesty, especially in physical appearance.

Yihus: Lit. "linage." The ability to trace a child back to his ancestors. Is loosely used to refer to having a distinguished Jewish family background.

Yoetzet halakha; yoatzot halakha, pl.: A female rabbinical adviser certified by a panel of Orthodox rabbis to be a resource for women with questions regarding *taharat hamishpa'ha*. This role was devised to assist women who are more comfortable discussing very personal issues with other women.

Yom Tov; Yamim Tovim, pl.: The Jewish festivals. Includes Passover, Sukkot, and Shavuot (Pentecost).

Zera: The seed, usually male. May refer to semen or to sperm.

Zt"l: Acronym for *zekher tzaddik(im) levrakha*, lit. "May the memory of the righteous be a blessing."

Useful Organizations

AMERICAN FERTILITY ASSOCIATION

The American Fertility Association is a national organization dedicated to supporting women, men, and families facing infertility and decisions related to family building and reproductive health, from prevention and treatment to social, psychological, and financial concerns. Through educational symposia and forums, free publication, interactive media, and advocacy for research funding and policy, the American Fertility Association serves as a lifetime resource for men and women needing reproductive information and support and forwards the causes of adoption and reproductive health.

> Contact information:
> Tel: (888) 917-3777
> www.americanfertility.org.

AMERICAN SOCIETY FOR REPRODUCTIVE MEDICINE

This is the premier society for reproductive specialists in the United States. The ASRM also serves as an umbrella organization for several special interest societies, such as the Society for Reproductive

Surgeons, the Society of Reproductive Endocrinologists and the Society for Assisted Reproductive Technologies. The society is active in promoting physician education but also publishes a wealth of material of interest to patients and the public.

Contact information:
Tel: (205) 978–5000
www.asrm.org

ATIME

A Torah Infertility Medium of Exchange was established specifically to help those in the Jewish community experiencing infertility. Volunteers provide a listening ear and a caring heart to help couples through this arduous journey. The following services are available: A telephone helpline, peer support network, insurance support and advocacy, 24-hour nurse helpline, educational and inspirational symposia, an interactive website, a comprehensive library, the ATIME quarterly magazine, medical referrals, weekend retreats, and more.

Contact information:
Tel: (718) 686–8912 USA
(416) 638–4618 Canada
(052) 862–1436 Israel
www.atime.org

MAKHON PUAH

Makhon Puah (the Puah Institute) in Jerusalem is an organization devoted to helping childless couples fulfill their long-awaited dream of bringing home a child of their own. The organization trains rabbis and other counselors to give advice and referrals regarding reproductive technologies. Counselors at the Puah Institute embody a unique synthesis of rabbinical wisdom and dedication combined with specialized training in modern reproductive medicine. Couples receive personal counseling, free-of-charge, in a sensitive, caring, and discreet environment.

Among its many activities, the Puah Institute trains *mashgi-hot*, or female supervisors, to act as rabbinical representatives and overseers in fertility laboratories across Israel. The Puah Institute is dedicated to sharing its professional experience with rabbis, health-care providers, and the general public though its array of lectures, seminars, and training courses, with the goal of raising awareness of reproductive health issues on the societal level.

> Contact information:
> Tel: (02) 651–5050 Israel
> www.puah.org.il

NISHMAT

Nishmat, the Jerusalem Center for Advanced Jewish Study for Women, trains *yoatzot halakha*. The program consists of two years (over 1,000 hours) intensive study with rabbinic authorities in *taharat hamishpa'hah,* supplemented by training from experts in modern medicine and psychology and related topics including gynecology, infertility, women's health, family dynamics, and sexuality.

Upon completion of the program, the *yoetzet halakha* is certified by a panel of Orthodox rabbis to be a resource for women with questions regarding *taharat hamishpa'hah* (an area of Jewish law that relates to marriage, sexuality, and women's health). This role was devised to assist women who are more comfortable discussing very personal issues with other women.

The *yoatzot halakha*, who speak Hebrew and English, answer questions on women's health and halakha (primarily *taharat hamispa'hah*) via two venues—a hotline and a website. The website (www.yoatzot.org) provides relevant articles and answers to frequently asked questions, as well as the opportunity to privately ask individual questions.

Contact information:

Tel: (02) 642–0102

(877) YOETZET Toll free from the United States and Canada

RESOLVE

RESOLVE is a nationwide infertility association established in 1974. It is a dynamic organization with an established, nationwide network of chapters mandated to promote reproductive health and to ensure equal access to all family building options for both men and women experiencing infertility or other reproductive disorders.

The mission of RESOLVE is to provide timely, compassionate support and information to people who are experiencing infertility and to increase awareness of infertility issues through public education and advocacy.

Contact information:

Tel: (617) 623-1156

Help Line: (888) 623-0744

www.resolve.org

ZIR CHEMED

Zir Chemed is a non-profit organization dedicated to assisting infertile Jewish couples throughout the world experience the miracle of birth. It aims to achieve this by introducing the basic components of a comprehensive treatment infrastructure—counseling, information, clinical treatment, and financial planning—at a communal level.

Contact information:

www.zirchemed.org

Bibliography

Halakha and Infertility

Auerbach, S.Z. "Artificial insemination." *Noam* 1:145–166, 1958, (Hebrew).

Bakshi-Doron, E. "A serious question regarding storing [frozen] semen in order to be able to fulfill the [commandment] of procreation." *Assia* 11 (44:34–29), 1988, (Hebrew).

Bick, E. "Maternity in fetal transplants." *Crossroads: Halakha and the Modern World*. Alon Shvut-Gush Etzion: Zomet, 1987, pp. 79–85.

Bick, E. "Ovum donations: A rabbinic conceptual model of maternity." *Tradition* 1:28–45, 1993.

Bleich, J.D. "Test-tube babies." *Tradition*, Summer 1978.

Bleich, J.D. *Judaism and Healing: Halakhic Perspectives*. New York: Ktav, 1981.

Bleich, J.D. "Maternal identity revisited." *Tradition* 28 (2):52–57, 1994.

Bleich, J.D. "In vitro fertilization: Questions of maternal identity and conversion." *Tradition* 25 (4):82–102, 1991.

Brander, K. "Gynecological procedures and their interface with halacha." *Journal of Halacha and Contemporary Society* XLII:30–45, 2002.

Broyde, M. "The establishment of maternity and paternity in Jewish and American law." *National Jewish Law Review* 3:117–158, 1988.

Broyde, M. "Cloning people: A Jewish law analysis of the issues." *Connecticut Law Review*, 30:2, 1998.

Clark, E.D., Silverman, Z. "Surrogate motherhood in the case of high-risk pregnancy." *Journal of Halacha and Contemporary Society* 38:5–38, 1999.

Dichovsky, S. "When is testicular piercing permissible?" *Assia* 23(5): 13, Feb. 2001.

Eliyahu, M. "Pregnancy reduction." *Tehumin* 11:272–274, 1991.

Ellinson, G., Snyder, M. "Early ovulation as an impediment to conception: A halakhic problem and some suggested solutions." *Proceedings of the Association of Orthodox Jewish Scientists*, vol. 6, 1980.

Goldberg, Z.N. "Maternity in fetal transplants." *Crossroads: Halacha and the Modern World.* Alon Shvut-Gush Etzion: Zomet, 1987.

Goldberg, Z.N. "On egg donation, surrogacy, freezing sperm from an unmarried man, and postmortem sperm retrieval." *Assia* 17 (65–66):45–49, 1989.

Grazi, R.V., Wolowelsky, J.B. "Donor gametes for assisted reproduction in contemporary Jewish law and ethics." *Assisted Reproduction Reviews*, 2: 154–160, 1992.

Grazi, R.V., Wolowelsky, J.B. "Preimplantation sex selection and genetic screening in contemporary Jewish law and ethics." *Journal of Assisted Reproduction and Genetics*, 9:318, 1992.

Grazi, R.V., Wolowelsky, J.B. "Multifetal pregnancy reduction and disposal of untransplanted embryos in contemporary Jewish law and ethics." *American Journal of Obstretrics & Gynecology*, 5:165, 1991.

Halevi, H.D. "Multifetal pregnancy reduction and the halakhic status of embryos in vitro." *Assia* 12 (47–48):14–17, 1991.

Halperin, M. "In vitro fertilitzation, embryo transfer, and embryo freezing." *Jewish Medical Ethics* I (1):25–30, 1988.

Kahn, S. *Reproducing Jews: A Cultural Account of Assisted Conception in Israel.* Durham, North Carolina: Duke University Press, 2000.

Rosner, F. "Artificial insemination in Jewish law." *Judaism*, Fall 1970.

Rosner, F. "Judaism, genetic screening and genetic therapy." *Mount Sinai Journal of Medicine* 65: 406–413, 1998.

Shafran, Y. "Fertility procedures on the Sabbath." *Tehumin* 17:335–339, (Hebrew).

Shavran, Y. "Halakhic considerations of testicular sperm aspiration for fertility therapy." *Badad* 4:56–71, 1997.

Sinclair, D. *Jewish Biomedical Law: Legal and Extra-legal Dimensions*, Oxford: Oxford University Press, 2003, pp. 68–120.

Teitelbaum, J. "Responsum on donor artificial insemination." *HaMaor* 15:3–13, 1954 (Hebrew).

Zilberstein, Y. "Fetal reduction." *Assia* 12 (45–46):62–68, 1989 (Hebrew).

Zilberstein, Y. "Selecting fetuses for implantation." *Assia* 13 (51–52):54–58, 1992 (Hebrew).

Zohar, N. "Artificial insemination and surrogate motherhood: A halakhic perspective." *S'Vara* 2:13–19, 1991.

Waldenberg, E. "In vitro fertilization: A medical halakhic discussion." *Assia* 33:5–13, 1982 (Hebrew).

Landmark Publications in Reproductive Medicine

Asch, R.N., Ellsworth, L.R., Balmaceda, J.P., Wong, P.C. "Pregnancy after translaparoscopic gamete intrafallopian transfer," *Lancet* 2:134, 1984.

Buster, J.E., Bustillo, M., Thorneycroft, I.H., et al. "Nonsurgical transfer of in vivo fertilised donated ova to five infertile women: report of two pregnancies." *Lancet* 2:223, 1983.

Barritt, J.A., Willadsen, S., Brenner, C., Cohen, J. "Epigenetic and experimental modifications in early mammalian development: Part II. Cytoplasmic transfer in assisted reproduction." *Human Reproduction Update*, 7(4):428–435, 2001.

Bunge, R.G., Sherman, J.K., "Fertilizing capacity of frozen spermatozoa." *Nature* 172:767, 1953.

Chang, M.C., "Fertilization capacity of spermatozoa deposited in the fallopian tubes." *Nature* 168:697, 1951.

Devroey, P., Braekmans, P., Smitz, J., et al. "Pregnancy after translaparoscopic zygote intrafallopian transfer in a patient with anti-sperm antibodies." *Lancet* 1:1329, 1986.

Edwards, R.G., Donahue, R.P., Baramaki, T.A., Jones, H.W., "Preliminary attempts to fertilize human oocytes matured in vitro." *American Journal of Obstetrics and Gynecology* 1:1163, 1981.

Gemzell, C.A., Diczfalusy, E., Tillinger, K.G., "Clinical effect of human pituitary follicle-stimulating hormone." *Journal of Clinical Endrcrinology and Metabolism* 18:1333, 1958.

Gianaroli L., Magli, M.C., Ferraretti, A.P., et al. "Preimplantation genetic diagnosis increases the implantation rate in human in vitro fertilization by avoiding the transfer of chromosomally abnormal embryos." *Fertility and Sterility* 68:1128–1131, 1997.

Gleicher, N., Friberg, J., Fullan, N., et al. "Egg retrieval for in vitro fertilization by sonographically controlled vaginal culdocentesis." *Lancet* 2:508, 1983.

Handyside, A., Lesko, J.G., Tarin, J.J., Winston, R.M.L., Huges, M.R. "Birth of a normal girl after in vitro fertilization and preimplantation genetic testing for cystic fibrosis." *New England Journal of Medicine* 327:905–909, 1992.

Kruger, T.F., Menkveld, R., Stander, F.S.H., et al. "Sperm morphological features as a prognostic factor in in vitro fertilization." *Fertility and Sterility* 46:1118–1123, 1986.

Malter, H.E., Cohen, J. "Partial zona dissection of human oocytes: A nontraumatic method using micromanipulation to assist zona pellucida penetration." *Fertility and Sterility* 51:139, 1989.

Ng, S.C., Bongso, A., Ratnam, S.S., et al. "Pregnancy after transfer of multiple sperm under the zona." *Lancet* 2:790, 1988.

Oktay, K., Aydin, B.A., Karlikaya, G. "A technique for laparoscopic transplantation of frozen-banked ovarian tissue." *Fertility and Sterility* 75:1212–1216, 2001.

Oktay K., Buyuk E., Rosenwaks, Z., Rucinski, J. "A technique for transplantation of ovarian cortical strips to the forearm." *Fertility and Sterility* 80:193–198, 2003.

Palermo, G., Devroey, J.S., Van Steirteghem, A.C. "Pregnancies after intracytoplasmic sperm injection of single spermatozoon in to an oocyte." *Lancet* 340:17–18, 1992

Porcu, E., Fabbri, R., et al. "Birth of a healthy female after intracytoplasmic sperm injection of cryopreserved human oocytes." *Fertility and Sterility* 68:724–726, 1997.

Rubin, I. "The nonoperative determination of patency of fallopian tubes: By means of intra-uterine inflation with oxygen and the production of an artificial pneumoperitoneum." *Journal of the American Medical Association* 75:661, 1920.

Steptoe, P.C., Edwards, R.G. "Birth after reimplantation of a human embryo." *Lancet* 2:366, 1978.

Trounson, A., Leeton, J., Besanko, M., Wood, C. "Pregnancy established in an infertile recipient after transfer of a donated embryo fertilized in vitro." *British Medical Journal* 286:835–838, 1983.

Publications of General Interest in Reproductive Medicine

Burkman, R.T., Mei-Tzu, C.T., Malone, K.E., et al. "Infertility drugs and the risk of breast cancer: Findings from the National Institute of Child Health and Human Development Women's Contraceptive and Reproductive Experiences Study." *Fertility and Sterility* 79:844–851, 2003.

Guzick, D.S., Carson, S.A., Coutifaris, C., et al. "Efficacy of superovulation and intrauterine insemination in the treatment of infertility." *New England Journal of Medicine* 340:177–183, 1999.

Hansen, M., Kurinxzuk, J.J., Bower, C., Webb, S. "The risk of major birth defects after intracytoplasmic sperm injection and in vitro fertilization." *New England Journal of Medicine* 346:725–30, 2002.

Kashyap, S., Davis, O.K. "Ovarian cancer and fertility medications: A critical appraisal." *Seminars in Reproductive Medicine* 21:65–71, 2003.

Levi, A.J., Raynault, M.F., et al. "Reproductive outcome in patients with diminished ovarian reserve." *Fertility and Sterility* 76:666–669, 2001.

Porcu, E., Fabbri R., et al. "Clinical experience and applications of oocyte cryopreservation." *Molecular and Cellular Endocrinology* 169:33–37, 2000.

Oktay, K. "Ovarian tissue cryopreservation and transplantation: preliminary findings and implications for cancer patients." *Human Reproduction Update* 7(6):526–534, 2001.

Retzloff, M.G., Hornstein, M.D. "Is intracytoplasmic sperm injection safe?" *Fertility and Sterility* 80:851–859, 2003.

Schieve, L.A., Meikle, S.F., Ferre, C., et al. "Low and very low birth weight in infants conceived with use of assisted reproductive technology." *New England Journal of Medicine* 346:731–7, 2002.

Schwartz, D., Mayaux, M.J. "Female fecundity as a function of age: results of artificial insemination in 2,193 women with azospermic husbands." *New England Journal of Medicine* 18:404–406, 1982.

Index

A

Abdominal
  area 141
  bloating 173
  cavity 168, 209, 252
  fat 141
  intra-abdominal pressure 262
  surgery (laparotomy) 15, 307
  wall 152, 168–169
Abortion 149, 415
  selective 415
  spontaneous 70
Abraham xi, 104
Prof. Abraham, Abraham S. 201, 204,
  212, 430, 431
Acid sphingomyelinase 148
Acrosomal cap 256
Acrosome 256–257
Adam 430
Adhesions 152, 180, 209, 313, 325, 360
  ovarian *see* Ovarian, adhesions
  pelvic *see* Pelvic, adhesions

post-surgical 316
uterine *see* Uterine, adhesions
Adoption 86–87, 89, 93, 98–99, 104,
  156, 416, 419, 421
  adopted child/son 96, 104
  On Adoption (R. Soloveitchik)
    vii, xxix, 101
  pre-adoption 93
Adrenal
  glands 149, 151, 172
  hormones 150
  hyperplasia 172
Adultery 417–421
Aetius 8
Aggadah xxi, 48, 101, 103
Agglutination *see* Sperm,
  agglutination
Agonadal individuals 434–435
Agonist 174
Aharonim 9, 11, 20, 48–51
AIDS 14
Al-Jazzar (10th cent) 46

499

Aldabi, Meir ben Isaac (Tashbetz
  1310–1360) 38, 42
Amenorrhea (absent menses) 143, 322
American Fertility Association 92,
  487, 501
American Fertility Society (AFS)
  15–16, 416
American Society of Reproductive
  Medicine 176
Amma 42
Ammon 430
R. Ami 44
Amoraim 8
Amudei Gola *see Sefer Mitzvot Katan*
Amylase suppositories 264
Anal tone 261
Anaphrodesia 13
Anathema 138, 415
Anatomical 197, 199, 203, 207, 208, 210
  279, 317
  abnormalities 134, 152, 158, 178
  anomalies 13
  boundaries 194
  detail 162
  disease 180
  disorder 171
  dissection 10
  distortion 305
  fact 199
  impediments 12
  infertility *see* Infertility,
    anatomical
  irregularities 325
  landmarks 194, 325
  obstructions 128
  problem 136, 264
  source 197
  variation of the cervix 350
  work 40
Anatomy 8, 162, 164, 192, 194, 204, 268
  and physiology 9, 32–33, 38, 252
  female 8–9, 15, 129, 192–193

  intrauterine 167
  male 253
  pelvic 168, 359–360
  reproductive 9, 32, 38, 194
  tubal 162, 166
  uterine 152, 162, 164, 166–167, 300
Anatomy and Physiology *see*
  Physiology
Androgen 143–144
Andrology laboratories 265
Anemia 300
Anesthesia 268
  ether 15
  general 168, 210, 273, 336, 342
  local 270
Aneuploidy 351–352, 435
  embryo *see* Embryo, aneuploidy
  embryonic *see* Embryonic,
    aneuploidy
Animalcules 10–11
Animalculists 35, 40, 43, 54
Anovulation *see* Ovulation,
  anovulation
Anovulatory *see* Ovulatory,
  anovulatory
Antagon 174, 295, 323–324
Antral follicle count 152
Aphrodisiacs 8
Aquinas, Thomas (d. 1274) 46
Arayot 22–23, 48, 355–356
ART *see* Assisted reproductive
  technology
Artificial insemination 416, 427
  and child's status 416
  and female factors 279
  and gender selection 422
  and ovulation occurrence 215
  and rabbinical supervision
    396–397
  early 294
  in halakha 45, 234, 281, 292, 393
  in history 14, 20–22, 33, 45–52

with husband's sperm (AIH) 14,
279, 284, 416
when it's used 177–178
Aristotle (384–322 BCE) 7–8, 34,
36–39, 43
Asch, Dr. Ricardo 23, 347–349
R. Asher ben Yehiel *see* Rosh
Asherman's Syndrome *see*
Syndrome, Asherman
Ashkenazic
and hereditary diseases 145–149
Jewish Community 148
Jews 89, 145–146
Aspartoacylase 146
Aspiration
epidydimal sperm 343
micro epidydimal sperm (MESA)
262, 272, 275, 396
microsurgical epidydimal sperm
(MESA) 272, 396
needle 270, 343
percutaneous epidydimal
sperm 273
pneumonia 147
testicular 270
Assisted hatching 346–347
Assisted reproduction xxviii, xxxi,
184, 281, 304, 311–362, 408
and COH 292–293
and embryo transfer 324, 335
and fertility history 18, 20
and high process
gonadotropins 183
and medical, halakhic overlap 248
and ovarian failure 304
and rabbinical supervision
368, 399
and treatment algorithm 182
and varicocele litigation 272
and Y-deletion study 267
definition and explanation
179–180

Assisted reproductive technology
(ART) 101, 312, 318, 346, 409, 412
and cancer 174
and child status 415–416
and embryo transfer 325
and ethics 409
and GIFT 348
and gonadotropins 293
and halakha 357–358, 408, 412
and IVF 315
and miscarriage 333
and rabbinical consultation 358
and recombinant FSH 286
and SART 335
and Shabbat 341
and semen analysis 158
definition and explanation 179–181
Assur 25, 26, 431
Astringents 12
Astroglide 260
ATIME (A Torah Infertility Medium
of Exchange) 92, 488
Atresia 176–177
R. Auerbach, Shlomo Zalman 195,
199, 201, 212, 215–216, 235, 396,
420, 431
Autosomes 266, 351
Averroes (d. 1198) 46
Avicenna (980–1037) 46
Avot see Ethics of the Fathers
Azospermia 251, 312–313, 343
complete 261
non-obstructive 343
obstructive 343
Azospermic 236, 269
Rabbi Azulai, Haim Yosef David
(1724–1806) 51

B

"Be fruitful and fill the earth" 73
"Be fruitful and multiply" *see Peru
u'revu*

R. Bahya ben Asher (1255–1350) 37
Barrenness xi, 14, 98, 104, 140,
    247, 409
Basal
    FSH levels 319
    levels 295
    temperature charting 283
Basal body temperature (BBT)
    214–215, 374
    charting 215, 300, 302
    testing 214
Bava Kama 74
BBT *see* Basal body temperature
Beit HaMikdash 370
Ben Ish Hai (Rabbi Hayyim, Yosef
    [1833?–1909]) 50–51
Ben Sira, Shimon 20, 47–50, 417
Ben Zoma 50
Berakhot, Tractate 430
Beriah 431–432
Beth Shmuel 235
Betulim see hymen
Biah 48
    gemar 50, 52
    shello k'darkah 232
    rishona 50
Bimanual exam 151–152, 203–204
Biochemical testing 158
Biological Testing 170
Biopsy 161–162, 206–208, 210, 214,
    236–237, 269, 297, 300, 343, 350
    blastomere 351
    confirmatory 297
    embryo xxvii
    endometrial 161–162, 206–207,
        213–215, 297, 300, 302, 304
    testicular 236–237, 269, 396
Birth
    birthing process 198, 201
    canal 192
    Cesarean 143
    childbirth *see* Childbirth

control 233
control pills 300–301, 303, 324
defects 143, 330
dry 197–198
live 146, 333–334, 354, 435
mother 356–357, 432–433
stillbirth *see* Stillbirth
vaginal *see* Vaginal, birth
Bitahon 75
Bladder 152, 177, 192–193, 258, 263,
Blastocyst 326, 330–332, 334, 337–338,
    344–346
Blastomere 350–352, 428
    biopsy *see* Biopsy, blastomere
Bleeding
    awareness or sensation of 190
    cervical 194–195, 204
    continuous 296, 299
    cyclic 128, 162, 166
    estrogen-withdrawal 303
    halkhic 197
    hymenal 200
    internal flow of 190
    irregular 290
    Lupron-induced 296
    menstrual 190–191, 200, 208, 212,
        298, 301, 340
    midcycle 284, 298–299
    minor bleeding disturbances 304
    niddah 197, 201, 207, 210
    physiologic 211
    post-operative 342
    postcoital 233, 235
    superficial 206
    transient 200
    traumatic 201
    uterine 128, 194–196, 198–199, 201,
        208, 210–211, 284, 307, 338
    vaginal xi, 189, 195, 233, 337
R. Bleich, J. David 432
Blessing xviii, xxvii, 5, 67, 69–70, 74,
    82, 101, 409, 424, 438

Blindness 148
Blood
    chemistries 262
    circulation of 10
    components 8
    flow 262
    pressure 142, 147
    sugars 290
    test/testing 213, 228, 262, 296, 375
    uterine xviii
    vessels 192, 228, 253, 256
Bloom Syndrome *see* Syndrome,
    Bloom
R. Blumenkrantz, Avrohom 194, 204
Brain 5, 7, 34, 36, 42–44, 126, 253, 322
    see also Hypothalamus
    base of 155, 254
    central area of 173, 254, 294,
    dead 423
    spongy degeneration of 146
Brain-dead 423
Brain tumors 228
Bravelle 286
Brit 88–90
Bromocriptine (Parlodel) 150, 172
Brown, Louise 17, 311, 335
Broyde, Michael 431–432
Brush 203–204
Buserilin 324
Buster, John 16

C
Cadavers 320
Cain 430
Canavan's Disease (Spongy
    Degenerative Disease) 146
Cancer 79, 146–147, 174–175, 258, 332,
    353, 438
    breast 175–176
    female 174
    head/neck 147

    ovarian 174–175
    uterian 300
Cannula/cannulate 207–208, 210, 350
Capacitation 16, 257
Carbergoline (Dostinex) 150
Carbon dioxide 168–169, 210
Cardiovascular
    disease 142
    instability 147
Catheter 166, 177–178, 205, 208, 211,
    271, 280, 289, 325, 333, 338
Caucasians 146
Cell
    inner cell mass 326
    membrane 258
Celsus 228
Centers for Disease Control (CDC)
    313, 318, 335, 348
Centrifuge 377
Cervical
    alterations in secretion of cervical
        mucus 302
    canal 122, 161–162, 192, 194–195,
        203–207, 210, 280, 285, 325
    dilation 192, 197, 201, 206–207 *see
        also* Cervix, dilation of
    environment 124
    intracervical insemination 179
    mucus 123–124, 129, 159–160, 205,
        284, 288, 302
    stenosis 325, 350
Cervix
    anatomical variation of 350
    bleeding/blood from 194–195, 203,
        206–207, 210
    blood supply to 206
    diameter of 193, 199, 201, 204,
        206–208
    dilation of 153, 199, 203, 207,
        209–211 *see also* Cervical,
        dilation
    disease of 160

opening of 197–198
portion of 199
trauma to 161
visualization of 203, 206
Cesarean delivery 143
Cetrotide 174, 295, 323–324
Chalibeats 12
Chang 17
Charity 84, 95, 354, 430
Chemotherapy 178, 228, 258, 437–438,
    chemotherapeutic drugs 258
Chicken Pox *see* Varicella
Childbearing 5, 153, 417
Child/children
    biological 83–84, 92, 251,
        305–306, 356
    female 7, 235, 330
    genetic 267, 270, 421, 435
    male 7, 235, 267, 330
    orphaned 98
Childbirth xiii, 89, 102, 175, 277
Childless couple 89, 102, 104, 234, 411
Chlamydia 145
Cholesterol 142
Chromosomal
    abnormalities 259
    defects 154
    instability 147
Chromosome 256, 266, 351–352, 436
    cilia 125–126, 432
    sex 266, 351
    X 256
    Y 252, 266–267
Clitoris 192
Clomid 172, 283
Clomiphene 16, 170–173, 176, 178,
    181–182, 283–285, 287–288,
    290–294, 297, 302–303, 360, 362
    clomiphene citrate 156, 172,
        283, 375

clomiphene citrate challenge tests
    (CCCT) 156
prolonged exposure to 171
Cloning xxvii, 19, 22–23, 424, 426–435
    "clone" 429
    embryonic 428
    human 426, 431, 433–434
    reproductive 428–429, 431, 433
    somatic cell 428, 433
    stem cell 429, 431
Clonor 429, 432
Cloth 191, 213
Clotting
    blood clotting 300
    clot formation 173
CO$_2$ 325, 327
Coagulating lesions 169
R. Cohen, Dovid 217
Coital 140
    ability 260
    adequacy 260
    frequency 140, 260
    non-coital 52, 235
    postcoital bleeding 233, 235
    postcoital diaphragm 235
    postcoital examination 230
    postcoital test/ testing (PCT)
        159–161, 205, 213–214, 215,
        261–263, 268, 302, 304, 393
Coitus interruptus 230–232, 236, 281,
    294, 341, 413
Coloring 215–216, 375
Compartment
    inner compartment 194–195
    outer compartment 194, 196
Conception
    artificial 416
    assisted 117, 120, 431
    Ben Sira's 20
    genetic 20
    keys to 74
    natural 133, 416

non-coital 52
non-natural 45–46
preconception testing 145
predecessor's 32
rabbinic vii, 31
spontaneous 262
virginal 45–46, 49
Condom 230, 235–236, 266, 281,
    294, 341
    medical 266, 341
    perforated 230
Congenital 305
    abnormality 164, 167
    absence 261–262, 305, 343
    adrenal hyperplasia 172
    anatomic abnormalities 227
    malformation 147
    syndromes 228
Conjugal
    privileges 140
    relations 40, 48, 281
    union 229
Contraceptive 232
    oral 15, 319
Contrast dye 162, 164, 210
Controlled ovarian hyperstimulation
    (COH) 291–293, 315, 320–321
Conversion 355, 357, 421
Corneal clouding 147
Coronary angioplasty 210
Corpus luteum 128, 298
Cramping 147, 163, 280
Crinone 283
Cryopreservation 331, 338, 345 *see also*
    Freezing
    embryo 312, 315, 331, 338, 345, 396,
        402, 423, 437
    oocyte 437
    sperm 273, 332, 342, 396, 402, 423
Cryptorchid testes 252
Cryptorchidism 252
Culture 17, 330–331

blastocyst 344
conditions 330
dishes 325
egg 325
embryo 325, 327, 331
laboratory 311
media 315, 337, 400
techniques 321
Cumulus 328
Curette (scraping device) 206–207
Cycle cancellation 333–334, 341
Cyclic hormonal functioning 65
Cyst 128, 143, 152, 169, 289, 307
    ovarian *see* Ovarian, cysts
    ovulation *see* Ovulation, cyst
Cystic fibrosis 146, 261, 276, 343,
    351, 363
Cytoplasm 329, 435–436
    donor *see* Donor, cytoplasm
    egg 329, 429, 435
Cytoplasmic
    factors 436
    transfer 435

D

"Day 3 testing" 318
R. da Trani, Isaiah
dan lekhaf zekhut 83
R. Danzig, Abraham (1748–1820) 198
De Graaf, Reinier 10, 34–35
    Graafian follicle 10
Deafness 148
Decalogue 98
Dehydration 173
Demyelination 146
Delivery 20, 141, 143, 180, 197–198,
    289, 352, 414
Deuteronomy 75, 101, 103
Developmental
    age 148

delay 146
stage 330, 425
Dexamethasone 360
Diabetes 142–143, 177, 258, 263, 290
Diagnosis 108, 114, 118, 159, 170,
    184, 236
    "unexplained infertility" 169, 292
    and treatment 65, 108, 116–117, 374
    fertility *see* Fertility, diagnosis
    infertility *see* Infertility, diagnosis
    luteal phase insufficiency 297, 299
    male factor problems 109
    male infertility xxx
    medical 51
    preimplantation genetic (PGD) 18,
        23, 149, 180, 350–351, 394, 422
    prenatal *see* Prenatal diagnosis
Diagnostic 165–166, 169, 181, 208, 213,
    263, 312, 367
    accuracy 170
    capacity 347
    diagnostically heterogeneous 228
    evaluation viii, xxxi, 105, 161,
        169–170
    laparoscopy 168–169
    modalities 210
    procedures viii, 189, 192, 203,
        213–214, 413
    test/testing 108, 183, 292
    ultrasound *see* Ultrasound,
        diagnostic
Diaphragm 233, 235
    Postcoital *see* Coital, postcoital
        diaphragm
Dietary laws *see* Kashrut
Differentiation 256, 330, 428
Dilation 207
    abnormal dilation of veins 228
    cervical *see* Cervical, dilation *and*
        also Cervix, dilation of
    of external OS 199, 204–205
    of internal OS 204, 207

pretreatment 325
Dilatation and curettage (D&C) 306
Dilator 206–207
Diploid 428, 433
Distal part 164
Divorce 23, 234, 394
    grounds for 418–419
Divrei Shimon Ben Sira see Ben Sira
DNA 121, 256, 329, 350–352, 428–430,
    432–433, 435
    mitochondrial DNA 430, 434, 436
    molecule 350
    nuclear 430, 433, 435
    recombinant DNA technology 287,
        321, 339
    repair disorder 146
    testing 23, 397
Donor
    cytoplasm 32, 435
    egg *see* Donor egg
    gametes 416–417, 425
    gene 32
    ova 420
    sperm 21, 48, 416, 419–420
Donor egg *see also* Egg Donation
    and genetic/halakhic mother 421
    and nuclear transfer 435
    and ovarian reserve 156, 319
    and supervision 400
Dor Yesharim 148–149
Dorsal ridge 252
Dostinex *see* Carbergoline
Ductal obstruction 236
Dying 215–216 *see also* Coloring
Dyspareunia 268

E

R. Edinger, Yosef 50
Education 81, 102, 115
Edwards Dr. Robert G. 17–18, 311, 439
Eating disorders 136, 140

Egg
cytoplasm *see* Cytoplasm, egg
developing/development 126, 128,
170, 173, 282–283, 286, 288,
293, 298–299, 302–304, 307,
319–320, 324, 332, 336
donation *see* Egg donation
donor *see* Egg donation
excess eggs and disposal 394
fertilized 126, 128, 427,
follicles 35, 143, 152, 173, 176
genetically abnormal 135
harvest 336
healthy 154, 319
mature/maturation 10, 124, 126,
128, 160, 172–174, 193, 256, 283,
295, 319, 328, 336, 353
multiple egg development 336
multiple mature 347
presurgical egg extraction and
storage 437
production 126, 288, 293, 295, 319
recruitment 128
retrieval 18, 173, 320–321, 323, 334,
336–337, 340–343, 353, 358, 378,
394–395, 401–402, 427, 438
Egg Donation/Donor 32
and ART 180
and cloning 426, 432–433
and gestational surrogacy 356–357
and GIFT 349
and nuclear transfer 436
and oocyte cryopreservation 437
and ovarian failure 312
definition and explanation
353–356
halakhic mothers 432
history 16, 18, 24
R. Eider, Shimon 194
Ejaculate 123, 139, 157, 177, 230, 259,
266, 269, 273, 337, 343

Ejaculation
anejaculation 139
delayed 260
electro 268 *see also*
Electroejaculation (EEJ)
frequency of 257
non-coital 235
premature 260
retrograde 177, 227, 263–264
urine after 263
Ejaculatory
duct 228, 257, 262, 273, 361
dysfunction 260
mechanism 273
Electrocautery 169, 289
Electroejaculation (EEJ) 273–274,
342, 396
vibratory assistance, with 268
Electrofusion 436
R. Eliezer 231
R. Eliezer ben Ya'akov 44
Elkanah 98
R. Elyashiv, Yosef 22, 431
Embryonic
aneuploidy 352–353
cell 428
cloning 428
development 328, 343, 429, 433
growth 327
implantation *see* Implantation,
Embryonic
life 252
non-embryonic cell 426
precursor 252
shell 428
stem cells *see* Stem cells,
Embryonic
wastage 135
Embryo
aneuploidy 436
cleaved 331
cloned 428–429

cryopreservation *see*
    Cryopreservation, embryo
donation 345, 426
eight cell 326, 351
fertilized 31, 126, 129, 330–331,
    423, 428
four cell 326
freezing 17
growth 327, 331, 349
human 18, 429, 437
human embryo research 345
implantation *see* Implantation,
    embryo
microscopic 338
preembryo 193
pronuclear 326
quality 347
selection of 330
transcervical embryo transfer 350
transfer 16, 315,
    324–325, 333–335, 337–338, 340,
    343–344, 349–350, 358, 378,
    395, 402
tubal embryo transfer (TET) *see*
    Tubal embryo transfer
twin 332
untransplanted 345
Embryological
    debate 37
    development 35
    emergencies 345
    progression 252
    theory 32, 35, 40–41, 45, 345
Embryologist 24, 327–328, 330, 338,
    352, 358
Embryology 32–34, 36–37, 39–40,
    52–54
    human 33
    laboratory 24, 391, 437
Emmenagoga 12
Encephalo-myelogenic doctrine 34, 42

Endocrine 254
    glands 149
    neuroendocrine 253
    testing 149
Endocrinologists, reproductive *see*
    Reproductive, endocrinologist
Endometrial
    Biopsy 161–162, 206–207, 213–215,
        297, 300, 302, 304
    lining 193
Endometriomas 307
Endometriosis 132, 136–137, 152, 164,
    168, 171, 180–181, 209–210, 304,
    306–308, 313, 316–317, 353, 360
Endometrium 127, 161, 193–194,
    197, 208
Enzyme 146–148, 257–258, 264
Epidemiology 136
Epididymal sperm 343
Epididymal tubules 272
Epididymis 252–253, 257, 261–262,
    272–273, 275, 337
Epididymitis 228, 261
Epigenesis 35, 39, 43–44
Er 231, 233
Erectile dysfunction 139, 233
Erection 259, 274
Estradiol (E2) 154–156, 299, 303, 319
    see also Estrogen, natural estrogen
Estrogen
    anti-estrogen 283–284, 290
    blood 173, 303
    conjugated 303
    cyclic 300
    deficiency 298
    dose of 299, 303
    elevated level 332
    estraderm 284, 299
    level 173, 293, 295–296, 298–299,
        340–341
    low estrogen environment 172
    midcycle estrogen drop 299

natural estrogen (estradiol)
299, 303 *see also* Estradiol (E2)
patch 303
transdermal estrogens 299
transdermal patch 284, 296,
303, 308
Ethical xvii, xxvi, 16, 25, 32, 249,
416, 424
and religious 400, 437
challenges 409
debate 429
dilemmas 438
discussion 434
guidelines 21
issues xxxii, 73, 409–410, 422, 424
motivation 422
norms 76
principle 11
problems 415, 424
standards 119
system xvii
unethical 398, 423, 426, 427
Ethics 17, 411, 416
and cloning 426
First Ethics Committee Report 16
Jewish 410
Jewish law and xxiii, 4, 28, 409
medical xxix, xxxii
science and xxvii
Ethics of the Fathers 103
Euclid 40
Exodus, Book of 74, 409, 431
R. Eybeschutz, Yehonatan
(1690–1764) 51

F
Facial erythema (redness) 146
Fallopian Tubes
architecture and function 208
damaged 311
Gabriel Fallopius (1523–1562) 8

Gamete intrafallopian transfer
(GIFT) *see* Gamete
intrafallopian transfer (GIFT)
Zygote intrafallopian transfer
(ZIFT) 312, 349
Falloposcopy 210–211
Familial dysautonomia 147
Family Purity xi, xviii, xxvi, 108, 118,
140, 393
Fanconi anemia 147
Fatherhood and posthumous 423
FDA 15, 17
Fecundity 67
R. Feinstein, Moses 199–202, 204, 207
209, 212, 215, 231, 233, 237, 281,
417–418
Feldman, David 233,
Female factor 136, 156, 178, 261, 263,
272, 277, 279, 281, 313, 316–317
Femoral heads 147
Fertile time 124, 299, 302
Fertility
care 109, 184, 275, 399
diagnosis 116, 121
disorders 133
drugs 128, 143, 152, 162,
174–176, 347
innate 156
interventions 19, 133, 164
male, *see* Male, fertility
medication 154, 156, 333
natural fertility rate 312
normal 131–132, 150, 158, 316
peak fertility potential 140
problem 65, 75, 77, 112–113, 251,
275, 412
specialists 92, 307, 344, 438
subfertile 157, 227, 251, 266
therapy *see* Fertility therapy
treatment *see* Fertility treatment

Fertility therapy xxviii, xxxi, 114, 118,
133, 216, 439, 501
and artificial insemination 279
and blood tests 375
and hormonal disorders 150
and multifetal pregnancy 183
and ovarian reserve 156, 320
and posthumous reproduction 423
and rabbinic supervision 391–403
and Shabbat xxxi
brief history of 5–29
centrality of the woman 278
hormones used in 320
professional management of 189
Fertility treatment ix, xxiv, 14, 109,
124, 144, 176, 179, 249, 285,
377–379
algorithm 180
and breast cancer 175
and ethical issues 410, 414
and obesity 143
and Shabbat 369–379
Fertilization
human-17, 311
in vitro *see* In vitro, fertilization
in vivo *see* In vivo, fertilization
normal 256, 317, 326, 328, 337
Fertinex 286, 322
Fetal
damage 145
death 352
development 252
genetic anomalies 435
heartbeat 333
life 122
reduction 344
Fetus *see also* Fetal
"excess" 414
"fetus-sitter" 421
developing 7, 252, 285
diseased 351
female 8

genetically defective 149
preformed 41
Fiber optic endoscope 211
Fibroids 166–167, 169, 200, 300
uterine 168, 196
Filtration systems 327
Fimbriae 125
Fink, Nathan and Vivian 217
Flagellum 256–257
Fluorescent in situ hybridization
(FISH) 352
Fluoroscopy 162, 208, 210–211
Follicle stimulating hormone (FSH)
127, 303
and anovulation 282
and clomiphene 172, 283
and early ovulation 303
and GnRH analogs 174, 295–296,
322–323
and gonadotropins 173, 285,
287–288
and halakha 339
and hCG 287
and hMG 285
and hormonal testing 262
and natural hormones 320–321
and ovarian reserve 154–156
and patient selection 318–319
and pituitary-testicular axis
254–255
and polycystic ovary 143, 150
recombinant 286–287
urinary 286
Follicular
maturity 340
monitoring 340
Follistim 287, 322
Foster
care 92
parents 104

Freezing 294, 332, 345, 402
  (tanks), 427, 437–438 *see also*
  Cryopreservation
  egg xxvii, 437–438
  embryo 17
  oocyte 438
  ovarian tissue 438
  rabbinic supervision of 402
  sperm 395, 437
FSH *see* Follicle stimulating hormone
Functional abnormalities 134

G

Galactorhea 150
Galen (130–200 CE) 11, 33, 36–38
Gamete 22–24, 32, 179, 315–316, 327,
  337, 349, 396–397, 408, 416–417,
  425, 427
  donor 435 *see also* Donor, gamete
Gamete intrafallopian transfer (GIFT)
  16, 312, 347–349
R. Ganz, David (17th Cent.) 47
Gastrointestinal 146, 290
Gaucher's Disease 147
Gemilut hasadim 22
Gender selection 422 *see also* Sex
  selection
Gene
  BLM 146
  sex-linked 422
Genesis xviii, xxv, 68, 412
Genesis Fertility & Reproductive
  Medicine xxxi, 340, 501
Genetic
  abnormalities 31, 135
  complexity 135
  codes 427
  copy 426
  damage 135
  diseases 19, 145–149, 180, 351–352,
    433–434
  disorder 146, 353

duplicate 426–427
  father 19, 282, 419, 423, 432
  fetal genetic anomalies 435
  health 350
  histories 139
  information 121, 135, 350, 428
  instructions 428, 436
  makeup 350
  manipulation 434
  material 121–122, 350–351, 355, 436
  parents 24, 120, 357, 416, 421, 429
  sex-linked genetic disease 422
  splicing 32
  testing 149
Genetically
  abnormal 135
  defective 149
  normal 134, 352
Genetics 31, 130
Genitalia 203, 237, 261
Genital 8
  abnormality 147
  exam 248
  organs 34
  seed 231,
  tract 121, 124
Genitourinary trauma 258
Gentile 49, 370, 420
Germ cells 253, 428, 433–434
German Measles *see* Rubella
Germes 11
Gestation 31, 35, 432
  multifetal 332
Gestational 411, 421, 432, 435–436
  mother 421, 435–436
  sac 333
  surrogacy 305–306, 356–357, 425
  surrogate 23, 180, 305, 357
GIFT *see* Gamete intrafallopian
  transfer (GIFT)
Glucocerebrosidase 147
Glucose utilization 290

Glycolipids 147

GnRH *see* Hormone, gonadotropin releasing hormone (GnRH)
  agonist 295, 315, 323–324, 336, 340
  analogs *see* Hormone, gonadotropin releasing hormone analog
  antagonist 295, 315, 323–324
  receptors 323

Gomel, Victor 16

Gonadal failure 433–434

Gonadotropin 173–174, 176, 178, 182–183, 228, 285–288, 290–296, 301, 321, 323, 336, 339–340, 342, 360, 362 *see also* Hormone
  hCG *see* Human Chorionic Gonadotropin
  Human menopausal (hMG) 16, 285–287, 320–322
  stimulation 336, 340
  therapy 173, 286, 288, 296, 340–341

Gonal F 287, 322

Gray, Dr. John 114

R. Grodzinski, Haim O. 235

Groin 271

Guillemin, Roger C.L. 322

Gynecologic
  consultation 247
  surgeon 15

Gynecological
  cancer 147
  exam 202

Gynecologist xxx, 15, 17, 113, 115, 145, 152, 157, 162, 171, 247, 275, 311, 410

Gynecology 8, 152, 278, 501

H

Hadash assur min haTorah 25, 431

Hakhmei haMasorah 102

Halakha xvii-xviii *see also* Halakhic

and intrauterine insemination (IUI) 284–285, 394

and in vitro fertilization (IVF) 183, 234, 339, 394, 408

and ovulation induction (OI) 395

and paternity 20–22, 432–433

and semen analysis 69, 118, 392

pesakei 120

reproductive xxiv, 23, 119, 248, 276

Halakhic
  analysis 49, 432
  authority 77, 86, 120, 281–282, 339, 343, 352, 377, 379, 392, 408, 411, 419, 436 *see also* Posek/Poskim
  barriers 299
  cases 423
  community xxv, xxxii, 191, 407
  concerns 108, 118, 121, 159, 230, 236, 249, 306–307, 349, 356, 408, 416
  conflicts 115
  decision (*pesak din*) 118–119, 212, 400
  decisor (*morei halakha*) 248, 392–393
  difficulties 434
  dilemma 32, 52, 119, 345, 436
  extra-Halakhic Kabbalistic 233
  factors 411
  factors in male infertility, 109
  grounds 117, 233, 282
  hurdles 70, 425
  infertility *see* Infertility, halakhic
  intricacies 412
  issues xxx, 32, 75, 77, 86, 108–109, 290, 293, 339, 344, 357, 395, 431
  limits 411
  medical ethics, xxix, 32
  mother 355, 421, 432–432, 436
  objection 408, 418
  options 412

paternity *see* Paternity, halakhic
permissibility 27, 425
permission *see heter*
process 32, 118, 358
question 76, 355, 357, 394, 399, 408
ramifications 46, 49
relative 356
restrictions 109, 247, 251, 293
solution 118
source xxix, 118, 409, 430
status 345, 355, 373, 416, 431
supervision *see* Supervision,
    halakhic *and also* Rabbinic
    supervision
supervisor 379
verdicts *see Pesakei halakha*
will 420
Halakhist 235, 411–412, 415–417, 419,
    423–424
HaLevi, R. Yehuda *See Kuzari*
Halitza 420, 423
Haller, Albrecht (1708–1777) 46
Hannah 74, 83, 98
Hannah's Prayer xiii
Hanukah 89
    candles 82
Haploid 428, 433
R. Harari, Tzvi 217
Haredi 22, 25, 112, 115, 317
Harvey, William (1578–1657) 10–11, 34
Hasidic 138
Hashga'ha 395–397, 399, 402–403
    see also Rabbinical supervision,
    Supervision
Hatching, assisted 346–347
R. Hayyim, Yosef *see Ben Ish Hai*
Hazal 32, 38, 40–43, 45, 57
hCG *see* Human Chorionic
    Gonadotropin
Heape, Walter 16
Heder 38
Hei, Hebrew etter 104

Hematogenic Doctrine 34, 43
Hematospermia 235
Hepatitis 145
Hernias 258
R. Herzog, Isaac 233
Hesed 112, 432
Heter 23–24, 292, 294, 396
Hexosaminidase 148
High Holiday services 70
High Priest *see Kohen gadol*
Hippocrates 7–8, 33–34, 36, 43
Hippocratic corpus 7
Hirsutism 144, 290
HIV 14, 145
Holeh she'ein bo sakanah 373, 377–378
Holocaust 84, 88
Home Ovulation-Prediction Test Kit
    see Ovulation, Home Ovulation-
    Prediction Test Kit
Homeostatic needs 255
Homunculus 10, 11, 35, 41, 248
Hormone
    adrenal 150
    agonist 174
    antagonist 174
    bioengineered 321
    follicle stimulating (FSH) *see*
        Follicle stimulating hormone
    gonadotropin 228
    gonadotropin releasing hormone
        (GnRH) 128, 173–174, 255, 289,
        295, 301, 322–324, 336, 340
    gonadotropin releasing hormone
        analogs (GnRH analogs)
        173–174, 294–295, 307–308,
        315, 322
    hCG *see* human chorionic
        gonadotropin
    human 287, 321
    internal 295
    levels 227, 375

luteinizing (LH) *see* Luteinizing
  hormone
male 255, 290
master 174, 295
natural 285, 315, 320
ovarian 176, 306
pituitary 150, 173, 285, 319
reparative 298
testicular 262
thyroid 150, 172
thyroid stimulating (TSH) 150
treatment 375
tropic 319
urinary LH kit *see* Urinary, LH
  kit 1
Hormonal
  "surge" 215
  abnormal hormonal
    stimulation 124
  assessment 262
  basis 162
  disorders 150
  dysfunction 176
  effects of ovulation 214, 374
  environment 289
  evaluation 360
  output 161, 291, 301
  medications 285
  pretreatment 438
  problem 262, 268
  production 128
  secretion 128, 134, 252
  signal 128, 298
  status 284
  stimuli 128
  support 298
  system 129, 254
  testing 262
  therapy 117, 289
  treatment 170, 306
Hospitalization 168
Hot flashes 307–308

HSG *see* Hysterosalpingogram (HSG)
Human Chorionic Gonadotropin
  (hCG) 173, 287, 322, 336, 339 *see
  also* Hormone
  and biochemical pregnancy 333
  injection 341, 376, 378
Humagon 322
Human follitropin 285, 322
Human genome xxvii, 19
  Project 434
Hunter, John 14, 45, 51
Hydrosalpinx 153, 359
Hymen 47, 192, 200
Hyperinsulinemia 144
Hyperpolactinemia 172, 268
Hypertension 258
Hypospadias 45
Hypothalamus 126–128, 173, 254–255,
  283, 289, 294, 322–323
Hypotonia (poor muscle tone) 146
Hysterectomy 305
Hysteria 8
Hysterography 359
Hysterosalpingogram (HSG) 162–164,
  166, 208–209, 211–212, 300,
  359, 375
Hysterosalpingography 359
Hysteroscope 166–167, 210, 306
Hysteroscopy 166–167, 209–210, 300,
  325, 375
  operative 167

I

ICSI *see* Intracytoplasmic sperm
  injection
Idiopathic (unexplained) 228 *see also*
  Infertility, idiopathic
Illegitimate 19, 418–419 *see also
  Mamzer*
Illicit relations *see Arayot*
Immune system 307
Immunodeficiency 146

Immunological disorders 313
Immunology 130
Implantation 31, 128–129, 134, 170,
    193, 206, 283, 311, 315, 317, 324, 328,
    330–331, 338, 343, 346–347, 352, 435
    embryo 161, 351–353, 357
    failures 343, 352
    rate 325, 331, 337, 343–344, 436
Impotence 81
    psychogenic 273
    sexual *see* Sexual, impotence
Impregnation xii, 7, 45
    artificial 45–46
    bathhouse 47, 49–52
In utero 35, 432
In vitro fertilization (IVF) xi, 21–24,
    153, 180, 184, 275, 292, 314–315, 343,
    346, 424
    and blastocyst transfer 331, 350
    and child status 415
    and cloning 427, 432
    and counseling 335
    and cryopreservation 331–332, 342
    and cytoplasmic transfer 435
    and egg donation 353–355
    and egg retrieval 336, 395
    and embryo transfer 324–325
    and endometriosis 309
    and expected high failure
        rates 320
    and fallopian tube diseases
        179, 305
    and fertile women 316
    and genetic father 282
    and GIFT 347–348
    and GnRH 323–324
    and gonadotropins 173
    and halakha 183, 234, 339, 394, 408
    and ICSI 270, 273, 275, 313, 317,
        327–330
    and live birth 333
    and looking forward 439
    and MESA or TESE 262
    and multifetal pregnancy 183,
        344, 414
    and natural hormones 320–321
    and nuclear transfer 436
    and oocyte cryopreservation 437
    and ovarian reserve 156, 318–320
    and ovary stimulation 174, 335–336
    and parental relationship 431
    and preimplementation genetic
        diagnosis (PGD) 351–352
    and sex/gender selection 352,
        395, 422
    and Shabbat 340, 378
    and sonohysterogram 166
    and sperm procurement 341
    and supervision 401–402
    and surrogacy 357
    and uteras, vagina absence 305
    and *yamim tovim* 358
    and ZIFT 349
    as treatment of 1st choice 314
    clinics 328, 331, 437
    cycle 316, 344, 355
    definition 281
    development techniques 312, 315
    expanded indications for 316–318
    history 16–18
    human 17
    lab 24, 327, 358
    Louise Brown 311, 335
    pregnancy *see* Pregnancy, IVF
    program 340, 354, 357
    statistics 332–334
    success 314, 315, 318, 320
    treatment 339, 378
    treatment algorithms 182, 359–362
In vivo 163, 347
    fertilization 293, 330
Incubation 337, 347, 349
Incubator 325, 327, 331, 345, 349,
    402–403

Infants, prematurely born 344
Infertility
    anatomical 304–305
    causes of 13, 17, 170–171, 180, 203,
        282, 313–314, 316–317
    curing 277
    diagnosis 69, 79, 154
    epidemiology of 136
    evaluation 109, 141, 145, 157, 161,
        169, 412
    female viii–ix, 6, 8, 13, 125, 131,
        140, 248, 263, 268, 277, 282,
        315, 317, 394, 433
    halakhic 299, 301
    human 428
    idiopathic 316
    longstanding 259
    male *see* Male, infertility
    male factor *see* Male factor
        infertility
    management of xxvi, 181, 229, 374
    modern infertility techniques 17
    most common cause of 137
    most common female cause of 143
    origins of 136
    ovulatory 175
    patriarchs' and matriarchs' 93, 96
    permanent 126
    primary 163
    secondary 88
    sources of 317
    testing 69, 230
    treatment *see* Infertility
        Treatment, *see also* specific
        names of treatments
    tubal 15, 145, 304
    tubal factor 137, 312, 316
    unexplained 136, 169–170, 178,
        180, 182–183, 292, 313–314,
        347–348

Infertility drugs and medication *see*
    specific drugs: Bravelle, Clomid,
    Clomiphene Citrate, Crinone
    Progesterone, Fertinex, Follistim,
    Gonal F, Humegon, Metrodin,
    Pergonal
Infertility treatment 12, 15, 81, 92
    algorithms 315
    and artificial insemination 279
    and hMG 285
    and IUI 281
    and marital pressures 85
    and ovarian cancer 174–175
    and rabbinic consultation 86
    and supervision 392
    and technological advances xxv
Inguinal canal 252
Inhibin 155, 255
Initiated cycle 333
Injection
    gonadotropin 288, 293
    hCG *see* Human chorionic
        gonadotropin
    intracytoplasmic sperm injection
        see Intracytoplasmic sperm
        injection
    intramuscular (IM) 286–287, 289,
        321, 336, 339, 376
    intravenous injection 289
    subcutaneous (SQ) 286–287, 289,
        340, 376
Insemination xi,
    artificial *see* Artificial
        insemination
    bathhouse 20, 40, 50, 52
    cervical 179, 301
    donor (DI) 15, 23, 416–420, 424
    early 292
    in vitro 395
    insulin 142, 144, 172, 290–291
    intracervical 301

intrauterine *see* Intrauterine
  insemination
sensitizing agents 290
Intercourse
  daily 260
  ejaculation during 260
  first 50, 192, 200
  forbidden 418
  hasty 260
  natural 265, 279
  normal 47, 200, 232, 280, 341
  orgasm during 268
  sexual *see* Sexual, intercourse
  time of 161
  unnatural 232–233 see also *Biah,
    shello k'darkah*
  unprotected 131
Internal examination 151, 190–191, 195,
  199, 202, 212
Intimacy 85–86, 138
Intracytoplasmic sperm injection
  (ICSI)
  and assisted hatching 347
  and cryopreservation 270, 273
  and first birth 18
  and IVF 267, 313–317, 337, 343
  and MESA or TESE 268, 275
  and rabbinical supervision 395
  and treatment algorithm 361
  as scientific advances 312
  definition and details 327–330
Intrauterine insemination (IUI)
  and clomiphene 182, 285
  and COH 291–292
  and cryopreservation 332
  and GIFT 347–348
  and gonadotropins 182
  and halakha 284–285, 394
  and OI 178–179, 183, 314, 348
  and rabbinical supervision 396
  and Shabbat 377

and treatment algorithm 181,
  360–362
and viscosity 264
definition and explanation
  177–178, 280–281
Iodine 162
Isaac 74,
Isaiah 68, 99
R. Israel, Abraham 49
R. Isserles, Moshe (c. 1520–1572) *see*
  Rama
IUI *see* Intrauterine insemination
IVF *see* In vitro fertilization

J
Jacobson, Dr. Cecil 23
Jeremiah 20, 47–48, 417
Jew xxvii, 19, 25, 27, 32, 73, 93, 99,
  117, 355–356, 369–371, 373, 376,
  379, 409
  Ashkenazi/Ashkenazic 89,
    145–148
  haredi see Haredi
  non-Jew 36, 73, 355, 372–374,
    376–379, 419, 421 *see also*
    Gentile
  observant xxv, 6, 25, 68, 317, 379
  traditional 25, 27
Jewish chain 88-
Jewishness 355–356
Johnson, Dr. Abraham (Lucina Sine
  Concubito) 46

K
K-Y Jelly 260
Kabbbalistic 42, 233–234
Kaddish 84
Kal d'aved ra'hamana l'tav aved 25
R. Karelitz, Abraham (1878–1953)
  194, 201
Karet 370

R. Yosef Karo see *Shulhan Arukh*
Kashrut 26, 397–398. 416
Kedusha 80
Ketubah 23
Klinefelter's disease 433
Kohen gadol 20, 47, 102
Kollel students 137
Kruger, Tineas 158, 265
Kuzari (R. Yehuda HaLevi) 98

L
Labia majora/minora 192
Labor 82, 198
La-erev 68
R. Lampronti, Isaac see *Pahad Yitzhak*
R. Landau, Ezekiel (1713–1793)
  198–199
Laparoscope 17, 169, 210, 311
Laparoscopic 16, 271, 312
  evaluation 169
  instruments 169
  surgery 16, 305, 337
Laparoscopy 289
  and egg retrieval 336
  and endometriosis 307
  and GIFT 347–348
  and intrapelvic pathology 164
  and pelvic ultrasound 152
  and Shabbat 374
  and surgical repair 171
  and TET 349
  and tubal infertility 305
  and ZIFT 349
  definition and explanation
    167–169, 209–210
  diagnostic 168–169, 181
  operative 168–169, 181
Laparotomy 171, 307
Lashevet yitzrah 22, 68, 235, 431
Leah 83, 117
Leukemia 147
Leuprolide acetate 324

Leviticus 36–37, 75
Leydig cell 252–253, 255
LH see Luteinizing hormone
Libido 139
R. Libschitz, Barukh Mordekhai ben
  Ya'akov (1810–1885) 52
R. Lichtenstein, Aharon 411, 422
Likutei Maharil 48
Liver 147–148, 262
Long, Crawford 15
Lubricant/lubrication 260
Lucretius (96–55 BCE) 8
Lupron 174, 295–296, 301, 323
  gonadotropin 296, 301
  therapy 296
R. Luria, Judah see Maharal of Prague
Lusitanus, Amatus (1511–1568) 46,
  49–50
Luteal phase
  defect 291
  deficiency 297
  insufficiency 297, 299–300
Luteinizing hormone (LH) 375
  and anovulation 282
  and clomiphene 283
  and early ovulation 301–302
  and GnRH analogs 174, 295–296,
    322–323
  and gonadotropins 173, 285, 288
  and hCG 287
  and hMG 285–286
  and hormonal testing 262
  and medical therapy 269
  and natural hormones 320
  and ovulation monitoring 283
  and pituitary-testicular axis
    254–255
  and postcoital test 159–160
  and Shabbat considerations
    214–215
  and ovarian stimulation 335
  and ovulation 127

and urinary FSH 286
Home ovulation-predication test
  kit 375
levels in the urine 215
recombinant 288
Lysosomes 148

M

Ma'aseh Tuvia see Tobias Cohn
Macrocephaly (large head) 146
Macrosurgery
  and testicular biopsy 269
  and varicocele ligation 271
Magen Avot 38
Maharal of Prague 432
Maimonides *see* Rambam
Maimonides Medical Center xv, xxvi,
  xxx, 501
Makkah (wound or lesion) xviii, 169,
  192, 199–202, 205, 207, 210–211
  and uterine lining, 134
Male
  factor *see* Male factor
  fertility 14, 156–158, 160, 248,
    263, 329
  infertility *see* Male infertility
Male factor / Male factor infertility
  14, 156
  and GIFT 348
  and ICSI 327–329, 337
  and infertility sources 317
  and IVF 180, 313, 316, 327,
    341–342, 348
  and OI and/or IUI 178, 183, 281
  and PCT 160
  and postcoital test 263
  and sperm procurement 337
  and surgical procedures 269
  and the physician 117
  and the woman 113
  and treatment algorithm 359–362
  halakhic issues 109

impeding fertility 108
percentages 136–137
Male infertility xxx–xxxi, 278
  and a brief history 13, 16
  and artificial insemination 279
  and choosing right caregiver 275
  and hormonal problems 268
  and ICSI 329
  and the emotional aspect 81
  and varicocelectomy 16
  and varicoceles 262, 272
  and ZIFT 349
  evaluation and treatment of
    251–276
  general overview of 227–237
  recalcitrant male infertility 328
  treatment 8
Malignancy/malignancies 175
Mamzer 19, 21, 26, 48–49, 355
Marital
  counseling 92
  life 27, 112–114, 120
  relationship 22, 84, 86, 113
Marriage xii, 19, 68–70, 79, 84–87,
  90, 93, 98, 113–114, 116, 136–137,
  139, 232–233, 291, 392, 417–419,
  423, 438
  contract see *Ketubah*
Mashgiach/Mashgiha/Mashgihim
  25, 368, 397, 400–402 *see also*
  Rabbinical supervision *and also*
  Supervision
Masturbation 13, 230–236, 292, 294,
  342, 412–413, 422
Maternal 6, 435,
  age 352, 331, 435
  grandfather 425
  serum 325
Maternity 20, 22, 349, 438
Matriarch 70, 84, 93, 96–98, 373
Matriarchal paradigm 6
Matrilineal 356

Medical
  advances 97, 407
  advice xxix, 77, 119
  complaint 139
  ethics *see* Ethics, medical
  gospel 8
  help 70, 75, 97
  illness 80, 139
  information 86, 92
  issues xxvi, 118
  obstacles of cloning 432
  procedure 85, 198, 408
  protocol 118, 413
  reasons 183, 332, 340, 422
  therapy 3, 27, 112, 268–269,
    307–308, 434
  school 116
  solution 113
  treatment xxviii, 65, 74, 76,
    92–93, 170, 248, 292, 307, 357,
    370–371, 413, 437
Medical ethics
  halakhic xxix, 32
  Jewish xxxii
Medicine xv–xvi, 9, 14, 16, 24, 36, 39,
    46, 74, 116, 119, 229, 322, 346, 372,
    391, 410, 416
  emergency xvi,
  modern xii, 27,
  reproductive xxv, xxvii, xxx–xxxi,
    15, 20, 23, 31–33, 116, 120, 176,
    315, 391, 501
  western 9
Melakhah 371–372 *see also* Shabbat
*Men are from Mars, Women are from
  Venus see* Gray, Dr. John
Menopause/Menopausal 31,
    154–155, 304
  "medical" 307
  early 176, 353

human *see* Gonadotropins,
    human menopausal
  natural 307
  perimenopausal 319, 435
  postmenopausal 155, 285, 320, 426
  premature 312
  urine *see* Urine, menopausal
Menses 6–7, 154, 261, 322
Menstrual
  blood 11, 34, 36–39, 41
  cyclic menstrual pattern 128
  cyclicity 136, 277, 322
  disturbances 150
  flow xviii, 6–7, 12, 192, 194–195,
    212, 374
  fluid 34
  history 140
  period xviii, 86, 128, 140, 152, 190,
    283, 288, 305
  premenstrual staining 297
Menstrual cycle 85, 123, 140, 154–156,
    160, 172, 189, 193, 200, 212, 261,
    281, 302–304, 307, 318–319, 339, 374
  abnormality 113, 150
  atypical 393
  disorder 282, 304
  irregular 290
  normal 135, 176, 289, 298, 319
  regular 156
Menstruation 11–12, 191, 198, 201,
    205–208, 212, 215, 283, 288,
    296–297, 299, 306–307, 323
  cyclic 128
  normal 144, 283
Messianic
  era 370
  prophecies 99
Metformin 172, 290–291
Metrodin 286
Mezuzot 99

Micro epidydimal sperm aspiration
(MESA) *see* Aspiration, micro
epidydimal sperm
Microadenomas 150
Microfilaments 257
Micromanipulation of sperm and
eggs 18
Micropipette 328
Microsurgery
and fallopian tubes 16, 305
and testicular biopsy 269
and varicocele ligation 271
Midrash xxi, 48, 83, 96, 98–99
Devarim Rabbah 99
Tanhuma 74
Mikvah xviii, 115, 140, 190–191, 268,
283, 288–289, 292, 294, 296, 301,
303, 340, 374, 393
ovulation prior to 140, 268
Milex Corporation of Chicago 230
Milk 150, 231
Miscarriage 70, 135, 164, 197–198, 286,
352, 435
rates 135, 154, 352
recurrent 150, 162, 164, 352
repeated 129
spontaneous 70, 143
total 414
Mishnah xviii, xxi, 9, 36, 68, 97,
194, 410
mishnaic 25, 36
Mishna L'Melech R. Rosanes, Judah
(d. 1727) 50–51
Mitochondria 257
mitochondrial DNA *see* DNA,
mitochondrial DNA
Moab 430
Modesty see *Tzini'ut*
Moellin, Jacob (1360?–1427) *see*
Likutei Maharil
Molecular biology 130, 321

Monday 13–14
Moreh Nevukhim 430 *see also*
Rambam
Morgagni, Giovanni Batista 12
Morphology/Morphologically 157–158,
265, 337, 339, 345
sperm *see* Sperm, morpholoy
Mucolipidosis Type IV 147
Mucus 124, 159–160, 205
cervical *see* Cervical, mucus
plugging 325
problem 285
production 124–125
watery mucus discharge 124
Muktzeh xviii, 216, 371 *see also*
Shabbat
Mullis, Karry 350
Mumps 228, 261
Multifetal pregnancy 183, 290, 338,
344–345, 414–415
and aborting 394
and blastocyst transfer 331
reduction (MPR) 183, 344, 414, 415
Mutar 26, 430
Myomas 152, 164

N

N-acetylaspartic acid 146
Nafarelin 324
Nahmanides *see* Ramban
Nahum Ish Gamzu 96
Namon, Luis 10
National Institutes of Health of the
United States 345
Natural selection 328, 342
Navot et al 318
Necrosis, aseptic 147
Nedarim, tractate 232
Nehunia ben HaKana (a first century
Tanna) *see Sefer HaBahir*

Neonatal
　death 143
　outcome 334
Nervous system 13
　autonomic 147
　central 253
Neshama 36
Neurodegeneration 148
Neuroendocrine system 253
Neurological 261, 268
　progressive neurological
　　degeneration 148
　progressive neurological disease
　　146–147
Neuronal centers 254
R. Neuwirth, Yehoshua Yeshaya 216
Newborn 98, 352
Newton 13
Niddah xi, xviii, 281, 113, 189–202 see
　also Tahara, and also Makkah,
　and also Zavah
　and cervical dilation 207
　and gynecological exam 202–212
　and hysterosalpingogram (HSG)
　　208–209
　and laparoscopy 210
　and pelvic exam 203–205
　and ultrasound 210
　and uterine lining 194, 197, 204
　ben 21, 48
　introduction to laws of,
　　189–202, 413
　period of abstention xii
　seven clean days 190–191, 200,
　　202, 208, 212
　Tractate 5, 36–37, 40–42, 44,
　　234, 432
Niemann-Pick Disease 148
Nishtaneh hateva 51
R. Nissim Gaon 431
Nitrogen, liquid 339, 345
Noah 231

Novarel 322
Nuclear material 256, 258, 436
Nuclear transfer 23, 435–436
Nucleus 122, 258, 424, 429, 433,
　435–436
Nymphomania 13

O

Obesity 128, 137, 141–144, 317, 334
Obstetrician 145
Obstruction
　anatomical *see* Anatomical,
　　obstruction
　conception, to 299
　distal 359
　ductal *see* Ductal obstruction
　ejaculatory duct 262
　fertility, to 301
　intercourse, to 279
　mechanical 209
　proximal 359
Offering
　Grain (*Omer*) 25
　sin 370
OI *see* Ovulation induction
Oktay and colleagues 437
Oligomenorrhea (irregular
　periods) 143
Omer grain offering 25
Onan 231, 233
Onanism 47, 231
Oocyte 15, 17, 256–257, 324, 328–330,
　333, 353, 395, 436–438
　donor/donation of 353–354,
　　359, 362
　membrane 328
　recipient 353
　retrieval of 17, 330–333, 378
　unfertilized human 437
Oophorotomy 289
Optic atrophy 146
Oral tradition xvii, 103

Orchitis 261
   mumps orchitis 228
Orgasm 12, 123, 158, 257, 260, 268
Orthodoxy 80
os (mouth) 192
   external 192–194, 196, 199,
      203–207
   internal 192. 195, 199, 204,
      206–208
   internal cervical 210
Osteoarthritis 142
Ova 11–12, 154, 337, 420
R. Ovadia Yosef 22
Ovarian
   adhesions 291
   cancer *see* Cancer, ovarian
   capsule 126,
   controlled ovarian
      hyperstimulation (COH)
   cycle 127–128, 284
   cysts 128, 168, 353
   enlargement 152, 173
   failure 69, 304, 312–313
   follicles 154–155, 336
   function 144, 174, 206, 305, 317,
      323, 332, 357
   hormones *see* Hormones, ovarian
   hyperstimulation syndrome
      see Syndrome, Ovarian
      Hyperstimulation
   markedly abnormal ovarian
      reserve 359
   premature ovarian failure 180,
      353, 433
   reserve 154–156, 318–319, 323, 353
   reserve testing 315, 318, 320
   reserve screening 153, 155–156
   scarring 291
   stimulants 183, 322, 336, 427
   stimulation of 18, 312, 320, 331,
      335–336, 339–340, 358, 427
   suppressants 324

tissue 18, 437–438
tumors 171
Ovarist theory 11
Ovary
   Polycystic Ovary Syndrome
      (PCOS) *see* Syndrome, PCOS
Ovidrel 322, 339
Ovists 35, 43
Ovulation
   anovulation 143–144, 282,
      289–291, 359–362,
   cyclic 282
   cyst 128 see also Corpus luteum
   disorder 136, 282, 300
   early 288, 293–295, 301–303
   exposure to sperm at time of 134
   failed 144
   Home Ovulation-Prediction Test
      Kit (OPK) 159, 375
   induction (OI) *see* Ovulation
      induction
   monitoring 374
   natural 287
   normal 126, 172, 289–290, 292, 322
   oligo 282
   predictor kit (OPK) 159, 275
   premature 323–324, 336
   prior to *mikvah* 140, 268
Ovulation induction (OI) 184
   and anovulation 282
   and cervical insemination 179
   and clomiphene 172, 283
   and continuous bleeding 300
   and egg supply 176
   and endometriosis 309
   and GIFT 348
   and GnRH analogs 174, 323–324
   and gonadotropins 285
   and halakha 395
   and IUI 178–179, 183, 313–314, 348
   and IVF 315
   and laparoscopy 169

and multifetal reduction 414
and natural hormones 320
and PCOS 286
and premenstrual staining 297
and Shabbat 376
and treatment algorithm 181, 362
explanation 172
protocol 182
safety 174
Ovulatory 317, 360
agents 282, 291
anovulatory 283, 295, 316, 360
cycle/cycling 161, 176, 181–182,
290–292, 298, 304, 335, 360
disorders 136, 287, 313
disturbances 316
dysfunction 182, 313
infertility *see* Infertility, ovulatory
non-ovulatory cycle 298
problems 175
process 294, 303
response 182
stimulants 414
system 295
Ovulists *see* Ovists
ovum 12, 34, 102

P

Pad *see* cloth
Pahad Yitzhak (R. Issac Lampronti
[1679–1756]) 49
Palermo et al. 328
Pancoast, William 14, 23
Pancytopenia (bone marrow
failure) 147
Pangenesis Doctrine 34, 42–43
Papanicolaou (Pap) smear 203–205
Paralysis 148
Pardes 50
Parenting 86, 92, 99
posthumous xxvii
Parlodel *see* bromocriptine

Parturition (birth) 438
Paternity/Parenthood xxiv–xxv,
19–20, 22, 52, 68, 76, 88, 101,
104, 344
Abrahamic 104
genetic 397
halakhic 20–22, 432–433
posthumous 424
Pathalogic/Pathalogical 297, 299, 304
Patient advocacy organizations 92
Patriarchs 74, 84, 93, 96–97
Patrilineal 356
Passover 89, 213
four questions 82
seder 82
PCOS *see* Syndrome, Polycystic Ovary
(PCOS)
Pelvic 168
abnormal pelvic factors 360
abnormalities 168
adhesions 145, 316
anatomy *see* Anatomy, pelvic
cavity 17, 162, 168
contents 169
disease 169
disorders 168–169
exam 151, 153, 159, 167, 198, 203,
205, 210
infections 261
intrapelvic pathology 164
organs 151–152, 167, 169, 307
reconstructive procedures 209
surgery 164, 171, 304
ultrasound 152
Pelvis 152, 162, 166, 208, 257, 306–308
Penina 98
Penile 234, 236
Penis 192, 237, 257, 261, 263
Percutaneous 269
Percutaneous epidydimal sperm
aspiration (PESA) 273

R. Peretz ben Eliyahu of Corbeil
(c. 1295) *see Sefer Mitzvot Katan*
Pergonal 285–286, 322
Perineum canal 252
Period of abstention xii *see also
Niddah*
Peru u'revu xviii, 5, 22, 68, 80, 96, 99,
107, 120, 407, 412, 424, 431–432
Petri dish 17, 311, 347, 401–402
Petzuah daka 343
R. Pfoifer, Aharon 194, 201
PGD *see* Diagnosis, Preimplantation
genetic (PGD)
PH 327 *see also* Sperm, PH
Phlebotomy 11
Physiology 7, 9, 109, 121, 154
anatomy and 9, 32–33, 38, 252
human oocyte 17
reproductive xxvi, 33, 130, 277, 316
Pikuach nefesh 372
R. Pinhas Eliyahu Hurwitz
(1765–1821) *see Seifer HaBrit*
Pirkei Avot *see* Ethics of the Fathers
Pituitary 128, 149, 262, 320, 322–323
and testicular structures 228
function 128, 174, 295, 299
gland 127, 149–150, 155, 159, 172,
174, 215, 253–255, 258, 283, 287,
295, 302–302, 319–320, 322–323
hormones *see* Hormone, Pituitary
Pituitary-Testicular Axis *see*
Testicular, pituitary-testicular axis
production and release 174, 295
secretion 255, 303, 322–323
Placenta 298
Plato (c. 428–347 BCE) 8
Socratic-Platonic viewpoint 103
Platonic philosophy 103
Pliny 7
Polycystic Ovary Syndrome (PCOS)
see Syndrome, Polycystic Ovary
(PCOS)

Polymerase chain reaction (PCR) 52,
350, 352
Polyp 164, 166–167, 300
Pope Innocent x 46
Dr. Porcu, Eleonora 437
Posek/Poskim 22–24, 26, 32, 52, 119,
248, 249, 261–263, 266, 343,
345,352, 355, 357, 358, 374, 392–3,
396–397, 410–411, 417, 419, 422,
433, 436
Postcoital *see* Coital, postcoital
Postoperative 168–169, 171
Prayer xi, 19, 25, 70, 74, 84, 96–97
Pre-eclampsia (toxemia) 143
Preembryo *see* Embryo, preembryo
Preformation 10, 11, 35, 39–41, 43–44
Pregnancy
bathhouse 45
biochemical 333
clinical 333, 436
cumulative pregnancy rates 132
ectopic 325
expected pregnancy rate 178
expected pregnancy rate per cycle
178
first 18, 437
full-term 357
healthy 111, 139, 314
high pregnancy rates 334, 345
induced hypertension (PIH) 143
IVF 16, 319, 432
lower pregnancy rates 155
miscarried 135
monthly pregnancy rates 132, 154
multifetal *see* Multifetal
pregnancy
normal 125, 154, 415
ongoing pregnancy rate 352
overall pregnancy rate 331
per cycle pregnancy rates 179, 334
rate per couple 179
rate per cycle 178–179

rates 286, 319, 328, 330–331, 333–334, 337–338, 343, 348, 352, 358
rates and IVF 312, 333, 348
SART 348
second 231
tests 135
tubal 126, 316, 348
Pregnant 20, 45–48, 50, 82, 87, 89, 132, 145, 150, 181, 288, 355
not pregnant 85, 181
Preimplantation genetic diagnosis (PGD) *see* Diagnosis, Preimplantation genetic
Prenatal diagnosis 149
Procreation 21, 32, 67–68, 70, 74, 97, 99, 102, 234–235, 239, 241–242, 408, 417
artificial 407
as a positive commandment 97
mitzvah of 68, 76, 231, 233, 282
Profasi 322
Progesterone 128, 144, 160, 176, 283, 297–298, 200–301, 306–308, 353
cream (Crinone) 283
hydroxyprogesterone 151
injectable 283
levels 296–298
natural 283
production 296, 299
supplementation 291, 297
synthetic (Provera) 283
therapy 354
vaginal suppositories 283, 297
Prolactin 150, 262, 268, 300
Pronuclei 326, 337
Prostaglandins 280
Prostate 253, 257, 261–262, 273
Prostatitis 228
Provera 283
Proximal part 164
Prozdor 38

Psalm 67
Puberty 176, 253, 258
Pulmonary 146
Purim 89

Q
Quadruplets 344

R
Rabbanut 356
Rabbinic/Rabbinical 49, 189, 216
adviser xxv, 267
amendment 191
approval 86, 284–285, 292
authorities xii, xvii–xviii, 183–184, 191, 207, 212, 266, 276, 282, 339, 344–345, 356–357, 392, 395–396, 400, 410, 417
community xxvi, 51
Conception of conception vii, 31
concerns 25
consultation 73, 263, 292, 301, 358
counseling 412, 419
court 21, 418
derivation 68
discussions 36
doubt 249
guidance 412
input 108
law xvii, xviii
legislation 189, 197
level 197, 200
literature 9, 39, 99, 190
misgivings 24
objections 302
opinions 69
ordinances 213
organization 421
origin 231
oversight xxxi, 358, 368, 395, 399
permission 160

position 234
professionals xxvii
prohibition 189, 214, 371–374, 376
responsa vii, 11, 20, 45, 95
restrictions 213
rulings xviii
sources 32–33, 44, 73–74, 98
supervisor 397, 416
supervision *see* Rabbinical
    supervision
terms vii, xvii
theory 37
view 417
violation 214
writings 20
Rabbinical supervision ix, xxviii,
    xxxi, 24, 377, 391, 395–397,
    399–400, 416 *see also Hashga'ha,*
    Mashiach/Mashgiha/Mashgihum,
    Supervision
and human error 399
and semen analysis 395, 400
Rachel xi, xiii, 70, 83, 117, 373
Radiographic dye 208, 211
Radiological 210, 261–262
Radiologist 162, 164
Radiotherapy 228
Rama (Rabbi Moshe Isserles) 191, 234
Rambam (R. Moses ben Maimon
    [1135–1204]) xvii, 9, 38, 50, 68, 75,
    101, 103, 195, 197, 232, 248, 410, 431
    Mishneh Torah xvii, 50, 101,
        103, 410
    Moreh Nevukhim 431
Ramban (R. Moses ben Nahman
    [1194–1270]) 36–38, 41, 75
Rashi (Rabbi Shlomo Yitzhaki
    [1040–1105]) 9, 42, 74–75, 194
Rebecca 70, 74
Rectal exam 261
Rectum 192–193, 262, 273
Reform movement 356

Renal
    function 262
    vein 229
Reproduction
    artificial 393
    assisted *see* Assisted reproduction
    female 278
    human xxiii, 18, 129, 133, 135
    posthumous 423
    sexual 428,
    third party 23
Reproductive
    anatomy *see* Anatomy,
        Reproductive
    assisted reproductive technology
        see Assisted reproductive
        technology (ART)
    biologist 17
    capacity 237, 305
    care 25, 119
    cloning *see* Cloning, reproductive
    cycle 133
    disorder 113, 143
    endocrinologist 150, 153, 173, 183,
        267, 275, 288
    failure 108, 433
    functioning 407
    halakha *see* halakha, reproductive
    health 355
    laboratory 24
    life 123, 131, 177
    mammalian reproductive
        system 311
    materials 24
    medicine *see* Medicine,
        reproductive
    medicine and governing health
        authorities 391
    organs 9, 171
    performance 142
    physiology xxvi, 33, 130, 277, 316
    practices 31

problems 258
process 6, 109, 121, 125, 128, 407
reproductive-age women 123
scientist 17
seed *see* Seed, reproductive
services 334
signal 255
specialist 24, 116, 135, 141, 154, 157, 164, 166, 174, 180, 275, 317, 323
surgeon 171
surgery 305
system 75–76, 311, 322
techniques xxxi, 275, 392
technology xxvi, xxxii, 16, 25–27, 32, 101, 158, 174, 179, 286, 293, 312, 335, 357–358, 408–410, 426–427, 433–434
therapy 397
tract 13, 124, 162, 177, 191–192, 194–196, 257, 279, 281, 284, 305, 347
treatment 3
years 153, 171
Repronex 285–286, 322
RESOLVE 92, 501
Respiratory difficulties 8
Retardation
mental 147–148
psychomotor 147
Retinal degeneration 148
Rishonim 9, 11, 20, 45, 48–49, 52
Ritual
immersion 355, 357 *see also* Mikvah
impurity 197
pool *see* Mikvah
Rohleder, Hermann 45
R. Rosanes, Judah (d. 1727) *see* *Mishnah L'Melech*
Rosh 9, 38
Ruach 36, 48
Rubella 145

Rubin, Isadore 15

S

Sabbath *see also* Shabbat
and IVF 340, 378
Halakhic xviii
Jewish 213, 369
Salpingectomy 359
Salpingography 210
Sanguino-lymphatic 13
Samuel xiii
prophet 83
Sanhedrin, tractate 99, 104
Sarah xi, 70, 76
SART *see* Society for Assisted Reproductive Technology
R. Schachter, Hershel xxx, 217
Schally, Andrew 322
R. Schick, Baruch *see Tiferet Adam*
R. Schick, Moses 50
R Schick, Solomon 50
Schenk 16
Scrotal
skin 270, 273
ultrasound *see* Ultrasound, scrotal
vein 262
Scrotum 252, 257, 262, 272
Sedation 337
Seed
emission of 43, 231–233, 237
female 7, 33–42, 45
genital 231,
male 7–8, 33–34, 37, 39, 41–45
ovarian 39
plant 33, 37
planting 371
reproductive 46
spillage 232–233
wastage of 44, 231, 248
Sefer HaBahir 42
Sefer HaBrit 41, 43–44
Sefer Hahinukh 95

Sefer Hasidim 98
Sefer Mitzvot Katan 20, 46, 48, 417
Seizures 146, 148
Semen
  abnormalities 177
  analysis *see* Semen analysis
  Computer assisted semen analysis
    (CASA) 158, 264
  ejaculated 157, 266
  procurement 230, 234–235, 237,
    268, 393, 423
  specimen 23, 178, 264, 294, 393
  viscosity 263–264
Semen analysis 400
  and fertility potential 265
  and *halakha* 69, 118, 392
  and history 14
  and hormonal testing 262
  and inadequate sexual
    performance 268
  and limited sperm 266
  and postcoital test 159–160, 263
  and rabbinical supervision
    395, 400
  and radiological studies 262
  and Shabbat 365
  and sperm evaluation 157–158
  and treatment algorithm 183
Seminiferous tubules 252, 255
Seminal
  seminal collection device
    (SCD) 265
  fluid 7, 123, 178, 230, 235, 257, 264,
    280, 337
  function 227
  vesicle 257, 261–262, 273
Semm, Kurt 16
Semmelweis, Ignaz Philipp 15
Sephardic xxi
Serono 286
Serophen 172, 283
Sertoli cell 252–253, 255,

Sertoli Cell Only Syndrome (SCOS)
  see Syndrome, Sertoli Cell Only
  Syndrome (SCOS)
Seven clean days 190–191, 200, 202,
  208, 212 *see also Niddah*
Sex selection 352, 394 *see also* Gender
  selection
Sex therapist 139
Sexual
  ability 259
  activity 12, 108, 412, 422
  dysfunction xv, 137–139, 152,
    178, 268
  foreplay 260
  frequency 260
  impotence 233 *see also* Erectile
    dysfunction
  intercourse 138, 190
  maturity 330
  modesty *see Tzini'ut*
  needs 81
  pathology 138
  performance 65, 81, 259, 268
  physical sexual contact 418
  relations 85, 138–140, 191, 231–233,
    267, 299, 374, 412–413, 417
  relationship 85, 87, 113, 233
  satisfaction 260
Shabbat xviii, 369–370, 213 *see also*
  Melakhah, and also Muktzeh
  And *muktzeh* xviii, 216, 371
  diagnosis and treatment on
    213–216, 374–379
  laws of 370–373
Shalom Bayit 22
Shefihut damim 248
Shettles, Landrum 17
Shevet Yehuda (Solomon ibn
  Verga) 47
Shevilei Emunah 38
Shiddukh 113
Shiva 84

Index

Shulhan Arukh xvii, 9, 75, 196, 198–199, 233, 410
Simhat Torah 89
Simms, Marion 15
Society for Assisted Reproductive Technology (SART) 16, 335, 348
Socrates 103
Sodom 430
R. Sofer, Moses (1762–1839) 194
R. Sofer, Simcha Bunim 235
Solomon ibn Verga (15ᵗʰ to 16ᵗʰ cent.) *see Shevet Yehuda*
R. Soloveitchik, Joseph B. viii, xxix, 73, 101
Somatic cells 18, 428–429, 433–434
Sonogram 152
Sonohysterogram 166, 300
Sonohysterography 211
Soranus 8
Spallanzani 10
Spasticity 146
Spatula 203
Speculum 151, 166, 203, 206, 208
  exam 124, 203
Sperm
  abnormalities 182, 230, 263, 266, 312, 329
  agglutination 264
  antisperm antibodies 264
  artificial collection of 234
  aspiration *see* Aspiration
  capacitated 257
  cell 121–122, 248, 252, 256–257, 264, 280, 337
  characteristics 157, 230
  concentration 264
  count 137, 157–158, 177, 227, 251, 260, 275, 313, 316, 327–328, 347
  dead 178
  defective 235
  deficiency 329
  donor/donation 32, 48, 86, 88, 437
  dysmorphic 329
  evaluation 109, 229, 266
  excess 349, 394
  freezing/frozen 395, 423, 437–438
  gentile 420
  head 121, 256–257
  linearity 264–265
  mapping 270
  maturation 253, 256–257
  morphology 157–158, 177, 265
  motile/ motility 121, 124–125, 157, 177, 205, 257, 264, 328, 337, 343
  non-viable 235
  PH 264
  polyspermy 328
  potent 178, 416
  precursor 252, 255–256
  procurement 51, 109, 234–235, 281, 302, 337, 341–342, 392, 408
  production 126, 135, 158, 229, 252, 254–255, 259, 262, 268–269, 286, 291, 317
  retrieval *see* Sperm retrieval
  sorting 422
  specimen 342, 344, 402, 416
  testicular *see* Testicular, sperm
  washing 182, 264, 280
Sperm retrieval
  and ICSI 329, 343
  testicular 312, 316
Spermatozoa 10, 12, 35, 256
Spermatic
  cord 228
  duct 228
  vein 229
Spermatids 256
Spermatocytes 256
Spermatogenesis 255
Spermatogenic failure 236
Spermatogonia 252, 255–256
Spermicide 266, 341
Spinal

cord 34, 42–43
cord trauma 273
marrow 8
nerves 274
Spongy Degenerative Disease *see*
Canavan's Disease
Spontaneous generation 34
Spotting 191, 195, 288, 307
Stem cell
adult 429
cloning *see* Cloning, stem cell
embryonic 429
Steptoe, Patrick 17–18, 311, 439
Sterile 13, 17, 157, 280
Sterility 12–13, 15, 104, 126, 258, 261,
376, 417, 425
Steroids 172, 255, 259
Stillbirth 143
Strabismus (cross eye) 148
Stroke 142
Subcutaneous 289, 307, 339
injection, *see* Injection,
subcutaneous
route 287, 321, 339
Subzonal insertion (suzi) 328
Sukkah 82, 95–97
Surrogacy 357, 421
gestational 305–306, 356–357, 425
Surrogate 32, 357, 394, 411, 421
carrier 394
gestational 23, 180, 305, 357
Supervision 392, 396, 398–402
halakhic 346, 378, 399, 401
and insemination with husband's
sperm 401
and ivf 401–402
Rabbinical *see* Rabbinical
supervision
Support groups 73, 91
Surgical 267
correction 13, 133, 171–172, 229,
305, 361

cure 9
damage 237
interruption 229
irreparable 313
management 306
means 126
microsurgical 269–272, 275, 396
obliteration 229
post-surgical adhesions *see*
Adhesions, post-surgical
presurgical egg extraction 437
procedure 13–14, 126, 139, 167,
192, 200, 209, 262, 269,
305–306, 333
reconstruction 272, 305
removal 273, 437
repair 171, 314
resection 181
sequalae 227
treatment 15, 308, 309
tying 271
Survival of the fittest 70
Swab
alcohol 376
cotton 203–204
Synagogue 89, 98, 420
Synarel 174
Syndrome 143, 305
Asherman's 165, 306
Bloom 146
congenital 228
Down 351
Klinefelter's 433
Ovarian Hyperstimulation 173,
293, 332, 341, 378
Polycystic Ovary (pcos) 137,
142–144, 150, 172, 183, 286,
289–290
Sertoli Cell Only Syndrome
(scos) 270, 433
Turner's 353, 433

Index

T

Tabernacle 371
Tahara xviii, 281, 289, 367 see also
   Niddah
   hefsek 202
   hezkat 202
Taharat hamishpa'ha – see family
   purity, Niddah
Talmud Torah 101, 103
Tashbetz (Rabbi Shimon ben
   Tzemach Duran (1360–1444) 38,
   43, 49–51
Dr. Taub, Moshe 201
Tay-Sachs 148–149, 351, 415
Tazria 36–37, 41–42
R. Teitelbaum, Yoel 417
   (Satmar Rebbe)
Temple 25
   first 7
   Jewish 370
   second 7
Tenaculum 206–208, 210
Test tube baby 17
Testes 7, 228–229, 237, 343
   Cryptorchid 252
   normal-sized 236
   wounded 237
Testicle 37, 40, 43, 229,
   236–237, 252–255, 257–258,
   261–262, 269–271, 343
Testicular
   abnormality 361
   activity 255
   aspiration 270
   atrophy 228, 272
   biopsy 236–237, 269, 396
   descent 252
   development 252, 267
   drainage 229
   failure 69, 228
   function 272
   hormone 262

   mapping 270
   paratesticular tissue 261
   Pituitary-Testicular Axis
      253–254, 262
   post-testicular dysfunction 228
   potential 255
   sperm 237, 262, 268, 312, 316
   sperm extraction (TESE) 262,
      268–269, 275, 396
   sperm retrieval see Sperm
      retrieval
   structures 228
   surgery 178
   tissue 258, 269
   vein 262
Testis 121, 237, 286, 337
   rete 252, 257
Testis determining factor (TDF) 252
Testosterone 151, 253, 255, 262
TET see Tubal embryo transfer (TET)
Thermometer 214–215, 375
Thyroid 149
   function 150, 300
   gland 149–150
   hormone see Hormone, thyroid
   hypothyroid 150, 172
   hypothyroidism 150
   supplements 150
Thyroxine see Hormone, Thyroid
Tiferet Adam (Rabbi Baruch Schick
   (1744–1808) 40, 44
Tissue 206, 270, 286, 321, 429
   abnormal 307
   adipose 192
   adult 429
   connective 253
   diseased 169
   egg-containing 353
   extractor 269
   homologous 426
   ovarian see Ovarian, tissue

paratesticular *see* Testicular,
    paratesticular tissue
retransplanted 438
scar 136, 164, 167–169, 304, 316
soft 152, 162, 262
testicular *see* Testicular, tissue
uterine 209
Tobias Cohn (1652–1729) 39
Toladot 371
Torah Lishma 51
Tosafot 74, 232
Totipotent 428–429
Toxemia *see* Pre-eclampsia
Transabdominal ultrasound 18
Transurethral resection of the
    ejaculatory duct (TURED) 273
Transvaginal ultrasound *see* Vaginal,
    Transvaginal ultrasound
Treatment
    algorithm 180–183, 315
    cycle 24, 118, 133–134, 173, 182,
        283, 294, 314, 323, 325, 332, 335,
        341–342, 358
    fertility *see* Fertility Treatment
    infertility *see* Infertility Treatment
    see also specific names of
        treatment
    medical *see* Medical, treatment
    pathways 314
    reproductive 3
    strategy 170, 180, 182
Triglycerides 142
Trimester, first 354
Triplets 334, 344, 414–415, 427
Trisomy 21–351
Tubal
    abnormalities 136
    anatomy *see* Anatomy, tubal
    blockage 17, 22, 144, 153, 180, 313
    damage 145, 305
    disease 304–305, 307, 314

embryo transfer (TET) *see* Tubal
    embryo transfer
factor 313, 359–362
factor infertility *see* Infertility,
    tubal factor
infections 317
infertility *see* Infertility, tubal
insufflation 15
muscle 125
occlusion 163–164
patency 164
pregnancy *see* Pregnancy, tubal
secretions 126
wall 126
Tubal embryo transfer (TET) 312,
    349–350
Tuboplasty 359
Tzini'ut 27, 80, 87, 138, 202, 278,
    393, 412
Tzitz Eliezer 21–22, 69, 149, 196, 201,
    214, 236, 349, 396, 418
Tzitzit 99

U

Ultra-Orthodox *see Haredi*
Ultrasound 152, 166, 210–211, 262,
    312, 333
    diagnostic 213
    exam/examinations 152–153,
        166, 173
    guidance 166, 325, 336–337
    monitoring 293, 304
    pelvic *see* Pelvic, ultrasound
    picture 166
    probe 152, 262
    scan 375
    scrotal 262
    tracking 283
    transabdominal 18
    transrectal (TRUS) 262
    transvaginal *see* Vaginal,
        transvaginal ultrasound

transvaginal ultrasound probe 152
vaginal *see* Ultrasound, vaginal
Unnatural intercourse *see* Intercourse,
    unnatural
Urethra 192, 257
    prostatic 257
    transurethral resection 273
    urethral opening 192
Urethral opening *see* Urethra,
    urethral opening
Urinary
    bladder 192
    LH kit 215
    proteins 286
    tract infections 260
Urine 159, 215–216, 263, 286, 375
    menopausal 286, 321
    postmenopausal women 285, 320
    testing 263, 283, 301
Urological 115, 260, 263, 268, 275
Urologist 248, 261, 267, 275, 329, 337
Uterus
    and fusion defects 305
    bicornuate 8, 164–165
    septate 164–165
Uterine
    adhesions 165
    anatomy 152, 162, 164,
        166–167, 300
    anomalies 165
    bleeding xviii, 128, 194–196,
        198–199, 201, 208, 210–211,
        307, 338
    blood xviii, 37
    cancer *see* Cancer, uterine
    capacity for implantation 206
    cavity 125, 129, 162, 164, 166–167,
        177, 196, 206, 208, 211–212,
        280, 325, 330, 338
    contents 198
    environment 129
    factors 136, 305

fibroids *see* Fibroids, uterine
    intrauterine anatomy 167
    lavage 18
    lining *see* Uterine lining
    midcycle uterine bleeding 284
    mole 49
    pathology 211
    tissue *see* Tissue, uterine
Uterine lining 134
    and atrophy 307
    and continuous bleeding 301
    and disordered development
        128–129
    and disruptions 302
    and early ovulation 302–303
    and embryo selection 330
    and embryo transfer 325
    and endometrial biopsy 161, 206
    and estrogen 296, 308
    and irregular menstruation 283
    and *makkah* 199, 201
    and menstrual cycle 194
    and midcycle bleeding 298
    and *niddah* bleeding 194, 197, 204
    and ovulation 128
    and pelvic exam 203
    and pelvic ultrasound 153
    and premenstrual staining 297
    and scraping 306
    unilateral uterine abscess 8

V

Vagina 12, 122, 127, 129, 151–153, 160,
    166, 192–195, 203, 206, 208, 210,
    212, 230, 236, 305, 393, 417
Vaginal 153, 341
    birth 163
    bleeding *see* Bleeding, vaginal
    environment 159
    exam 152, 263
    intravaginally 236
    muscles 268

opening 192
probe 153
progesterone vaginal
    suppositories 283
secretions 260
suppositories 297
transvaginal ultrasound 18,
    152–153, 166, 211, 337, 340
ultrasound 210–211
wall 336–337
Vaginismus 139, 268
Van Leeuwenhoek, Antonie 10, 35, 39,
    43, 230
Vaporization (with a laser) 289
Varicella (chicken pox) 145
Varicocele 137, 228–229, 261–262, 264,
    271–272, 361
    varicocele ligation 271–272
Varicocelectomy 16
Vas deferens 252–253, 257, 275
    congenital absence of the vas
        deferens (CAVD) 261, 343
Vascular 229, 261, 263
Vasectomies 275
Vasoepididymostomy 275
Vasovasostomy 274–275
Vena cava 229
Venery 12
Venous
    channels 271
    system 229
Vestible 192
Vibratory stimuli 342
Vilna Gaon 40
Von Baer Ernst 15, 34

W

R. Waldenberg, Eliezer *see Tzitz
    Eliezer*
Weiss, R. 108
Wilson, Andrew 11
Womb xiii, 7, 12, 98, 122, 128, 311,
    357, 425
    artificial 31
World Health Organization (WHO)
    158, 265
Wound, artificially induced *see
    Makkah*
Wright Brothers 439

X

x-ray 150, 162–163, 166, 208, 271, 300

Y

R. Ya'akov Emden (d. 1776) 40–41, 235
Yad Vashem 99
Yallow, PhD. Rosalyn S. 16
Yamim tovim 340, 358, 370 *see also*
    Shabbat
Y-deletion study 266–267
Yehoshua ben Yehotzadak 47
R. Yehuda HaNasi 36
Yevamot, trectate 107, 232
Yihus 19, 22
R. Yitzchak 44, 232–233
R. Yohanan xiii
Yom Kippur 376

Z

Zacchias, Paolo (1584–1659) 46
Zavah 190–191 *see also Niddah.*
Zera 36–37, 40

hash'hatat 233, 266, 349, 413, 431–432

hotza'at zera l'vatala 21, 44, 235, 281, 392

Zohar 233

Zona drilling 328

Zona pellucida 258, 328, 346

Zygote 331 *see also* Zygote intrafallopian transfer (ZIFT)

Zygote intrafallopian transfer (ZIFT) 312, 349–350, 474

About the Author

Richard V. Grazi, MD is the Director of the Division of Reproductive Endocrinology and Infertility at Maimonides Medical Center in Brooklyn, New York and the founder of GENESIS Fertility & Reproductive Medicine. He is board certified in Obstetrics and Gynecology, and holds subspecialty certification in Reproductive Endocrinology and Infertility. As the author of numerous scientific and scholarly articles, Dr. Grazi is a well-known figure in secular as well as Jewish communities with an interest in infertility. He has been honored for his advocacy on behalf of infertile couples by national organizations, including RESOLVE and the American Fertility Association. For many years, he has been named as one of New York's "Top Doctors" by *New York* magazine, and he has been recognized consistently by the Castle Connolly Medical Guide as one of the America's top reproductive specialists. His previous book, *Be Fruitful and Multiply: Fertility Therapy and the Jewish Tradition*, has been acclaimed in Jewish communities internationally.

The fonts used in this book are from the Minion family